real time
ophthalmic
ultrasonography

S. N. Hassani

real time ophthalmic ultrasonography

(in collaboration with R. L. Bard)

includes 423 illustrations

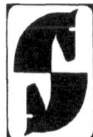

Springer-Verlag
New York Heidelberg Berlin

S. N. Hassani, M.D.
Assistant Professor of Radiology
State University of New York at Stony Brook and
Physician in Charge, Ultrasound Division, Department of Radiology
Queens Hospital Center
Jamaica, New York 11432

R. L. Bard, M.D.
Department of Radiology
Manhattan Eye, Ear, Nose, and Throat Hospital
New York, N.Y.

Library of Congress Cataloging in Publication Data

Hassani, S. N. 1938-
    Real time opthalmic ultrasonography.

    Bibliography: p.
    1. Ultrasonics in ophthalmology. 2. Diagnosis,
Ultrasonic. I. Title. [DNLM: 1. Eye diseases—Diag-
nosis. 2. Ultrasonics—Diagnostic use.   WW141 H353r]
RE79.U4H37   617.7′1   78-17197
ISBN-13: 978-1-4612-6297-8

9 8 7 6 5 4 3 2 1

ISBN-13: 978-1-4612-6297-8   e-ISBN-13: 978-1-4612-6295-4
DOI: 10.1007/978-1-4612-6295-4

To Our Families

foreword

by Dr. Nathaniel R. Bronson, II

This volume serves a two-fold purpose very nicely. For the ophthalmologist there is a presentation of the techniques and results of ultrasonic examination of the eye and orbit. For the radiologist or general ultrasonographer the essential ocular anatomy and pathology are described with these findings. Unlike conventional x-rays or static general body ultrasonograms, the examination of the eye by real-time ultrasonography must be done by an examiner with extensive personal knowledge of the eye and the orbit, both anatomically and pathologically. The student must realize that the Polaroid photographs can only show an example of what was transiently seen, such as spot films taken during fluroscopy. This is further complicated by the poor reproduction by Polaroid films of the actual gray scale seen during the examination.

Considerable work has been done to prepare this text. The author has done clinical ultrasonography of many eyes and presents the findings of his experience. As in most fields of medical diagnostic work this experience is essential to achieve the best results. The beginner in ophthalmic ultrasonography is encouraged to work with known pathology. Fortunately, pathologic changes in the eye can frequently be seen with a slit lamp or an ophthalmoscope. For example, a known retinal detachment is an ideal case with which to start. The sheet-like echoes leading to the optic nerve can be compared with ophthalmoscopic findings. One has more confidence then when similar sheet-like echoes are seen in an eye with opaque media, such as when a dense cataract or a vitreous hemorrhage is present.

The author describes what is one of the most important factors in real time ophthalmic, and I suspect general body, ultrasonography: three-dimensional thinking. On the screen one sees a two-dimensional image, but by angulation and rotation of the scan head this can and should be built up into a three-dimensional image in the examiner's mind. In the course of teaching this technique we have found this concept of three-dimensional thinking easy for some and difficult for others. For the latter I encourage them to work with test objects, such as a paper clip, in a dish of water constructing the three-dimensional image mentally.

The text describes the need to combine the ultrasonic findings with those of other examinations. While I feel confident in diagnosing a malignant melanoma of certain types and sizes in an eye, I would never suggest enucleation on that basis alone. This was brought out recently when we compared our ultrasonic diagnosis of orbital masses with those of the same patient done on a CAT scanner. In many cases both of us were wrong, but the combination of the two techniques significantly improved the diagnostic accuracy.

Ophthalmic ultrasonography has grown steadily over the years from the pioneering work of Mundt and Hughes, Oksala, Baum, and Purnell, but only in the last few years has its clinical use become widespread. The eye is an ideal organ for ultrasonic examination. The distances are short, and the acoustically clear vitreous is much easier than elsewhere where bone and gas are present. Ultrasonic advances in equipment are usually shown first in ophthalmology as a result of the acoustic environment. For example, gray scale has been in use in the eye for nearly two decades.

Enjoy your ultrasonic work. It is fun and interesting, and much pathology will be seen. For the ophthalmologist, learn the basics of ultrasonography. For the radiologist or ultrasonographer, work closely with your ophthalmologist to learn ophthalmic anatomy and pathology.

Nathaniel R. Bronson, II, M.D.
Director, Ultrasound Department
Manhattan Eye, Ear, Nose, and Throat Hospital

preface

Ophthalmic ultrasonic scanning has reached a stage of sophistication whereby detailed diagnostic information can be gained without discomfort to the patient. The procedure is quick, safe, noninvasive, and in many instances, supersedes and obviates more time-consuming procedures requiring catheterization, injection of contrast material, and serial radiographic imaging.

Real-time scanning is particularly useful in pediatric and geriatric patients. The adaptability of the scan head to any conceivable patient position and the portability of the machine smooth out many logistical problems in patient examination. The ability of the scanner to provide diagnostic findings in the presence of motion salvages many a study on an uncooperative patient. This advantage is not possible with a static B-scan unit. Indeed, the capability of evaluating the motility of a pathologic process is often the key to differentiating lesions that may have similar ultrasonic morphology. The motion of a linear segment of vitreous hemorrhage is far greater than a retinal detachment. This feature readily distinguishes the important disorders. Since this modality is noninvasive, it may be performed serially and at any given time. Multiple studies to optimally evaluate the biologic nature of a lesion are completely without morbid effects to the extremely delicate structures of the eye. The lens, in particular, is highly sensitive to ionizing radiation which results in early cataract formation. This undesirable consequence promotes the use of ultrasound when serial studies are considered.

The purpose of this book is to introduce the physician to the essential principles of ultrasound physics and the practical aspects of ophthalmic scanning procedures. Important concepts are clearly and thoroughly presented. Mathematical formulas and advanced physics principles beyond the scope of the clinician have been omitted. The text is limited to the eye and medially related areas in order to concentrate on each area in sufficient depth so as to be valuable to the specialist who must be familiar with the diagnostic capabilities of atraumatic scanning in his field. The methods of examination and diagnostic findings are sufficiently detailed to be useful to the radiologist and ophthalmic surgeon who are serious practitioners of ophthalmic scanning.

In the sections on physical and practical applications, precise directions for examination are given and scanning pitfalls with the production of artifacts are underscored. The scanning systems are presented so that the potential features and limitations of the imaging unit are recognized.

Examination of each area has been arranged so that the reader may review the pertinent regional anatomy before studying the ultrasonic presentation of normal structures. The pathology of each structure is presented as a disease spectrum and the evolution of the disorder is discussed. Correlation between sonographic findings and the histopathologic changes is emphasized.

Where controversy exists, the opinions of various authorities are cited and compared with our experience. The diagnostic versatility of the various imaging systems are evaluated for each organ complex and the investigative method of choice is suggested for each disorder.

Considerable attention is given to clinical and pathologic aspects. The practice of ultrasonic scanning requires a thorough knowledge of the diagnostic problems of ophthalmology and their related specialties. The text is designed as a bridge between sonographic imaging and general ophthalmic principles.

acknowledgments

We wish to express our deep appreciation to Drs. N. Finby, J. Smulewicz, Y. Chynn, R. Nuba, H. Zimmerman, R. Balkin, P. Ballen, D. Beards, J. Beards, W. Boockvar, M. Brody, S. Cahan, G. Chubak, J. Cook, Y. Fisher, R. Fleckner, D. Flug, K. Galician, P. Garber, R. Goldberg, S. Goodstein, D. Lerner, R. Malkin, P. Maris, I. Nasaduke, H. Perry, E. Pulice, W. Regan, I. Reizes, P. Schwartz, R. Stevens, R. Strome, E. Trayner, I. Udell, J. Shapiro, F. Theodore, N. Pickering, H. Skalka, M. Wohlstein, E. Weise, J. Dodick, G. Kretchman, and M. Bodian.

We are also very grateful to Akram Hassani, Joan Mark, Sonia Suga and Judy Sharpe, for their technical assistance.

The investigative efforts of our many colleagues in the field of ultrasonography have greatly facilitated the evolution of this textbook. The support of the publisher and the collaboration of the Editorial Staff are warmly acknowledged.

contents

introduction

The field of diagnostic ultrasound has expanded in application so rapidly over the past few years that it has become part of the routine diagnostic workup. The history of ultrasonography is vastly different from the evolution of x-rays. After the discovery of x-ray in 1885, it was rapidly accepted by the medical community and many radiologic societies soon appeared. The imaging potential of x-rays was so exciting that many patients and their physicians received massive exposure to this form of highly penetrating electromagnetic energy. The dreadful sequelae of radiation-induced injuries and malignancies subsequently appeared. The unforgettable tragic accidents of x-ray soon produced many advisory and protective agencies.

The history of ultrasonography is a long one and the procedure has suffered from many setbacks in its attempt for acceptance by the medical profession. Its inherently harmless nature has accounted for a significant portion of its popularity in modern medical practice. Whether the sophisticated electronic technology that spawned high resolution ultrasound will cause the growing field of ultrasound to supersede other diagnostic modalities, or create nonultra sonic imaging systems that will phase out ultrasonography, remains to be determined.

The pioneers of ultrasonography had much difficulty in applying sonar to diagnosis since they were using first generation scanners based on ultrasonic technology used in industry and military pursuits. In later years newer ultrasonic units designed to meet specific clinical purposes have been constructed. Cooperation of physicists, engineers, and physicians dedicated to ultrasonic imaging has led to the development of diagnostic systems of considerable practical value. Since the early days of the application of sonar principles in medicine, there have continually been new innovations in this field. The progress of acoustic waves in diagnostic imaging has been aided by the development of special ultrasonic transducers, sophisticated amplifiers, and sensitive electronic displays. The introduction of recently perfected scan converter systems adds a new dimension to the field of ultrasonography.

In spite of the absence of demonstrable side effects and the ease and accuracy of the study, its use did not become fashionable until very recently. The nature of the sound beam is that of mechanical energy and its possible long-term biologic effects still remain unclear. However, it is known that the ionizing effects of x-rays make even small doses potentially harmful. Sonar mechanical vibrations are such that energy below the level that breaks tissue bonds will not produce any tissue damage. In a large amount of documented data, no hazardous effects have been reported with low-intensity ultrasound energy up to now.

As mentioned, the field of ultrasonography has assumed such importance primarily as a result of the harmless nature of the modality. The tireless efforts of a large number of investigators from varied medical fields and allied services have developed sonography into one of the best diagnostic tools for the opaque and injured eye. The pioneers of ultrasound, using only A-mode to combat the skepticism of their colleagues must have been exceptionally dedicated and patient.

Scanning the eye and mentally integrating the A-mode spikes to give an answer to the clinician in need of a firm diagnosis must have produced great initial hope, but had a number of drawbacks due to inconsistency, time consumption, and interpretation. Many problems were alleviated by the introduction of B-mode scanning units. This technique was coupled with A-mode for optimal diagnostic information. After the development of the contact B-scan real-time scanner for ophthalmologic use, there have been sudden changes in sonography of the eye.

The true revolution in ultrasonography began with the development of the scan converter with its sophisticated logarithmic compression amplifiers. This presentation of a scan in various shades of gray-related to echo amplitude opened new horizons in the study of tissue signatures.

The fundamentals of ultrasound, like those of any other branch of medicine, require the user to be familiar with the effects and limitations of the method. By this technique we are able to locate different organs and tissues and measure the interfaces between them, and to cut in cross sections through different structures. In contrast to other examinations which yield indirect information, ultrasound enables us to outline the lesion directly and to investigate its relationship with neighboring structures. Ultrasound, both as a screening and diagnostic modality, is a noninvasive and atraumatic procedure and is complementary to angiography and CAT scanning in many cases.

The information gained through ultrasound, as in other imaging procedures, is optimized when coupled with the patient's clinical picture.

The word "sonar" is an acronym of sound navigation and ranging. Historically, ultrasound was developed during World War I. Langevin used the principle of sonar to detect and locate submarines. Sounding of the ocean floor to provide depth measurements was employed in 1918 to aid in shipping and navigation. Further improvement in technology created more extensive usage of sonar in industry and military situations. Military sonar used by the navy could measure the depth of a reflecting surface and also track an object in motion. In 1930 ultrasound was used in industry to detect flaws in iron castings. Prior to World War II, Dussik used ultrasound in the field of medicine. His attempt to visualize the ventricular system of the brain was unsuccessful. However, in 1937, he designed an ultrasonic device for application to the brain. The first ultrasonic instrument, called the supersonic reflectoscope, was introduced in 1940. This practical instrument, based on the pulse-echo technique, measured distance on the principle of transmission of very short pulses of sonic energy. During World War II the application of radar principles in military imaging further helped to develop the sonar technique. The conjoint use of both imaging systems speeded progress in each field and led to the availability of the first medical sonar units in the late 1940s and early 1950s.

Continuing new developments in ultrasound were spurred on by dedicated researchers. The application of new electronic circuitry and rapid reporting data, retrieval systems changed the use of ultrasound from that of a research tool to an essential diagnostic modality.

When the prototype of the contact ultrasonic scanner became more popular since the transducer could now be placed on the patient's eye with direct contact, many further advances in equipment design became possible. Water-bath scanning of the eye was another technical development, and was soon followed by the application of time—motion displays.

By using two-dimensional real-time scanning systems, the eye dynamically can be evaluated in addition to detection and evaluation of their three-dimensional images.

At present, ultrasonography usage is spreading into many branches of medicine. It has become an integral part of many subspecialties, such as obstetrics, gynecology, and urology, since it is one of the most accurate diagnostic tools in many disorders involving soft tissue pathology.

Modern electronics has given the medical sonographer high-resolution equipment that is relatively simple to use. The application of ultrasonography has been so rapid that it is now the preferred diagnostic test in many clinical problems. In certain disorders, such as opaque cornea and lens, it is virtually the only diagnostic tool available for visualization of vitreo-orbital disorders.

real time
ophthalmic
ultrasonography

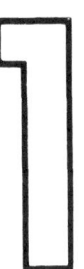

principles of ultrasonography

CHARACTERISTICS OF ULTRASOUND

NATURE OF ULTRASONIC WAVES

Sound is a mechanical vibration of particles in a medium around an equilibrium position. Sonic waves require a medium of a molecular nature in order to propagate. The highest frequency audible to the human ear is 20,000 cycles per second or 20 kilohertz (KHz). Sound waves above this frequency are described as ultrasound. Unlike electromagnetic waves, sound cannot travel across a vacuum.

The wavelength of audible sound in air varies from a few inches to a few feet. Ultrasonic waves are usually produced by a continuous series of contractions and relaxations of substances that have piezoelectric properties. The waves generated are carried as condensations and rarefactions in the transmitting medium. The frequency range used in diagnostic medicine is approximately 1 million cycles per second, with a wavelength of about 1.5 mm in water.

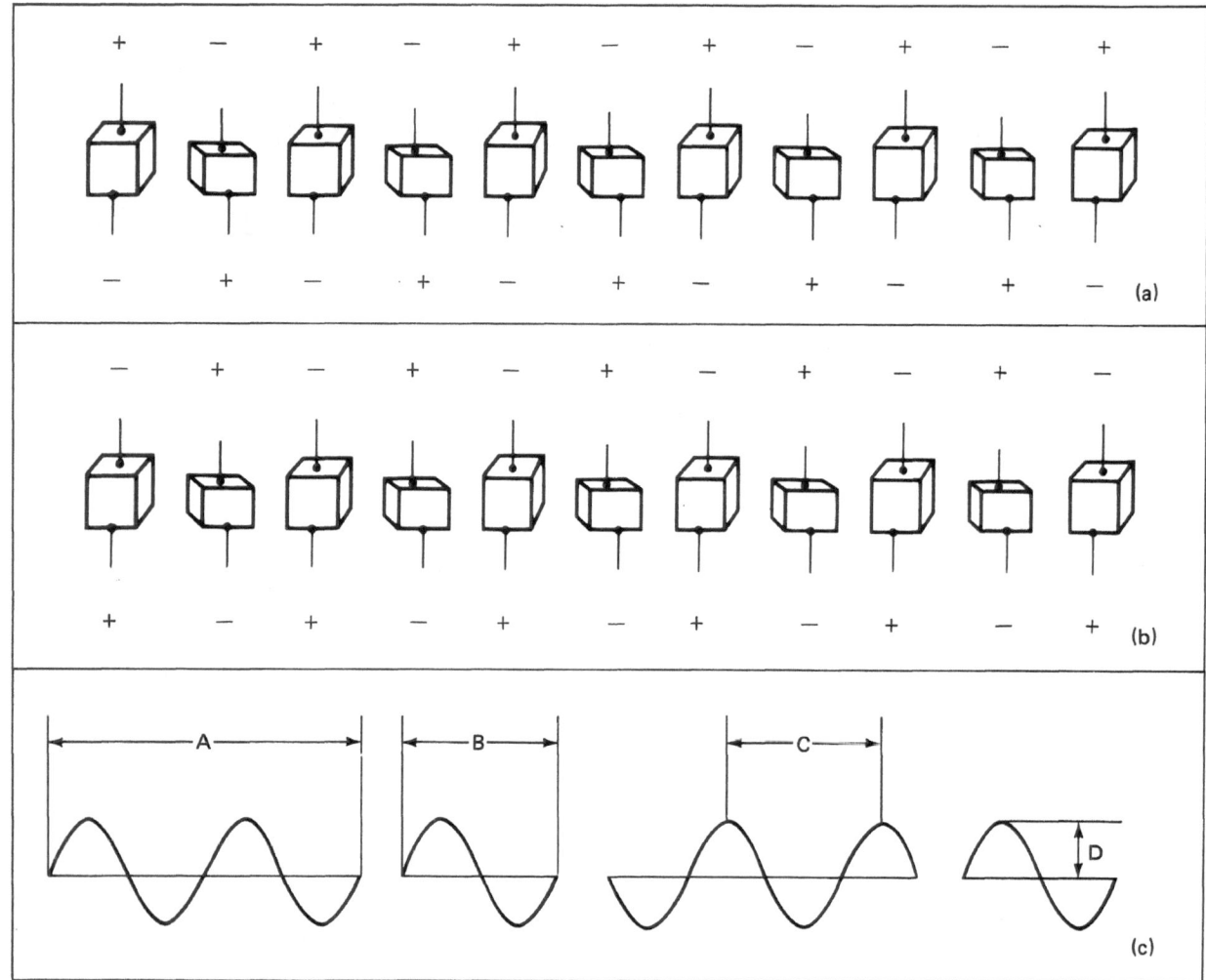

FIGURE 1.1
Piezoelectric effect. (a) Mechanical stress deforming crystal and producing current. (b) Expansion of crystal as current is applied and contraction of crystal as current polarity is reversed. (c) Wave pattern produced by alternate compressions and rarefactions. [*A*—spatial pulse length; *B*—full cycle; *C*—wavelength; *D*—amplitude.]

PIEZOELECTRIC PRINCIPLE

The piezoelectric effect is fundamental to the development of ultrasound. Piezo is derived from the Greek word *piesis,* "to press." Piezoelectric actually means "pressure electric." Quartz has piezoelectric qualities, since its size and shape change under the influence of an electric field. When an electric current is passed through quartz, the crystal expands and contracts according to the polarity of the current. Sound waves are generated as a result of these compressions and rarefactions. On the other hand, mechanical energy in the form of sound waves applied to the crystal produces an electric current. This is known as the piezoelectric principle (Figure 1.1a and b). Several other substances are known to have piezoelectric properties, such as barium titanate, lithium sulfate, and lead zirconate. The titanates are the more commonly used crystal for sonography.

SOUND WAVES

Sonic waves travel through a medium as alternate condensations and rarefactions. The following practical definitions are commonly used (Figure 1.1c).

1. *Cycle.* One cycle is the entire condensation and rarefaction phase.
2. *Wavelength.* The length of one cycle is a wavelength, or a complete condensation and rarefaction zone is a wavelength.
3. *Frequency.* The number of cycles per unit time; frequency of sound waves is described in terms of Hertz (cycles per second).
4. *Velocity.* Velocity is the speed of sound in the medium through which sound is propagated.

The relationship between velocity, wavelength, and frequency is as follows:

$$V = \lambda \times F$$
Velocity = Wavelength × Frequency

EFFECT OF MEDIUM

In any given medium the velocity of sound remains constant, but its frequency varies inversely with wavelength. The higher the frequency, the smaller the wavelength. High frequency sound waves are more directional than low frequency sound. However, the attenuation of high frequency waves is greater than that of low frequency waves, since the absorption of the sound is greater at high frequency. In medical work frequencies above 1 MHz are employed. At a frequency of 2 MHz, the wavelength of sound in water is approximately .75 mm.

Velocity depends on the density and elasticity of the medium. The elasticity of the medium is significant, since the velocity of sound changes in media of different inherent elastic properties. In a homogeneous medium, ultrasound travels in a straight line at a velocity dependent on the properties of the medium but independent of wavelength.

INTENSITY

The intensity of the ultrasound beam is a measure of the strength of its energy and is defined as power per unit area. The intensities used in commercially available medical units usually are between 1 and 40 milliWatts per square centimeter (mW/cm²). Tissue damage may occur at 4 W/cm²; thus, currently used intensity levels are roughly 100 to 1000 times lower in energy than the potentially damaging level. The safety margin is much greater, since the acoustic pulse is active less than 1% of the scanning time.

The decibel (dB) is the practical unit for the measurement of sound intensity. The ratio of signal amplitudes must be expressed logarithmically due to the wide range of echo energies.

BEAM WIDTH AND ECHO PATTERN

The beam width is related to the diameter of the crystal. Ultrasonic waves transmitted from the transducer have a diverging beam width. In this path, any echo received is registered as if it were in the central beam axis. A target on the edge of the beam is recorded in the same way as a target in the middle.

The appearance of the displayed point is important. The echo is registered as a dot or line. The dots lie in the center of the beam and the lines are perpendicular to the beam axis of the transducer. The length of each line is proportional to the width of the beam. The apparent beam width is wider if the target is located obliquely to the incident beam. The effective beam width changes with the sensitivity of the ultrasound machine. By increasing the sensitivity of the machine, low amplitude echoes from the edge of the beam are registered. However, the target is displayed as lines instead of dots and resolution is decreased. The geometry of the target is also extremely important (Figure 1.2a,b,c, and d). If the transmitted beam is stationary and at right angles to the target, the shape of the returned echo is specified by the electric characteristics of the transducer. If the transmitted beam is not

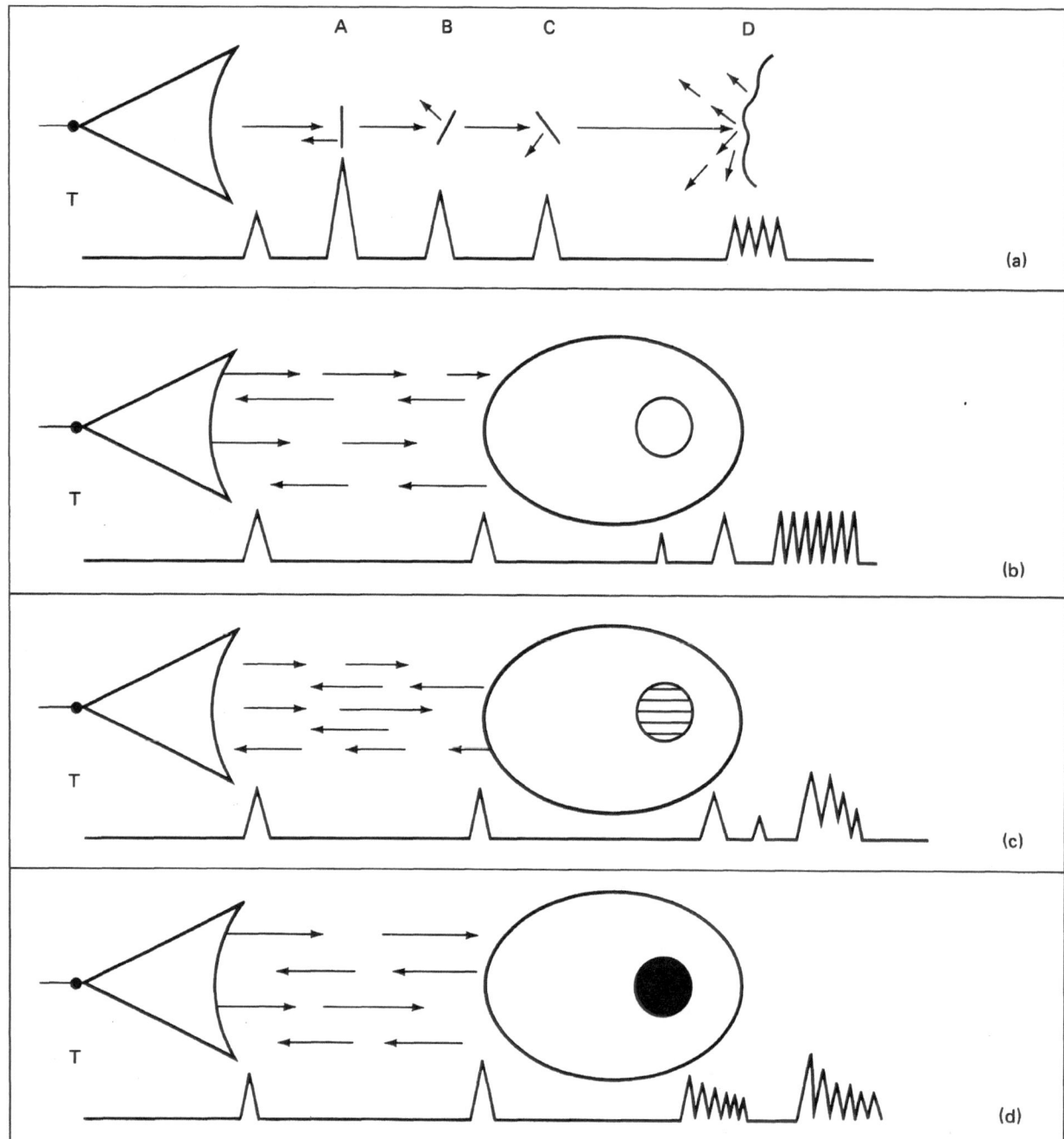

FIGURE 1.2

Reflection processes. (a) Strong echo generated by perpendicular interface (A). Weaker echoes due to sound reflected away from receiving transducer (B,C). Diffuse low level echoes from irregular reflecting interface (D). (b) No echoes produced as sound beam passes through homogeneous medium of cystic structure. Note high through transmission represented as multiple echoes distal to the posterior wall. (c) Echo production by inhomogeneous medium. Note poor through transmission with no echoes distal to the posterior wall. Low sensitivity. (d) Solid medium. Note extreme attenuation in sonic beam in the substance of solid mass due to absorption. High sensitivity. (T–transducer).

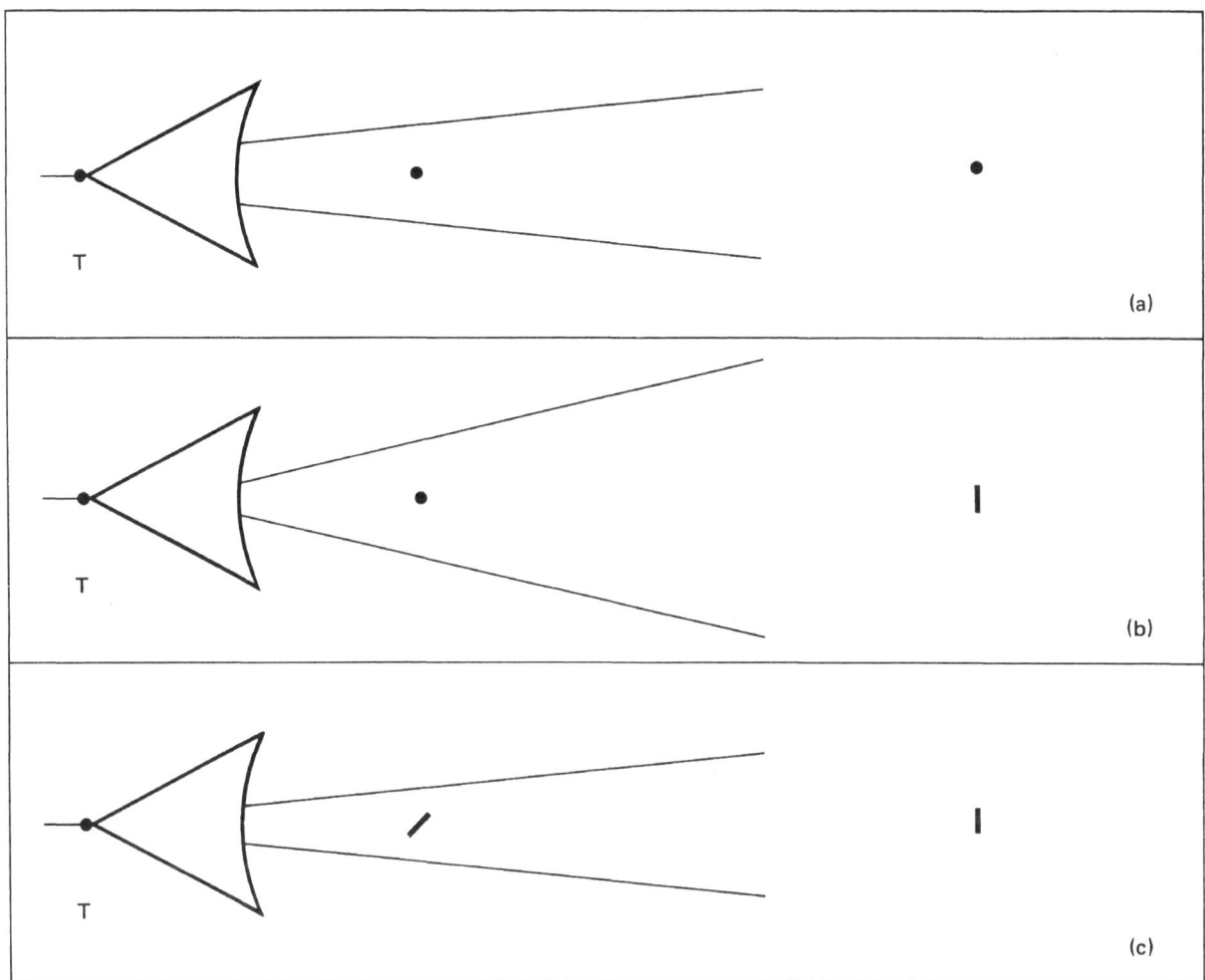

FIGURE 1.3
Echo shape and beam path. (a) Narrow beam. Point target displayed as sharp dot. (b) Wide beam. Point target displayed as short line perpendicular to beam. (c) Narrow beam. Oblique linear target displayed as short line. (T–transducer).

stationary or strikes the target obliquely, the shape of the returned echo is elongated due to a greater effective beam width with respect to the target. Thus, the echoes appear as small lines instead of dots (Figure 1.3a,b, and c).

ATTENUATION

When a sonic beam is passed through a medium, a decrease in the intensity of the sound, *attenuation,* may be expressed as a half value layer. The half value layer is the distance the transmitted sound must travel before its initial intensity is reduced by one half. For example, bone has a smaller half value layer than does soft tissue.

However, energy loss is also caused by beam divergence, scattering, and absorption of sound by tissue. The amount of sound absorbed is proportional to the depth of the tissue and the square of the frequency of sound. Attenuation of the sonic beam has many practical applications. For example, cystic and solid masses can be differentiated since cystic masses have a much greater half value layer than do solid structures. In general, soft tissue attenuation is 1 dB/MHz/ cm. Attenuation of bony structures is about 20 times greater than that of soft tissue.

ACOUSTIC IMPEDANCE

The transmissivity of the ultrasonic beam depends upon sound velocity (V) and the density (D) of the medium. The overall transmission is

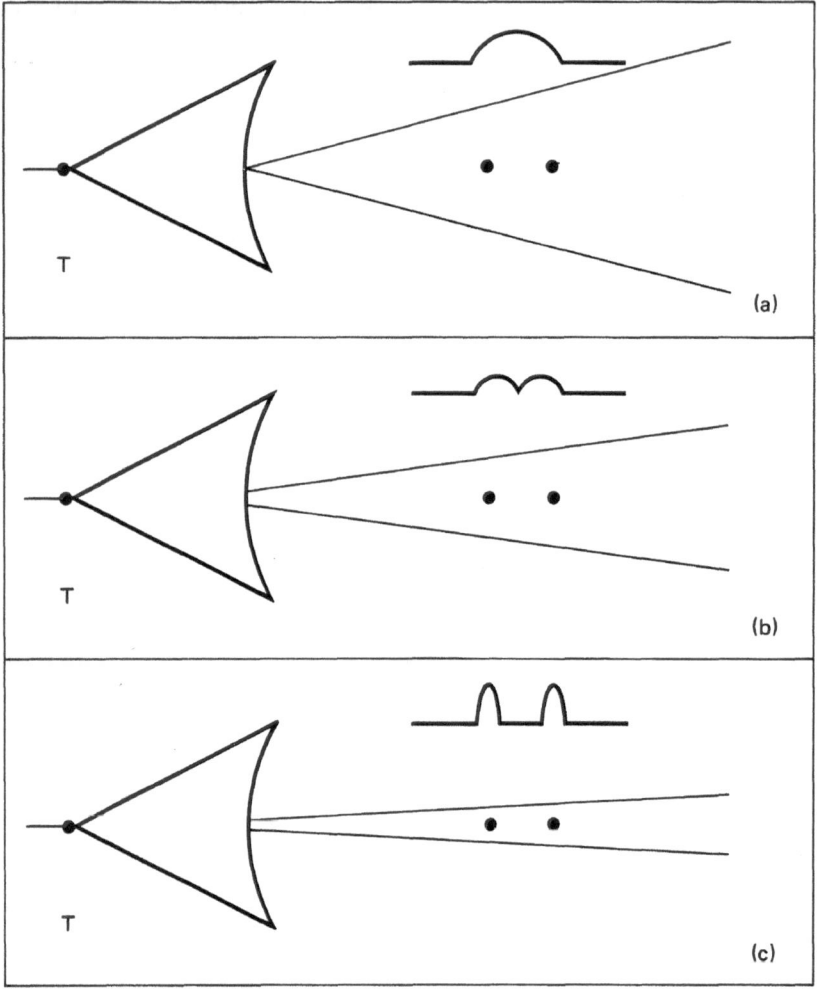

FIGURE 1.4
Axial resolution. (a) Two point targets displayed as one echo. (b) Two point targets partially resolved. (c) Two point targets resolved as two distinct structures. (T–transducer).

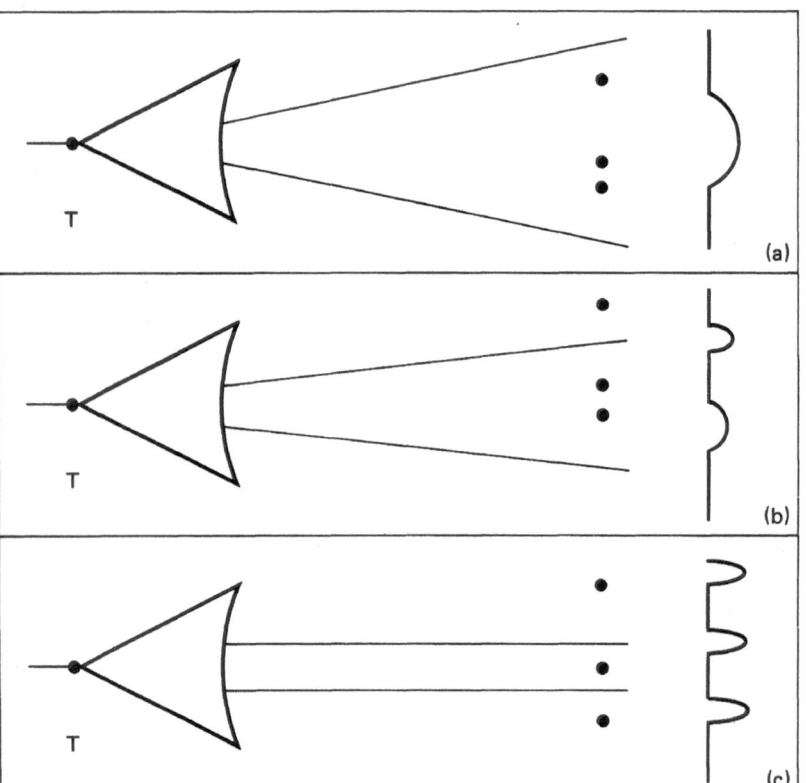

FIGURE 1.5
Lateral resolution. (a) Three point targets displayed as one point. (b) Two point targets shown as one point with better azimuthal resolution due to narrower beam width. (c) Optimal resolution distinguishing two closely spaced targets. (T–transducer).

defined as *acoustic impedance* (*Z*). Consequently, acoustic impedance is directly related to the product of the speed of sound in a given medium and to the tissue density.

$$Z = DV$$

Thus, where *Z* is the impedance, *D* is the density and *V* is the sound velocity. If the interface between two media is a region of acoustic impedance mismatch, a reflection will take place proportional to the impedance differential. Each tissue has a characteristic acoustic impedance.

RESOLUTION

Resolution is the minimum distance between two point targets required to register each point as a distinct entity. The greater the resolving power, the closer the two objects may be and still be individually recognized. The resolution of any wave form is directly related to the frequency of oscillation. Higher frequency sound usually has better resolution but its intensity falls off rapidly as it passes through a given medium. Lower frequency sound usually has excellent transmission but poor resolution characteristics.

In ultrasound we are concerned with axial and lateral resolution. Axial or depth resolution is the ability to distinguish two points along the beam axis (Figure 1.4a,b, and c). The minimum resolvable distance is measured as the axial resolution and depends on wavelength since objects separated by less than one wavelength cannot be resolved. Although the wavelengths of current transducers vary from .05 to 1.0 mm, the resolution of the oscilloscope, or scan converter tube, may not be sufficient to separate very closely spaced echoes. The display system must be sensitive enough to match the transducer frequency. Lateral or azimuthal resolution is the ability to distinguish two points located perpendicular to the beam axis (Figure 1.5a,b, and c). The minimum resolvable side by side distance between two objects is measured as the lateral resolution. This distance is inversely proportional to the width of the beam and depends on the diameter of the crystal, the wavelength, and the degree of beam divergence with distance.

REPETITION RATE

The rate at which bursts of ultrasonic energy are emitted is called the *repetition rate*. Most commercially available instruments emit 200 to 2000 repetitions per second. This high repetition rate requires extremely sensitive receivers capable of detecting a signal that has less than 1% of the incident ultrasonic beam energy reflected back to the transducer.

REVERBERATION

The face of the transducer may act as a reflecting surface to returning sound waves. Consequently, the sound beam may bounce back from the surface of the transducer, follow its original course, and, in return, hit the transducer a second time to be displayed on the oscilloscope at a distance twice as far from the transducer as the original echo. This pattern may be repeated with progressively weaker echoes. This phenomenon is called *reverberation* and may produce confusing and troublesome artifacts (Figure 1.6).

DISTANCE MEASUREMENT OF REFLECTING INTERFACE

By knowing the velocity of sound in the medium being examined and the time it takes for the sonic pulse to strike an interface and return as a reconverted echo, it is possible to measure the distance between the reflecting interface and the transducer. After the sonograph is calibrated for the velocity of sound in the medium examined, time is converted to distance automatically.

PULSE-ECHO RELATIONSHIP

Ultrasonography is based on the pulse-echo relationship. Short electric pulses produced by a generator are converted by a transducer into bursts of acoustic energy. The sound beam emitted proceeds in a typical divergent path and produces different echoes, depending upon interacting media.

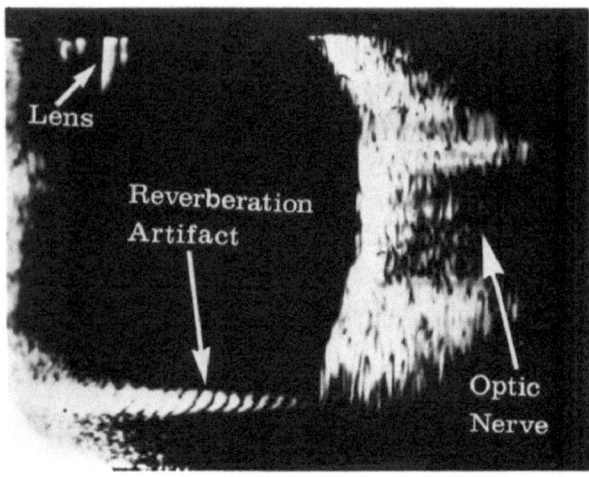

FIGURE 1.6
Reverberation phenomena. The face of the transducer acts as a reflecting surface to the returning sound beam. The echo bounced back appears on the oscilloscope as a series of progressively weaker echoes.

High frequency ultrasound has many similarities to light energy. In its course of travel, ultrasound will be reflected and refracted when it strikes an interface between two acoustically different media. If physiologic and geometric conditions are suitable, diffraction also occurs.

Reflection of ultrasound depends on the acoustic impedance mismatch of two media. The greater the difference in impedance, the greater the reflection. That portion of the sound wave not reflected is transmitted through the medium. If the incident beam is not perpendicular to the interface, sound will be reflected and refracted, depending on the angle of incidence. The incident beam should be normal to the interface studied to achieve maximum reflection back to the transducer. Snell's law of optical refraction applies to the refraction effect of the incident beam and Huygen's principle of optical diffraction applies to diffraction of the sonic beam.

The principal advantage of high frequency sound is that it can be aimed toward specific organs. Study by ultrasound is optimal when the beam strikes at an angle perpendicular to the reflecting interface. If the beam is not quite perpendicular to the object of interest, a portion of reflected sound will not return to the crystal. Therefore, correlation between directivity and reflectivity is necessary for a good examination.

Certain structures have high reflecting qualities for ultrasound waves. Flat and concave surfaces are specular reflectors and the reconverted waves return as a narrow beam. Proper angular relationships between transmitted waves and the reflected beam are required to receive echoes of maximum intensity from this narrow beam. For example, the posterior lens wall acts as a specular reflector. Structures that scatter the reconverted sound waves in a diffuse pattern are called diffuse reflectors. The orbital tissue is a typical diffuse reflector: the echoes produced do not depend on angulation and are usually of low amplitude.

Fluid filled structures transmit sound well and are detectable by the fact that reflection occurs at the boundaries, which are areas of differential impedance. The interface between a fluid filled cavity and bordering tissue yields a large impedance change and strong echoes are returned. Acoustic mismatch is much greater between tissue and bone. For example, at the interface between soft tissue and bone, more than 50% of the transmitted sound waves will be reflected. At an air soft tissue interface, 100% reflection occurs.

Different organs in the body have different acoustic impedances. Therefore, the transmissivity of sound will change as it travels through various tissues. Every time the transmitted beam of ultrasound strikes an interface, an ultrasonic wave (echo) is reflected back and displayed on an oscilloscope. The greater the acoustic impedance mismatch at the interface between two media, the greater the reflection. Consequently, in heterogeneous media many echoes are produced; in homogeneous media there are few or no echoes. Therefore, heterogeneous structures are said to be echogenic, whereas homogeneous regions are echo free or anechoic. A fluid filled cavity is homogeneous and thus echo free. Fluid filled cysts and solid masses are differentiated by the absence or presence of echo producing interfaces within the lesions.

The acoustic impedance of bone and high atomic number elements is very great, while that of air is low. Therefore, the incident beam at a soft tissue air interface is totally reflected. Since there is no beam penetration at soft tissue-bone interfaces, significant quantities of ultrasound are absorbed.

DISPLAY MODES

The reflected echoes may be displayed by A-mode, B-mode, or M-mode presentations and real-time scanning.

A-MODE (AMPLITUDE MODE)

The A-mode ultrasound system displays the electrically converted echo pattern as a vertical deflection (Figure 1.7a). The amplitude of each deflection is proportional to the reflected energy received by the transducer. The deflections occur at different points on a calibrated tracing, corresponding to the distance of the reflecting surface from the face of the transducer. The number, shape, location, and amplitude of the echo spikes furnish detailed information of the structure examined. The horizontal distance between registered echoes is proportional to the depth of the tissue which produced reflection.

B-MODE (BRIGHTNESS MODE)

With B-mode, echoes are displayed on the oscilloscope as a series of dots and lines, the brightness of which varies with the intensity of the reflected waves, since the echoes are projected as a linear series of bright dots (Figure 1.7b). The second dimension of the oscilloscope can be used for acoustic section or sectional study of an organ by moving the transducer in the desired planes. This technique is called B-mode. Consequently, a single section produces a two dimensional representation. In B-mode, a great deal of information is lost during the study.

M-MODE (MOTION MODE)

In M-mode, the motion of a pulsatile structure is recorded by moving the B-mode tracing across the oscilloscope at preselected speeds. Actually, the display of the amplitude of the echoes is changed to dots. The dots of moving organs on B-mode are swept across the oscilloscope in a vertical direction and registered. This motion can also be demonstrated in the horizontal direction by time exposure photography while the transducer is held stationary (Figure 1.7c).

Modification of the amplitude of echoes to dots is called intensity modulation. When the echo has been changed to a dot and the amplitude converted to intensity, the time factor may be introduced into the oscilloscope tracing. In most echograms the oscilloscope sweeps from bottom to top or from left to right on the display tube. When the M-mode sweeping has a vertical and horizontal motion, one dimension can be used

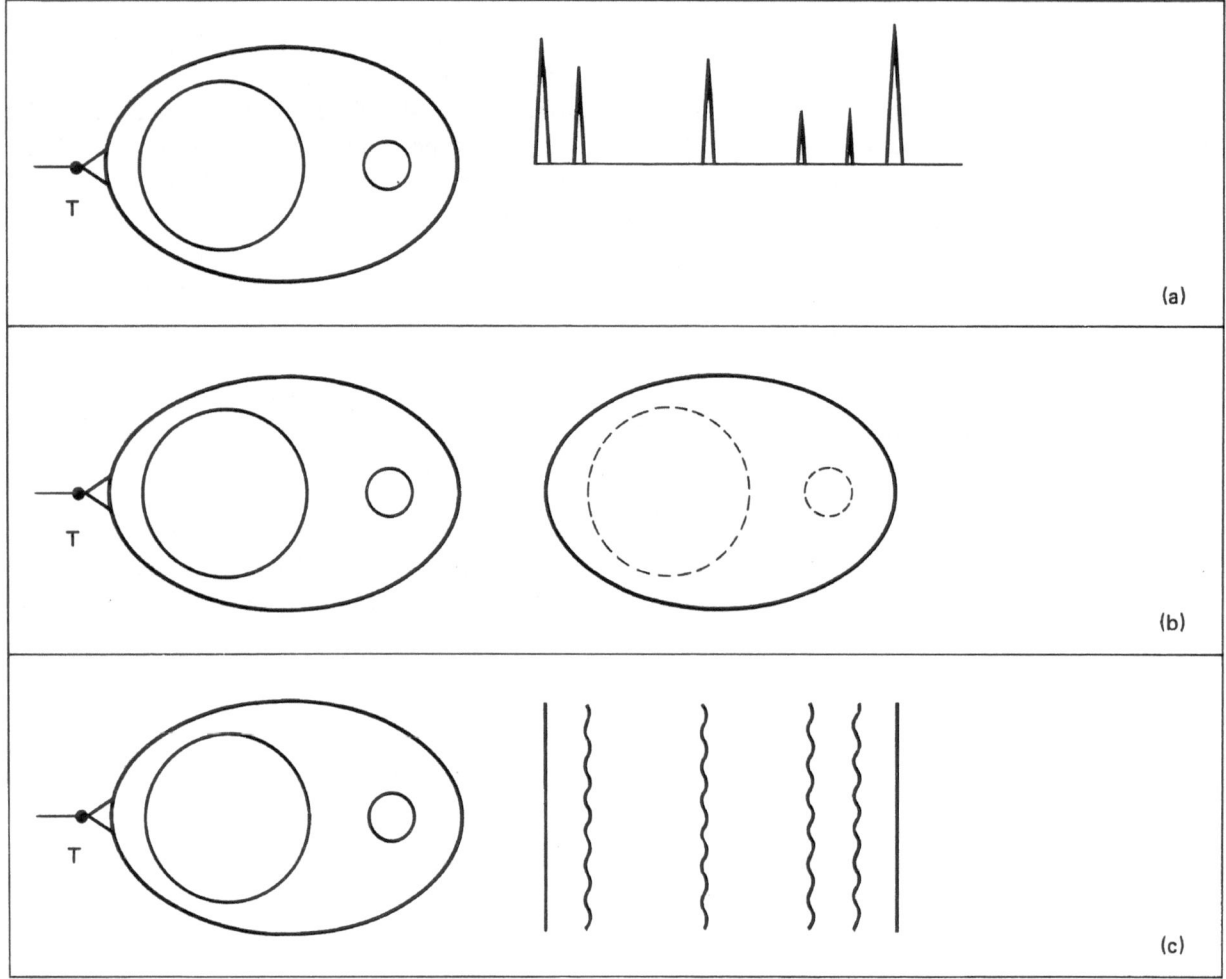

FIGURE 1.7
Display modes. (a) A-mode. Echo producing interfaces produce vertical deflections proportional to echo amplitude. (b) B-scanning. Vertical deflections converted into dots of brightness may be used for scanning. Brightness of dots is proportional to echo amplitude. (c) M-mode. Motion of objects recorded by moving the B-mode tracing along the time axis. (T–transducer).

for time and the other for distance. The tracing can be displayed on a regular television monitor as a black and white or a gray scale by using a scan converter.

The M-mode presentation may be recorded on Polaroid film or on a cathode ray tube. A strip chart recorder affords better detail.

MECHANISM OF CROSS-SECTIONAL IMAGE PRODUCTION

As the transducer moves over stationary structures, a cross-sectional image will be built up from the organ of interest. The scanning is performed through a specially designed housing that holds the ultrasonic transducer. The transducer motion is followed by a computer which spatially orients the transducer position and echo pattern on the monitor screen. As the transducer moves, the returned echo signals will appear on the oscilloscope. The final image is the representation of the outline of the scanned area.

With low sensitivity only the outline of the organs is visualized. At high sensitivity the internal texture is registered. With modern gray scale, different shades of gray are seen clearly without changing the sensitivity setting during the study.

GRAY-SCALE IMAGING

Conventional B-mode systems use threshold detection to register echoes on a phosphor storage oscilloscope screen. These echoes are recorded as dots of light and a large number of these dots are used to form an image on the screen. Echoes above a certain amplitude are displayed as dots with constant intensity, while echoes of a lesser amplitude below the detection threshold are not displayed. Final photographic record was taken in the form of a Polaroid picture of the storage screen. The resultant image showed dots of constant intensity although many echoes came from interfaces with varying echogenicity.

Gray scale displays a dynamic range of echo amplitudes simultaneously as varying shades of gray. High intensity echoes appear dark gray and low intensity echoes light gray. Anechoic areas are colorless with current registration methods. Usually, the sensitivity setting need not be adjusted to evaluate tissue echo characteristics.

Early gray-scale techniques used photographic film to record scans. Film was exposed to a scan pattern composed of amplitude modulated echoes presented to a short persistance oscilloscope. Usually four shades of gray were obtained with this method. Disadvantages included a complicated area scanning technique to prevent overwriting echoes, and a longer scanning time inherent with this maneuver. In addition, the camera F-stop setting, oscilloscope intensity, and film speed influenced the gray-scale effect. After the scan was completed, the film had to be developed before the picture could be interpreted. Current commercial systems in which a scan converter is used offer 8 to 10 shades of gray displayed on a television tube. The scan converter tube detects all echo intensities and is connected to a closed circuit television system providing an instant visual display of the area scanned. The technique is the same as for conventional B-scanning methods. Scanning time is reduced due to better resolution and simultaneous display of weak and strong echoes, eliminating the need to vary sensitivity settings during sectioning. The image developed on the monitor tube may then be recorded with Polaroid 70 or 35 mm film. Moderate differentiation of signal processing enhances contrast at tissue interfaces. Most scan converter systems offer information processing techniques for postscan image optimization.

REAL-TIME SCANNING

The real-time scanner has greatly increased the scope of information available from ultrasonic examination. This modality has been applied to numerous areas of the body. The two main advantages of real-time scanning are the rapidity with which the examination can be completed and the ability to observe motion. Real-time scanners usually employ many type of transducers (Figure 1.8a,b, and c). There are several commercially available real-time scanners.

We use the commercially available Bronson-Turner unit in the eye (Figure 1.9a) and in combination with the gray scale unit in the study of the thyroid. The scanning part consists of a handpiece and a small chamber which contains the transducer and acts as a water bag. The transducer has a 10 MHz frequency and is enclosed in a housing that is held against the closed lid. The transducer of the Bronson-Turner unit is about 1/4 inch in diameter and 1½ inches long. This unit has a rapid scanning rate of 11 sweeps/sec. This unit produces a dynamic display of successive cross sections, which appear on a T.V. monitor. The transducer moves in a sector scan and the image appears linearly. The scanning part is coupled through a flexible cable to the cathode-ray tube.

THE SCANNING PART

The cathode-ray tube resembles a 12 in television set. The section of the tissue being studied appears on the monitor as dark and light areas

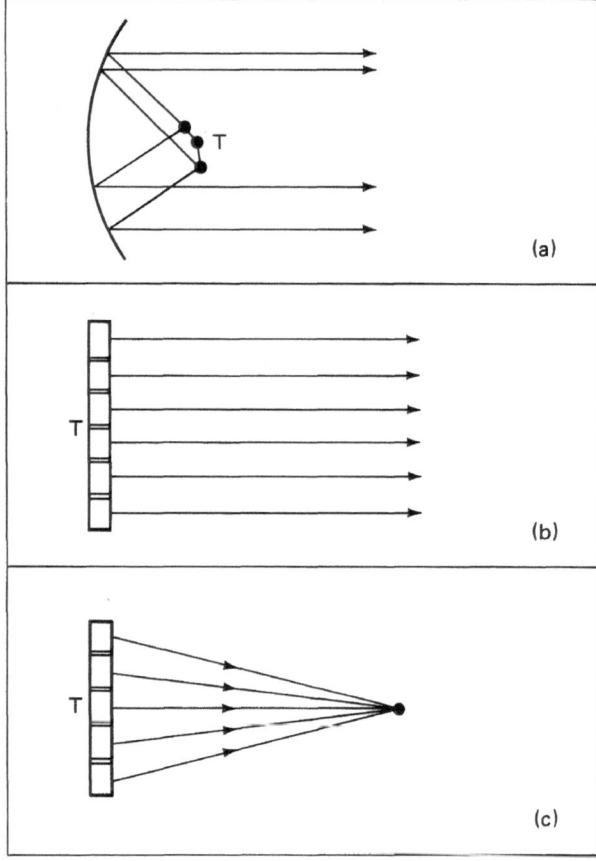

FIGURE 1.8
Real-time scanning systems. (a) Rotating transducer reflects sound waves from parabolic surface to generate parallel beam. (b) Linear Transducer Array. Multiple transducers being pulsed in sequence to produce parallel beam. (c) Phased Linear Array. Variable wavefront generated by coordinated pulsing of each transducer element. (T–transducer).

which directly correspond to the amount of the reflected beam. There are two controls, one selects the depth of field and covers the ranges of 0-3 cm, 1.5–4.5 cm, and 3–6 cm. The second varies the sensitivity setting of the unit (gain setting) and can be manipulated from 40 to 80 dB (standardized with reference of an echo returned from a plain glass plate) in calibrated gradations of 10 dB steps (Figure 1.9b).

PRACTICAL ASPECTS OF SONOLAPAROTOMY

SONOLAPAROTOMY

In sonolaparotomy, proper direction of the beam towards a specific organ is essential. Familiarity with ultrasonic sectional anatomy and knowledge of anatomical pathology and surface topography is extremely important. Comprehension of organ relationships and their normal ultrasonic pattern is necessary to evaluate the extent of disease and involvement of adjacent structures by the pathological process.

EXAMINER

In the field of ophthalmology it is essential that the eye be checked sonographically only by a physician. Sonography is similar to creating a painting. The art of the operator is to image the echoes of a lesion into existence and demonstrate its shape, location, and texture. Sonography is a very delicate test in the evaluation of eye disease, in the sense that pathology detection is more demanding of physician performance. The examiner must make a final interpretation before the procedure is terminated.

POSITIONING OF THE TRANSDUCER

The transducer acts as a transmitter and receiver. The time between the sonic emission and the returned echo measures the depth of the reflecting surface. The maximum reflection is achieved when the pathological area of interest

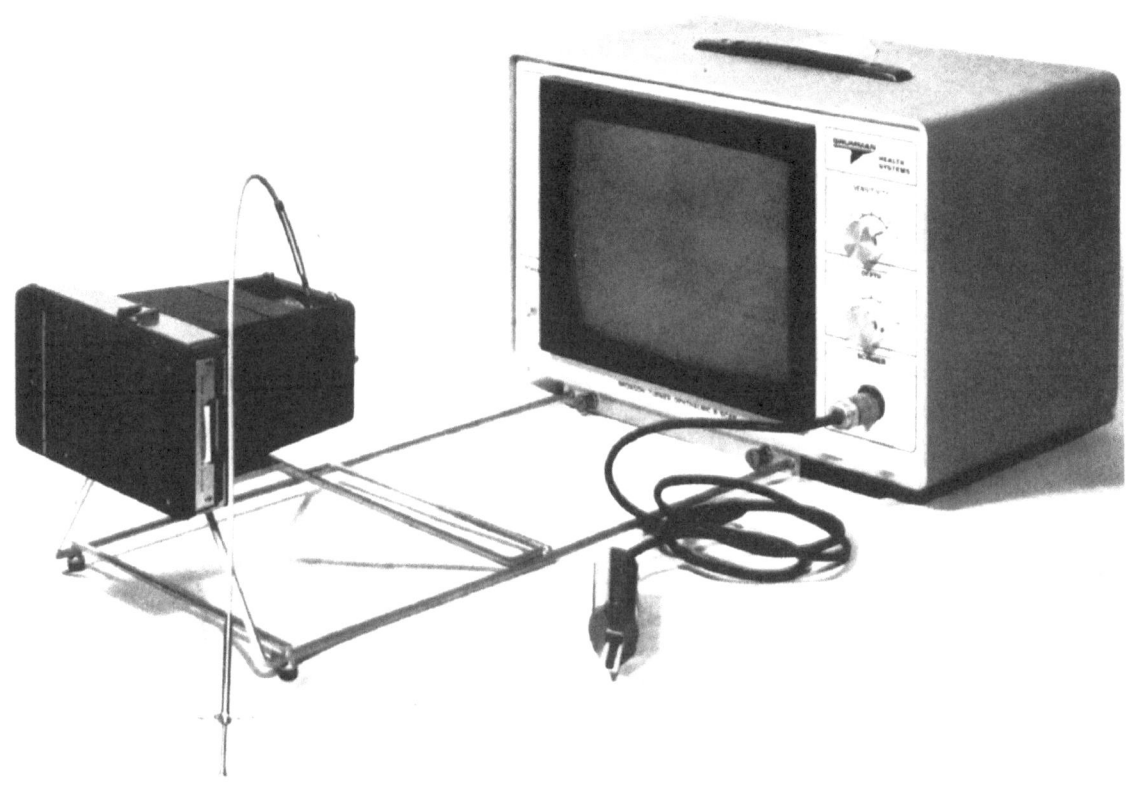

FIGURE 1.9a
The Bronson-Turner B-scan unit. (courtesy of the Storz Instrument Company)

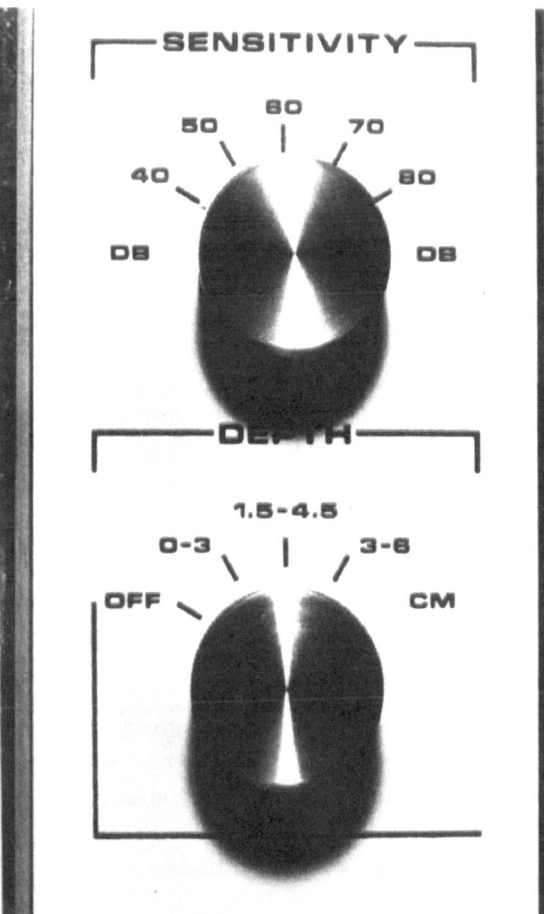

FIGURE 1.9b
Demonstration of two controls. One selects the depth of field and covers the ranges of 0–3 cm, 1.5–4.5 cm, and 3–6 cm. The second varies the sensitivity setting of the unit (gain setting) and can be manipulated from 40 to 80 dB (standardized with reference of an echo returned from a plain glass plate) in calibrated gradations of 10 dB steps.

13

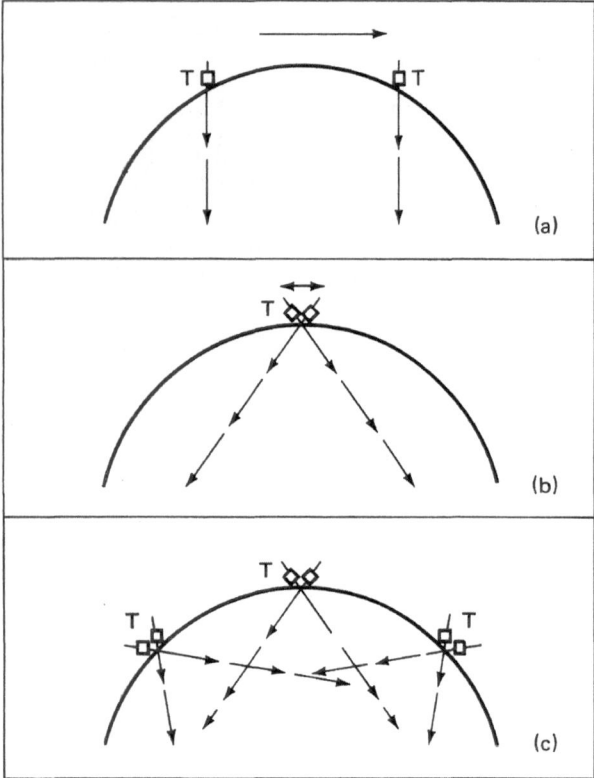

FIGURE 1.10
Types of scanning. (a) Linear Scan. Sound beam at right angles to the skin surface. (b) Sector Scan. Transducer rotated about a fixed axis. (c) Compound Scan. Combination of linear and sector scan. (T—transducer).

is perpendicular to the sonic beam. Any degree of tilt of the transducer or reflector diminishes echo intensity and may even cause loss of the signal.

TYPES OF SCANNING

There are several types of scanning (Figure 1.10):

1. Linear scan (Figure 1.10a)
2. Sector scan (Figure 1.10b)
3. Compound scan (Figure 1.10c)
4. Real-time scanning

PRINCIPLES OF SECTIONAL SCANNING

The evaluation of ultrasonic studies requires a complete three dimensional representation of organs and areas of pathologic significance. As the scan appears on the monitor the examiner builds up a three dimensional object which is the summation of two dimensional scan planes. For example, a retinal detachment with folds could be seen easily in one direction with its attachment, but by rotating the transducer it could be displayed as a circular or oval shape (Figure 1.11). As the application of ultrasound in medicine increases, more information can be obtained. Introduction of a precise and accurate identifcation system makes interpretation of an echogram easier. For this reason special scanning planes are needed in order to perform the study and obtain a corresponding sonic pattern for comparison with future studies.

TRANSDUCERS

TRANSDUCER COMPONENTS

The transducer has a lead zirconate crystal with piezoelectric properties which can expand and contract in response to electric pulses (Figure 1.1). The piezoelectric crystal has a small cylindrical shape and is generally 1 to 2 cm wide and 1 mm thick. The electrodes providing the electric

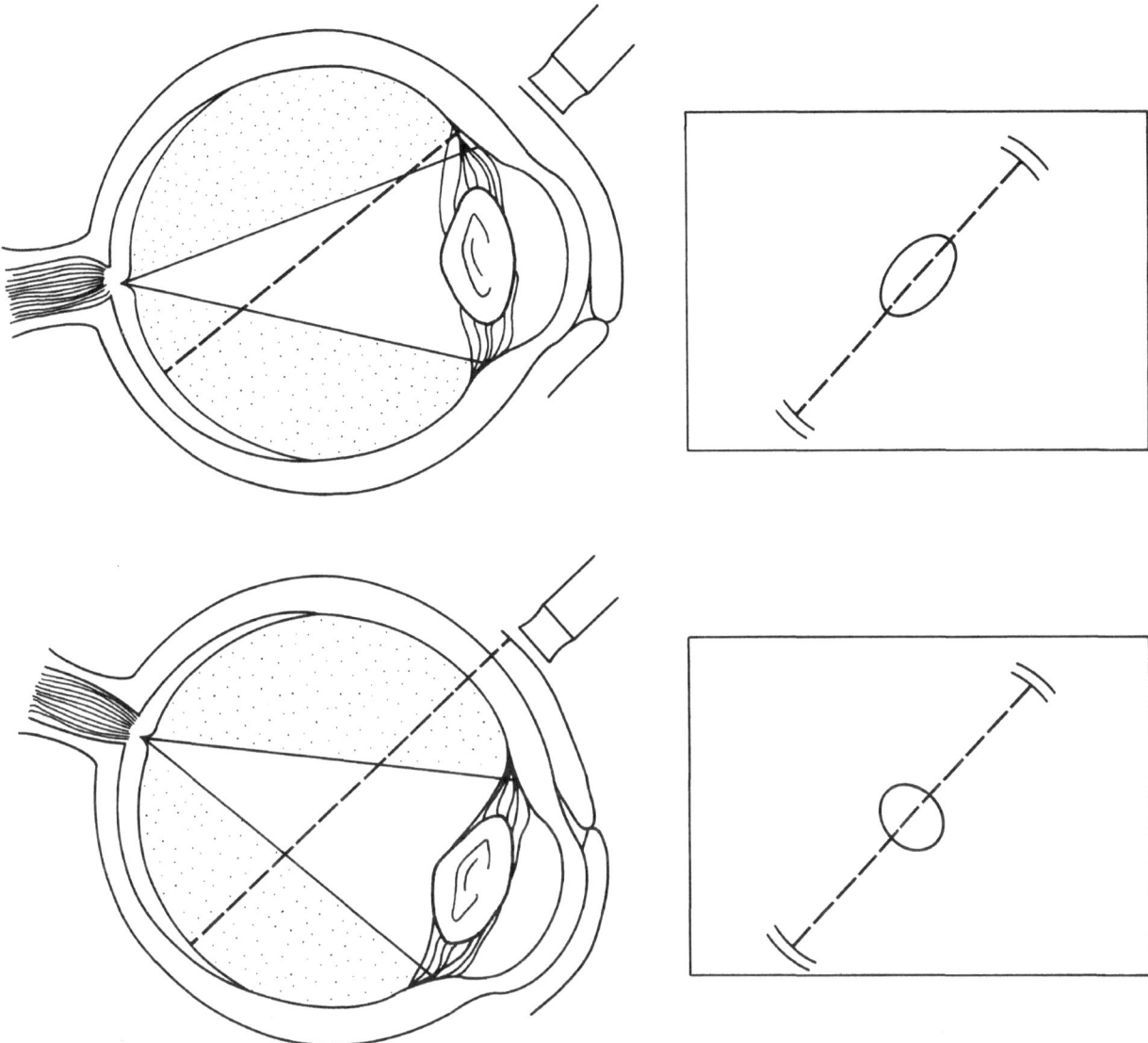

FIGURE 1.11
Retinal detachment and schematic representation of sonogram showing ovoid or circular echoes depending on transducer orientation.

potential are connected to both sides of the crystal. The vibrating crystal causes compressions and rarefactions in all directions. To provide a unidirectional ultrasonic beam, a backing material is used to absorb the waves in unwanted directions. The backing material acts as an acoustic as well as a mechanical damper for the crystal.

The frequency of oscillation controls the resolution capability of the system. After transmission, the acoustic energy of reflected sound is reconverted into electric impulses for data analysis, since the same crystal generates electric currents when exposed to returning high frequency waves. The transducers usually used in clinical work have different frequency ranges, from 1 to 25 MHz. Approximately 99.9% of the time the transducer acts as a receiver.

To vary the frequency of the sound, the transducer must be changed. Transducers of low frequency have longer wavelengths, resulting in greater beam penetration and better depth of study. However, increasing the wavelength decreases the resolution of the system. High frequency offers high resolution. In ophthalmology, the transducer frequency varies from 5 to 25 MHz. As a result, the higher frequency provides optimal definition of small objects but the depth of penetration is limited.

MOUNTING

The disc of piezoelectric crystal in the transducer has a suitable mounting arrangement for optimal resolution. To produce continuous waves a thin layer of a matching wave is used to improve the sensitivity. In the back of the transducer is a loading or backing material, which absorbs sound energy directed or transmitted backward. Consequently, the quality and shape of forward energy, especially of short pulses, are improved.

NEAR FIELD AND FAR FIELD

Divergence of the beam from the transducer is of extreme importance. In a circular transducer, the beam emitted from the face is cylindrical. During the course of propagation, the sound waves run parallel for a certain distance and then gradually begin to diverge. That portion of the

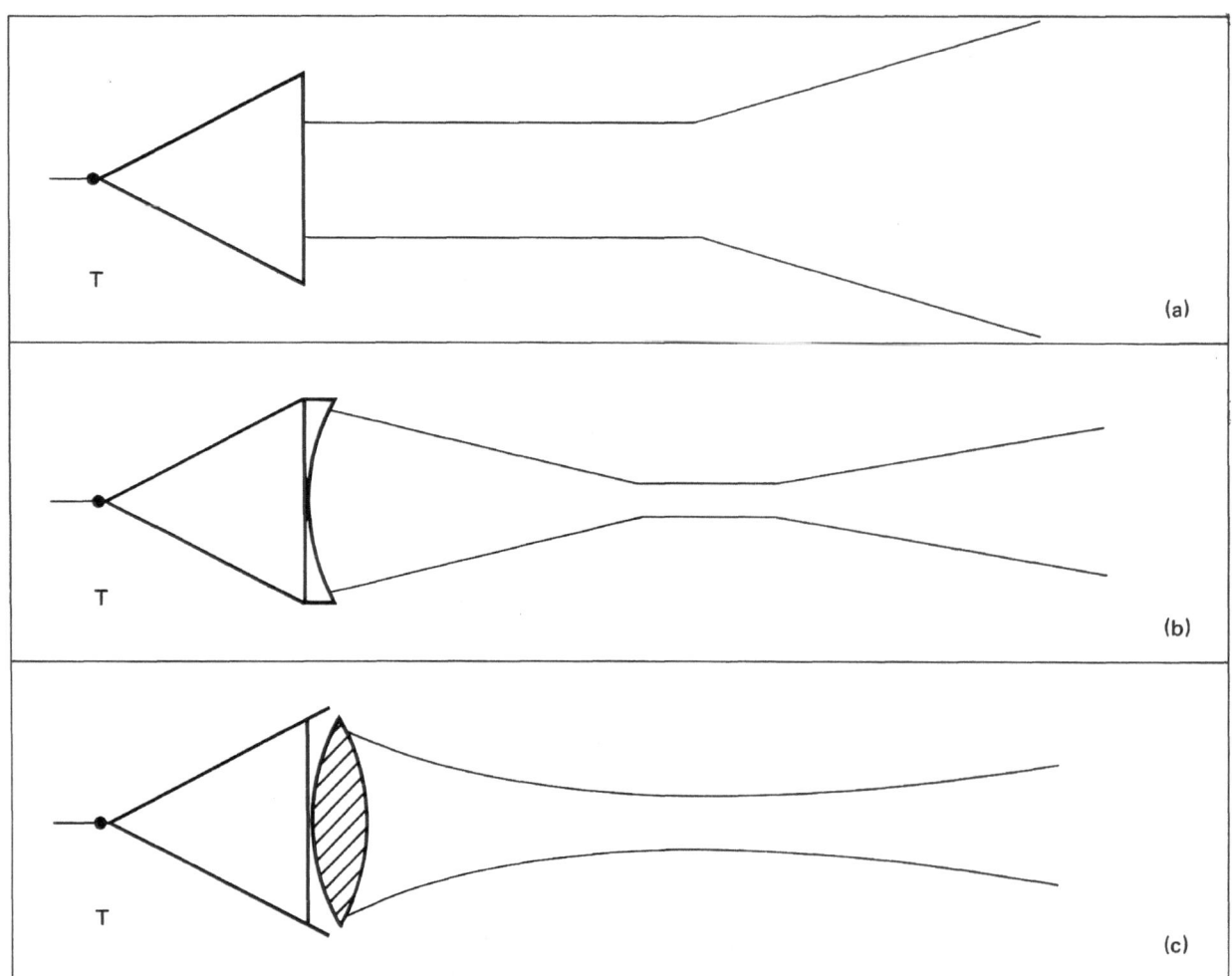

FIGURE 1.12
Transducer beam patterns. (a) Nonfocused transducer. Parallel wavefront forms the near field. Divergent beam in far field. (b) Focused transducer. Narrowest beam width at focal zone. (c) Collimated transducer. Elongated near field and less far field beam divergence. (T–transducer).

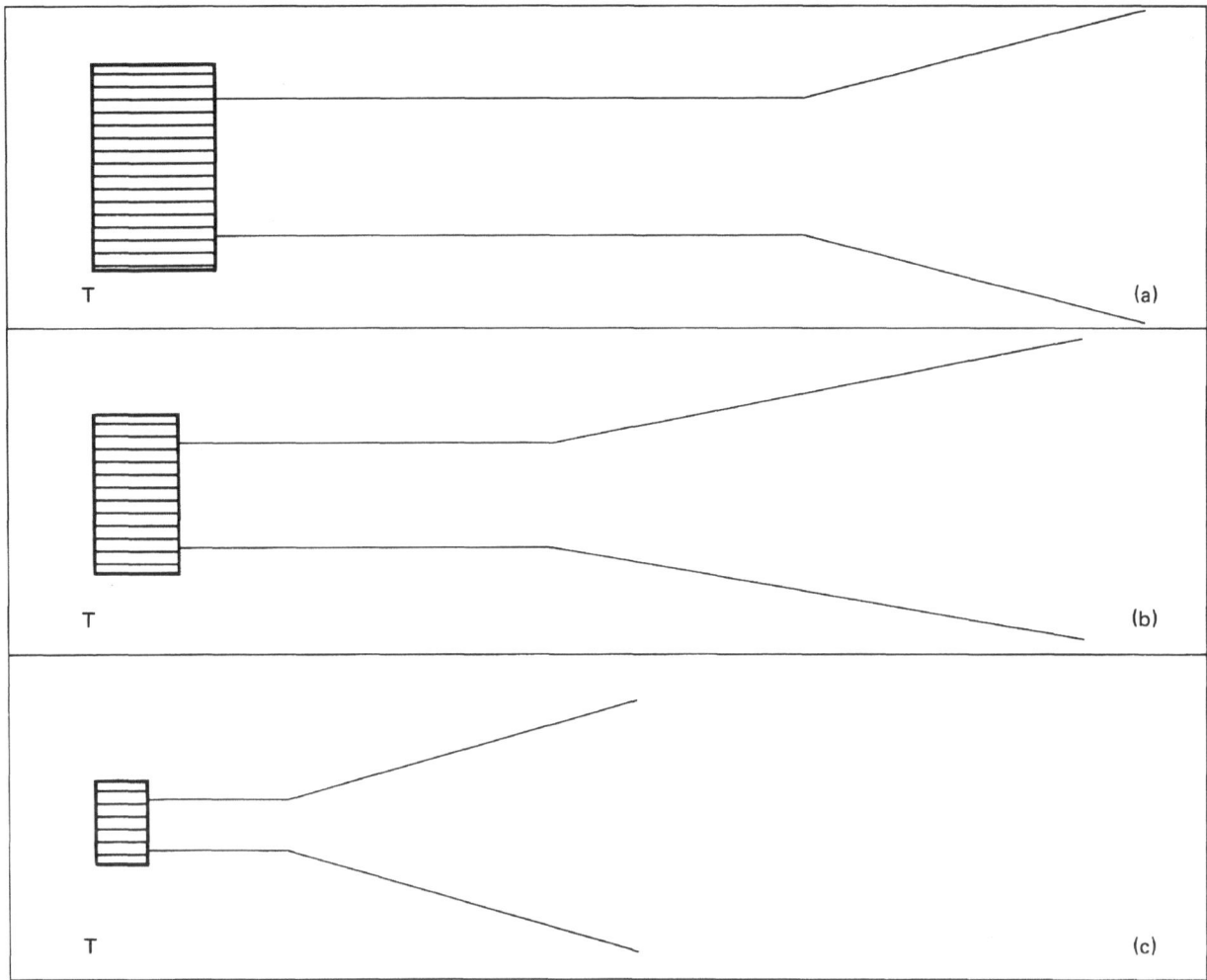

FIGURE 1.13
Beam width and crystal size. (a) Wide crystal with long near field. (b) Medium crystal with shorter near field. (c) Narrow crystal with short near field and great beam divergence in the far field. (T–transducer).

OPTIMAL CRYSTAL SIZE

To increase the resolution of the ultrasonic beam, its width should be as small as possible. To enlarge the near field and obtain better information, the size of the crystal is increased or wavelength decreased. Reducing the diameter of the crystal narrows the width of the beam but decreases the length of the near field and increases the divergent angle of the far field.

To obtain the optimum size of the transducer crystal, the beam width should be constructed in such a way that the near field is half the desired operating range of the transducer. To obtain higher resolution, frequency should be increased. In practice, the highest frequency consistent with maximum penetration for the required study is utilized (Figure 1.13a,b, and c).

beam close to and parallel with the transducer is called the near field and that extending from the divergent point is called the far field (Figure 1.12a,b, and c). At the end of the near field, the intensity of sound is maximal in the axis of the beam. Thus, maximum information is obtained when the object is located in the near field because the sound beam is parallel to the transducer and more perpendicular to the target. Consequently, the intensity of the reconverted echo is greater.

FOCUS

Resolution can also be improved by using a focused or collimated transducer to reduce beam width within the focal zone. By applying a focusing lens with a concave surface, the focus of the ultrasonic beam will be narrowed to a predetermined distance from the face of the transducer (Figure 1.12b and c). The focused transducer has helped to improve resolution of deep structures.

FUNCTION

As previously described, piezoelectric crystals emit ultrasound pulses as short as 1 microsecond in duration. After the sonic burst has been emitted, the transducer then acts as a receiver, picking up the reflected sonic waves. After this period of time, another burst of ultrasound is emitted and the cycle repeated. There are different types of transducers.

PULSE CHARACTERISTICS AND THE DAMPING SYSTEM

The optimal spatial pulse length is between 1 and 2.5 cycles. The excited crystal has a tendency to oscillate for a long time, producing a prolonged spatial pulse length too long to provide adequate axial resolution. The damping system controls crystal oscillation by mechanical and electronic means (Figure 1.14a,b, and c).

SIGNAL PROCESSING

Reconverted ultrasonic echoes produce an electric impulse when they reach the transducer crystal. This impulse is transmitted as an amplified radio frequency (RF) signal into the system. The RF mode appears as a series of signals above and below the baseline of the oscilloscope

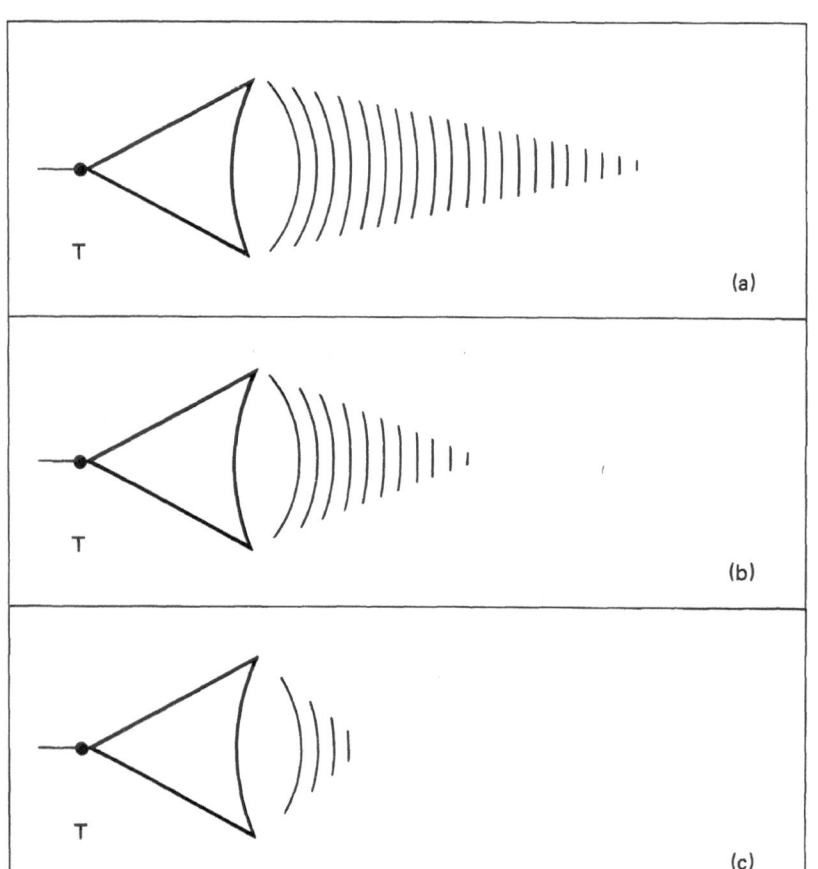

FIGURE 1.14
Damping effect. (a) Underdamping resulting in multiple oscillations of transducer crystal. (b) Proper damping producing optimal spatial pulse length. (c) Overdamping with insufficient pulse cycles. (T–transducer).

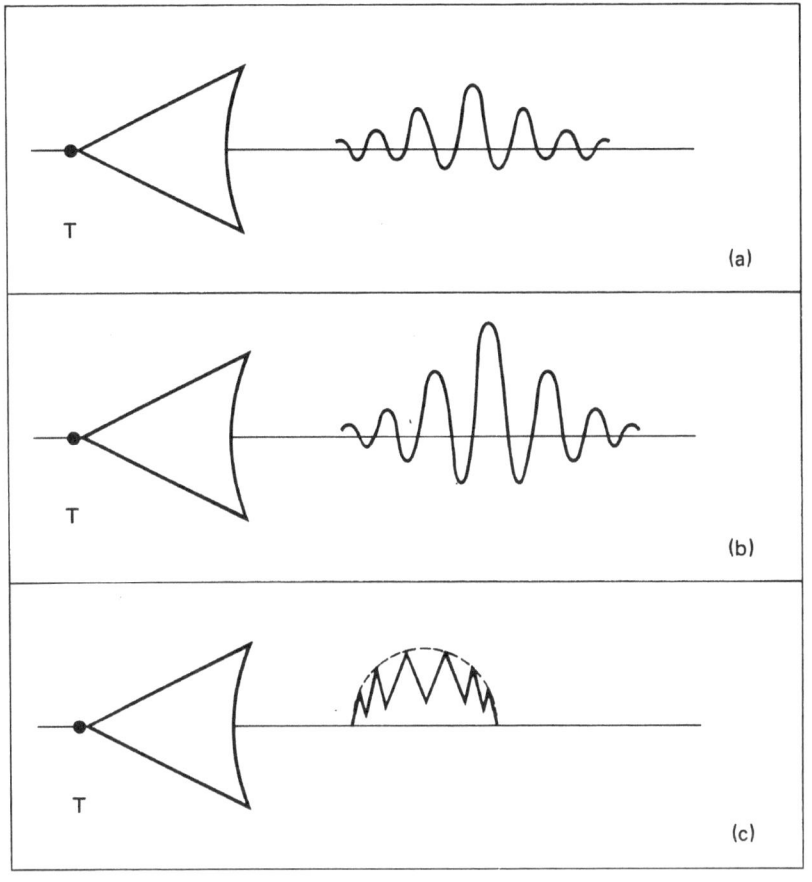

FIGURE 1.15
Signal processing. (a) RF signal produced by incoming echo on transducer crystal. (b) Amplification of RF signal. (c) Rectification of RF signal and envelope detection. (T–transducer).

(Figure 1.15a and b). Amplification increases the size of the signal without changing the information and is manually adjustable (gain control). Further modification depends on specific clinical use. Generally, after amplification, the waveform is rectified to remove all negative components so that only the upper half of the signal is presented. Further modification can be accomplished so that only the outline or boundary of the upper half of the electric signal is presented as an envelope detection (Figure 1.15c). This presentation is called video display. Envelope detection or video display with its multiple peaks can be converted into a smooth, single, large peak called the video signal (Figure 1.16a). This signal may be further amplified by accentuating the leading edge of the signal (Figure 1.16b) by taking the first derivative of the video signal that produces a thin echo. The small negative phase (Figure 1.16b and c) following the initial signal further accentuates the leading edge of the echo

by rectification, giving finer echoes and enhancing the resolution of the system. Another step in processing the video is to add a reject level so that only large amplitude echoes above a certain threshold will be detected (Figure 1.17a,b, and c). Rejection is very important to eliminate unnecessary echoes (Figure 1.17b) and electric noise or "grass" (Figure 1.17b and c). However, certain low level echoes are required for optimal information. The sonographer should adjust the rejection level as needed for proper ultrasonic examination.

ARTIFACTS IN ULTRASONOGRAPHY

Difficulties in scanning due to bone and air will be discussed in detail in Chapter 14. Echoes from internal structures vary according to acoustic impedance, size and shape, tissue attenuation from overlying structures, and structure depth.

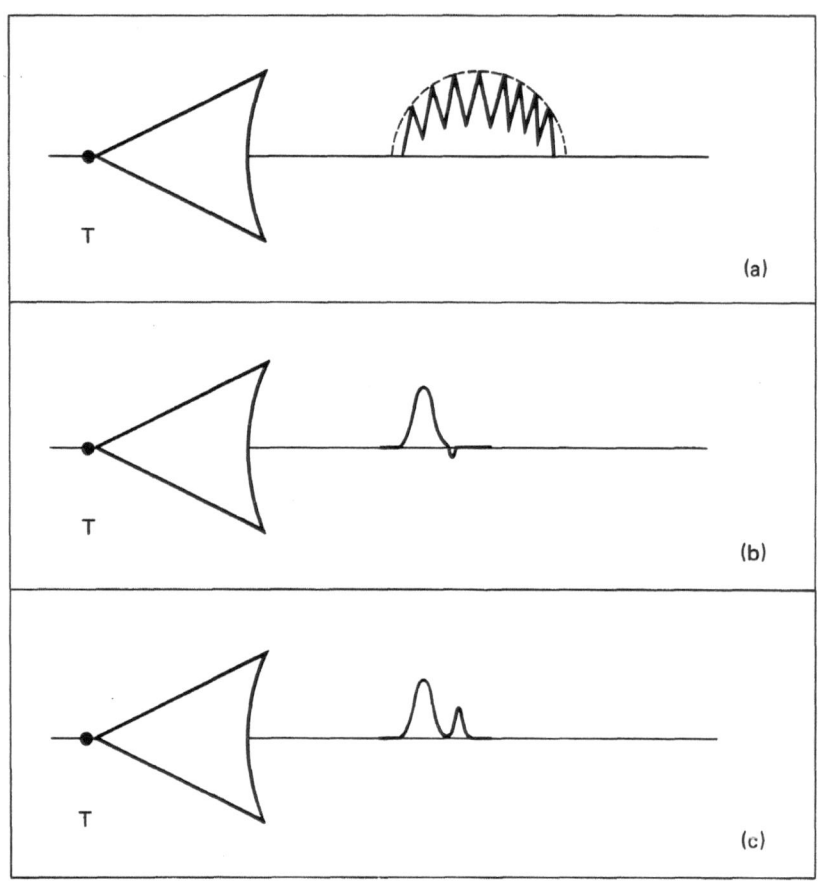

FIGURE 1.16
Signal processing. (a) Envelope detection of rectified RF signal. (b) Leading edge display or differentiation of signal. (c) Rectification and amplification of signal for oscilloscope display. (T–transducer).

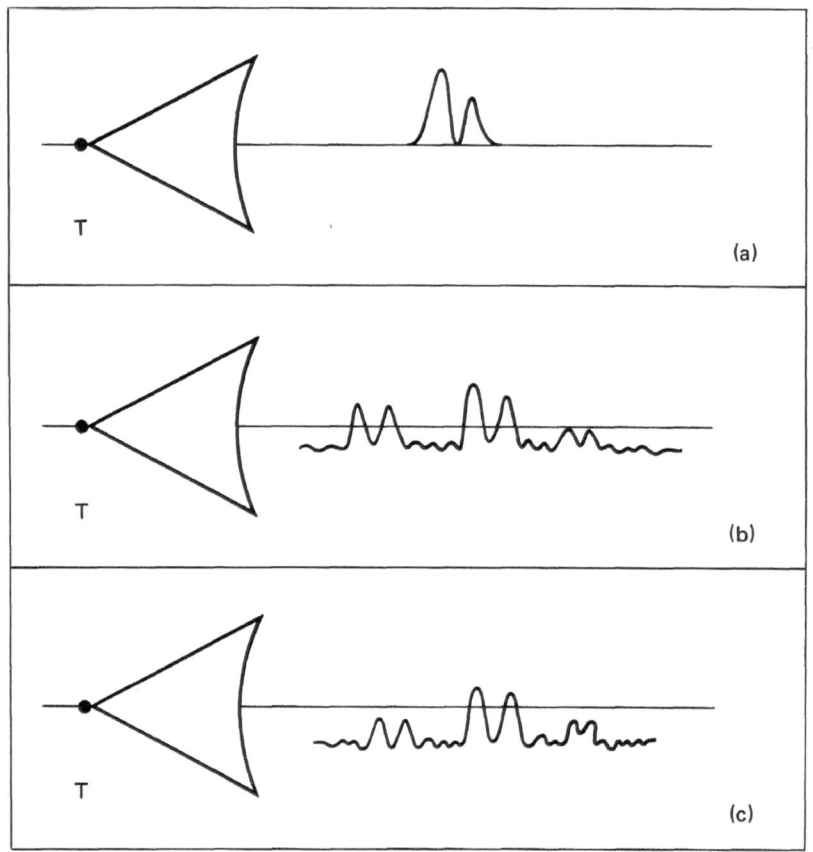

FIGURE 1.17
Rejection. (a) RF signal. (b) Amplified signal with unwanted echoes and electrical noise. (c) Elevation of baseline echo threshold displaying only amplified signal. (T–transducer).

Artifacts may result when the ultrasound beam is not perpendicular to the skin surface. Trouble from organ contour and image distortion due to beam width may occur. Echoes in the near field, close to the transducer, may be lost in the "dead zone" of the beam due to continued oscillation of the crystal during the receiving phase. Newly designed low pulse voltage units with effective damping systems compensate for this problem.

Reverberation artifacts are recognized by their periodicity and decreasing echo amplitude on the A-mode and B-mode. These occur when sound encounters a highly reflecting interface such as bone or air. The loud echo artifact, distal to a strongly reflecting surface and appearing as an echo free region immediately following the strong echo, is due to crystal reverberation. It is noted on the A-mode as echoes elevated from the baseline. Lowering the sensitivity permits the echoes to return to the baseline and the echo free artifact disappears.

Distortion caused by misalignment of potentiometers in the scanning system and changes in the present determination of acoustic velocity may be detected by frequent calibration with an acoustic phantom.

BIOPHYSICAL EFFECTS OF ULTRASOUND

The unexpected and tragic experiences resulting from the early applications of diagnostic radiology and the great physical and psychologic trauma produced by uncontrolled use of x-rays have alerted the ultrasonographer to extreme caution in the use of ultrasonic investigation in human beings. Ultrasonographers have carefully attempted to maximum their efforts to obtain diagnostic interpretations with minimal ultrasonic energy input into the adult and fetal organ systems.

During clinical applications, the possible genetic and somatic changes have been constantly monitored throughout short and long term periods. Many carefully controlled experimental studies have been performed to determine the various parameters of safe ultrasonic exposure. Even at this stage of the development of ultrasound, we have had limited experience with the long range effects. Whether the ultrasonographer's fingers will fall off in 20 years from excessive handling of ultrasonic equipment or whether he or she will show no detectable physical damage or definite chromosomal changes is totally unpredictable at present. However, according to the latest experimental reports and worldwide correlation of data on ultrasonic side effects, there is no substantiation of any harmful effects due to use of ultrasound at the energy levels encountered in current dianostic scanning units. The collected data of many investigators have revealed that there is an extremely large margin of safety at acoustic energy levels used in diagnostic ultrasound. Numerous publications based on clinical and laboratory findings have documented that to date there is no evidence that this level of ultrasonic energy has any genetic or physical deleterious effects.

Widely differing energy and power outputs are used in theropeutic ultrasound as compared with diagnostic insonation. In diagnostic work, the power of ultrasound is on the order of mW/cm². The energy levels used in physiotherapy are thousands of times greater and are sufficient to produce measureable heat in biologic tissues. Higher power is used in such surgical applications as ablation of nerge endings and destruction of normal and abnormal areas of the brain for neurosurgical therapy.

Tissue damage may occur at ultrasonic power levels many thousands of times greater than the diagnostic beam intensities currently used. Simple agitation may cause cellular membranes to rupture at high frequency. Elevation of tissue temperature and cavitation occur during prolonged exposure to high energy sonic waves. Chemical changes include a change in pH caused by the release of radicals and increased tissue oxidation rates. Also noted are increased membrane permeability and greater enzymatic activity. Since ultrasound is nonionizing, cumulative effects are not to be expected.

Ultrasonic waves with very high energy levels are used in cleaning mechanical devices, polishing metals, and drilling.

As mentioned, the damaging effect of ultrasound depends upon the energy range and physical characteristics of the sonic beam. The ultrasonic energy is the product of the measured radiation and the sonic beam velocity which is translated into watts. The intensity of the beam is the power per unit of specific cross-sectional area or, actually, watts per square centimeter (W/cm^2). The intensity or power of an ultrasonic beam usually is calculated from the electric input to the corresponding transducer. This measurement is an estimated value because the sound intensity suffers from complex variations of the pulse shape and spatial distribution of the beam energy.

There are many reports regarding the biologic effects of ultrasound in clinical application. The work of Hellman et al has revealed no evidence of fetal or maternal damage. In our experience over the past five years with a large number of patients who have undergone a variety of ultrasonic examinations involving such areas as the eye, thyroid, heart, brain, abdominal organs, and pregnant uterus: we have not found any deleterious effects thus far. However, we are still following our data.

Macintosh and Davey in 1970 reported an increased number of chromosomal aberrations after exposing human leukocyte cultures to low level diagnostic ultrasound, but in their second study they reported that chromosomal aberrations did not occur below the level of 8.2 mW/cm^2 intensity.

At present we conclude, on the basis of all existing evidence, that there are most likely no significant somatic changes produced by the energy level of the diagnostic range of ultrasound. The possibility of delayed genetic effects remains questionable.

GENETIC EFFECTS OF ULTRASOUND

The increased use of ultrasound in fetal and maternal disorders and its recent application to the male testis require investigation into the potential genetic hazards of clinical ultrasonography. An excellent *in vivo* study of mouse gonads insonated at levels up to 20 times the intensity of currently used ultrasound energy revealed no evidence that dominant lethal mutations or sterility are induced in male mice. Follow-up for eight weeks demonstrated no drop in testis weight or sperm count and no induction of translocations or chromosone fragments in spermatocytes. Although the risk of genetic derangement from ultrasound appears to be slight, its potential carcinogenic effects may not have been fully evaluated in humans at this early stage in the widespread application of ultrasonography to the general population.

TISSUE ECHO PATTERN

We use the following definitions for the evaluation and differentiation of echoes from different biologic tissues:

ECHOGENIC

The term *echogenic* is used to denote the presence of internal echoes within organs with complex interfaces of various anatomic heterogeneous structures, or strongly reflecting interface in homogeneous media (Figure 1.18).

ECHO-FREE

Echo-free areas have no internal echoes at maximum gain settings of the ultrasonic unit. The borders of the echo-free zone may be sharp or irregular. The distal boundary of the echo-free region must always be identified. Cysts are examples of echo-free structures (Figure 1.19).

ECHO-POOR

The term *echo-poor* signifies the presence of scattered, homogeneous or nonhomogeneous low amplitude internal echoes within a range of interest. The borders may be well defined or indistinct. This echo pattern is often seen in edematous tissue (Figure 1.20).

ECHO-RICH

The term *echo-rich* implies the presence of high amplitude echoes occurring at medium sensitivity settings. The outlines of the echo-rich area

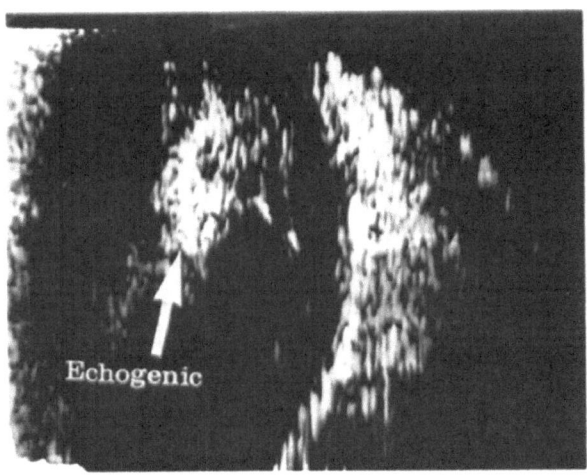

FIGURE 1.18

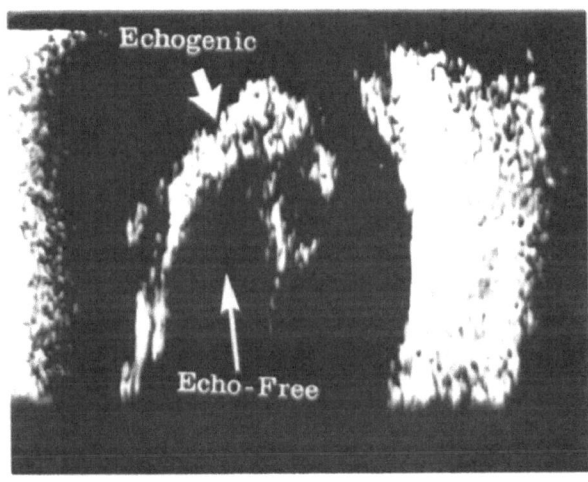

FIGURE 1.19

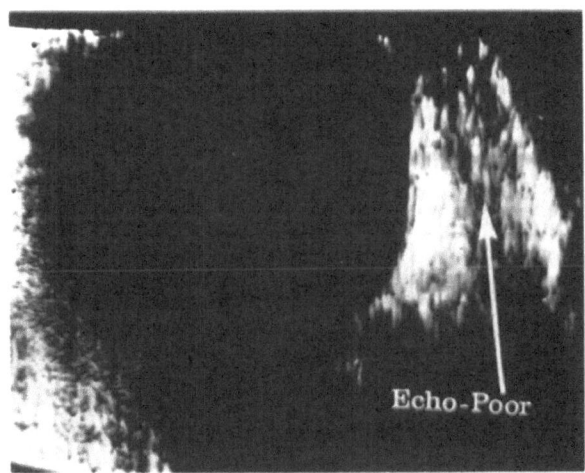

FIGURE 1.20

FIGURE 1.18
The normally clear vitreous body is filled with areas of medium and low amplitude echoes at high gain setting. This is an example of an echogenic area.

FIGURE 1.19
The acoustically homogeneous media of the vitreous body acts sonolucent and is the eye's cystic reference area. This anechoic region is called echo-free. This zone is interrupted by an echogenic focus of vitreous hemorrhage.

FIGURE 1.20
Echo–poor area. The rectus muscle sometimes has scattered echoes within it at high gain setting. This is designated echo-poor.

may be intact or interrupted. Echo-rich areas are found in many solid tumors in the rectus muscle at maximum gaze (Figure 1.21).

ECHO-DENSE

Echo-dense zones are filled with high amplitude echoes at low sensitivity. This is most commonly noted in areas distal to cystic lesions (Figure 1.22).

SONIC SHADOW SIGN

Ultrasonic waves are mechanical entities and will propagate at a rate depending upon the elasticity and density of the medium. The acoustic impedance and the velocity of propagation are two main factors in determining the nature of density of the medium. Water, soft tissue, and blood have similar velocities of propagation for sonic waves and similar acoustic impedances. Grossly, these media are homogeneous and practically no refraction of the beam will occur during passage through these media.

The velocity of ultrasonic waves in bone and their acoustic impedance therein is high. Thus, a large amount of refraction of the beam in a new direction will occur. There is a high absorption of sonic waves in bone. Similar conditions are also noticeable in heavily calcified organs or structures containing calcium, bone, or metal.

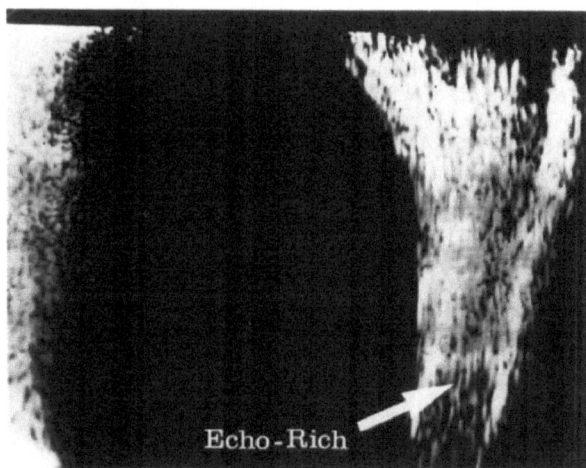

FIGURE 1.21
Echo-rich zone. The rectus muscle compared with the previous echo-poor muscle is full of homogeneous echoes and is termed echo-rich.

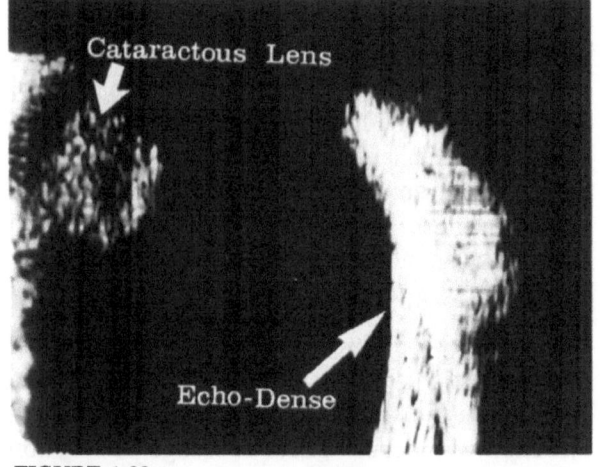

FIGURE 1.22
Echo-dense. The echo pattern of the orbital fat is of homogeneous high amplitude echoes. This echo-dense picture is often noted distal to cystic areas.

As a result of high absorption of the ultrasonic beam in heavily calcified areas or certain foreign bodies, there are no sonic waves beyond these structures (Figure 1.23). The acoustic impedance of air is low and, as a result, there is no propagation of ultrasonic waves at an air-fluid interface. This dominant interface causes complete reflection or bounces back all ultrasonic waves. Thus, air, bone, heavily calcified organs, and various foreign substances are barriers to ultrasound.

The absorption of osseous structures, metal, and heavily calcified regions or the complete reflection of sonic waves at an air-fluid interface causes a sonolucent area which is called a *sonic shadow*. The sonic shadow should not be mistaken for sonolucent or echo-free structures and be mistaken for a pathological condition. For better evaluation of this false impression, the transducer should be moved perpendicularly to the area of interest to investigate the through transmission properties.

DETECTION OF THROUGH TRANSMISSION PATTERN

Through transmission is the sound energy that passes through a structure and is then recorded by the receiving transducer. It is inversely proportional to the attenuating properties of the medium and is registered on the oscilloscope as the number of echoes and their amplitudes at the distal interface of the region insonated.

Characteristically cysts have posterior multiple echoes of high amplitude. We term this *high through transmission*. Large solid tumors tend to absorb significant sound energy and have few posterior echoes which are generally of low amplitude. This phenomenon is called *low through transmission*. In between these extremes, other levels of echo density will be appropriately defined as *moderate through transmission*. The combination produces the flood of echoes which we refer to as through transmission.

To evaluate transmission characteristics of a structure, the posterior border of that structure must be identified. The distal border is visualized

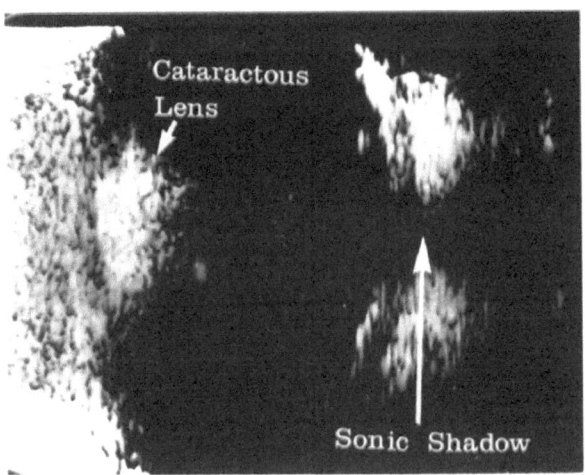

FIGURE 1.23
Sonic shadow. This cataractous lens highly attenuates the sonic beam so that the distal echoes from the posterior orbit fat are not registered on the receiver producing a typical uninterrupted funnel shape sonolucent or echo-free area posteriorly. This phenomenon is called the sonic shadow sign.

at low sensitivity settings when the medium is highly transonic, as in fluid structures and parenchymatous glands such as the liver and spleen. When the medium is poorly transonic, the sound beam is attenuated significantly and the sensitivity must be increased to amplify distal echoes. This is particularly true for solid, acoustically homogeneous tumors such as malignant melanoma and lymphomas. Indeed, maximum gain settings may be necessary to faintly image the distal wall. These masses may not contain sufficient internal interfaces to produce echoes and may appear as sonolucent lesions. In these cases, the echo-free region is differentiated from a cyst by a poorly delineated posterior wall, indicating poor through transmission.

Sonic shadowing is best appreciated during linear scanning with B-mode and by simultaneously noting the abrupt termination of A-scope echoes in a single high amplitude echo.

Tumors with internal degeneration permit better through transmission than do architecturally intact masses of the same histological type. The presence of fluid-filled necrotic spaces within a tumor increases beam transmission and the tumor appears on the oscilloscope as a lesion with multiple posterior echoes. At low sensitivity, anterior and posterior borders of a degenerating tumor may be outlined and the high posterior echo density may simulate a simple cyst. This error is avoided by sensitivity studies in which a characteristic echogenic mass is revealed as gain is increased.

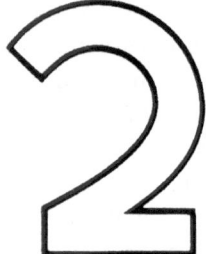

ophthalmic anatomy

INTRODUCTION

The sonographer must have a total understanding of the anatomy of the globe and orbit to understand the ocular functions and their modification in disease states. Certain structures must be considered in great depth as they are significant in the comprehension of the sonographic anatomy and sonopathology. This chapter will fully outline the anatomic structures and relationships basic to ophthalmological disorders and emphasize areas that are of key importance to the sonographer and eye surgeon.

ANATOMY

The eye rests in the orbital cavity and only its anterior aspect is exposed. The optic nerve originates from the globe and leaves the apex of the orbit in the optic foramen which also transmits the ophthalmic artery and sympathic nerve of the eye. The anterior one-third of the eye consists of a central

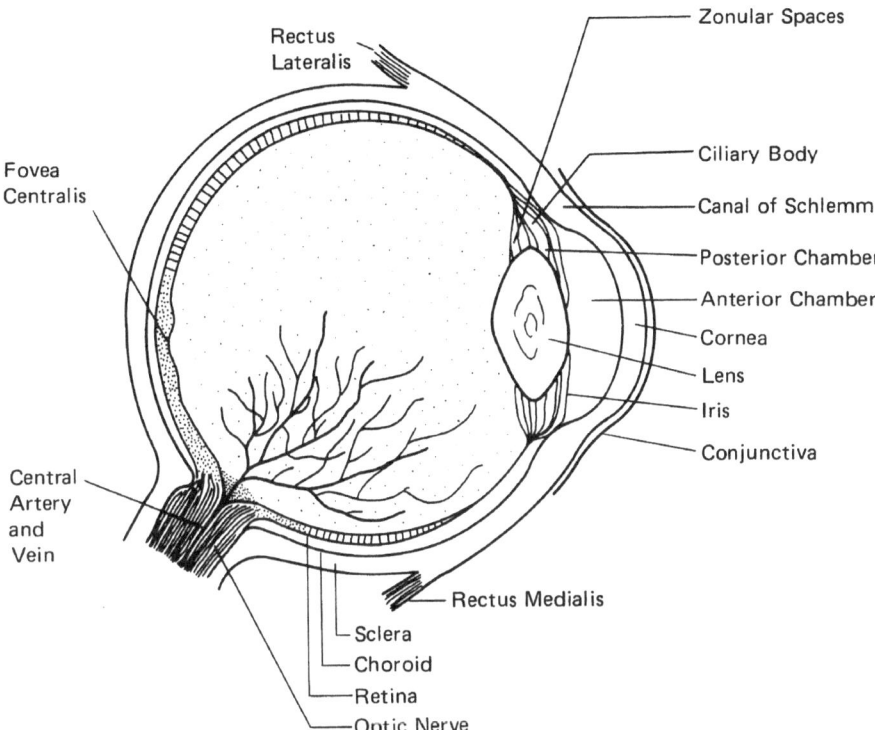

Zonular Spaces
Rectus Lateralis
Fovea Centralis
Ciliary Body
Canal of Schlemm
Posterior Chamber
Anterior Chamber
Cornea
Lens
Iris
Conjunctiva
Central Artery and Vein
Rectus Medialis
Sclera
Choroid
Retina
Optic Nerve

FIGURE 2.1
Cross-sectional anatomy of the eye.

transparent portion, cornea and a surrounding opaque portion, the sclera. The lacrimal gland is located in the upper portion of the bony orbit.

The anterior pole is the center of curvature of the cornea. The posterior pole is the center of the posterior curvature of the globe and is located at the temporal side of the optic nerve (Figure 2.1). The geometric axis is a plane which connects these two poles. The equator encircles the globe halfway between the two poles. The antero-posterior diameter of the normal eye is about 22 to 27 mm. The average eye is 24 mm. The equator is on the surface of the sclera and encircles the eye midway between the two poles (Figure 2.2). The circumference of the eye is approximately 69 to 85 mm.

GLOBE

The globe has three layers. The outer layer is composed of the cornea (transparent), sclera (opaque), and limbus (junction between cornea and sclera).

SCLERA

The white, opaque sclera constitutes the posterior five-sixths of the globe and is a dense, avascular, and fibrous structure. Posteriorly it is connected by fine collagen fibers to the dense bulbar fascia. This fascia is called "Tenon's capsule" which is a potential space separating the globe from the orbital fat and is the housing within the globe moves. Tenon's capsule extends anteriorly to the corneoscleral junction. Medial to the posterior pole of the eye, the optic nerve exits through the posterior scleral foramen and it is this area that the sclera is thickest. The anterior scleral foramen is the region into which the cornea fits. The vortex veins, which are the collecting channels for the choroidal veins, pierce the sclera about 4 mm posterior to the equator of the eye. The choroid is firmly fixed at the point of exit of the four vortex veins through the sclera.

CORNEA

The cornea forms the transparent anterior pole of the eye and is slightly oval in shape. The central optical portion is one-half mm thick and

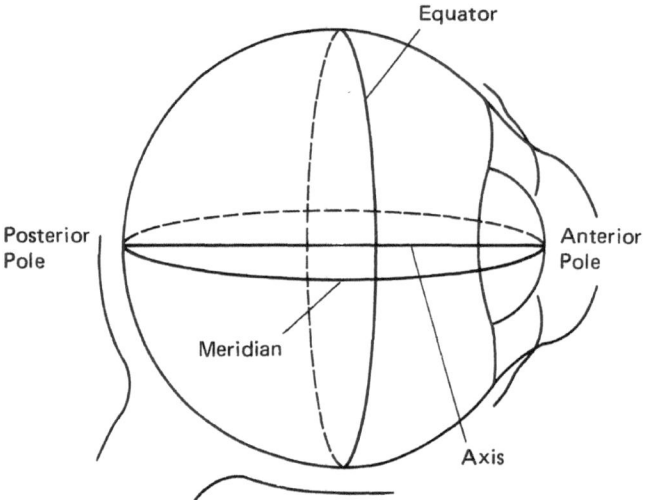

FIGURE 2.2
Coordinates of the eye, depicting the equator and the meridian. The visual axis, which connects the observed object and the fovea centralis, does not correspond to the antero-posterior geometric axis.

has parallel anterior and posterior surfaces. The cornea is the main refracting portion of the eye and is composed of five layers; from anterior to posterior these are:

1. Epithelium
2. Bowman's membrane
3. Stroma
4. Descemet's membrane
5. Endothelium

The central cornea is avascular, but the region of the corneoscleral limbus is supplied by the anterior ciliary arteries.

LIMBUS

This junction is a transition zone between the cornea and the sclera. This region is important since the drainage system of the anterior chamber is located interiorly. The trabecular meshwork surrounds the entire circumference of the anterior chamber (Figure 2.3). The aqueous humor is transferred to the canal of Schlemm through the trabecular meshwork. Disease in this area produces glaucoma.

UVEA

The middle layer or uvea consists of the choroid, ciliary body, and iris. This layer is vascular and

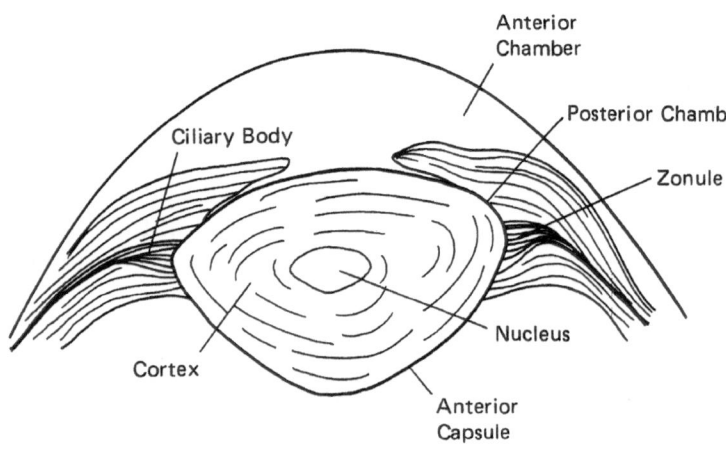

FIGURE 2.3
Cross-sectional anatomy of the anterior portion of the eye.

contains a central opening, the pupil. The choroid extends from the optic nerve posteriorly to the ciliary body anteriorly. It is attached firmly to the sclera in the regions of the optic nerve and vortex veins. Uvea comes from the Latin word *uva,* meaning grape. The vascular choroid nourishes the retinal pigment epithelium and the sensory retina. The choroid is divided into three layers of blood vessels. The membrane of Bruch is a tough fibrocollagenous structure separating the choriocapillaris (central vascular layer of choroid) from the retinal pigment epithelium which stops at the optic nerve.

The ciliary body is a ring of tissue between the base of the iris and the choroid which extends 6 mm back to the ora serrata. This marks the forward limit of the retina and choroid. The ciliary muscle adjusts the shape of the lens in accomodation.

IRIS AND PUPIL

The iris is a delicate diaphragm adjacent to the ciliary body and lies in front of the lens. This structure separates the anterior and posterior chambers. The iris inserts into the scleral spur through its connection to the ciliary body. The pupillary border rests on the lens and has a circular aperture, the pupil, which controls the entry of light into the eye.

RETINA

The retina is the inner layer of the eye. Embryologically, the retina develops from the invagination of the optic cup. This forms an outer layer, the pigment epithelium, and an inner layer, the sensory retina. The retina extends from the optic nerve posteriorly to the scalloped margin of the ora serrata anteriorly. The retinal pigment epithelium (RPE) is bound to the membrane of Bruch and extends from the optic nerve to the ora serrata anteriorly.

The sensory retina basically consists of a layer of photoreceptor cells connected to two neurons. The photoreceptor cells are the rods and cones.

The retina may be functionally divided into various regions. The optic disc is made of the axons of the ganglion cells that leave the eye through the sieve-like lamina cribrosa. The choroid and all layers of the retina, except the nerve fiber layer, terminate at the disc margin. There are no rods and cones in the optic disc. The nerve fiber layer has synaptic functions and contains the major retinal blood vessels, the central artery and vein of the retina. Frequently a physiologic cup is present in the central portion of the surface of the optic disk. The ora serrata is the anterior termination of the retina and consists of a scalloped fringe that parallels the ciliary processes. The central retina surrounds the fovea centralis, and is approximately 6 mm in diameter. This is the area of the macula lutea which has a high concentration of cones for greatest visual acuity. The extracentral peripheral retina is mainly composed of rod type photoreceptors and extends to the ora serrata.

The lens is located behind the iris and its position is supported by fine fibers, the zonule. These are attached to the ciliary body and the capsule of the lens. The crystalline lens is grossly transparent and biconvex with a diameter of 10 mm and a thickness of 4 mm. The lens continues to form fibers throughout life. Old fibers are compressed centrally to form an increasingly larger and less elastic nucleus. Normally, under microscopic examination, the lens contains multiple minute opacities and concentric areas of different indexes of refraction. The lens is composed of a lens capsule which completely surrounds it, and an anterior capsular epithelium. The lens substance consists of the cortex with newly formed soft layers of fibers and a dense central area of old compressed fibers called the nucleus.

GLOBE AND VITREOUS

The globe has three chambers (Figure 2.1): the anterior chamber, the posterior chamber, and the vitreous cavity.

The anterior chamber is located between the iris and the posterior surface of the cornea and communicates with the posterior chamber through the pupil.

The posterior chamber is a very small cavity and is located between the iris anteriorly and lens zonule posteriorly.

The vitreous cavity is the largest chamber and is located behind the lens and zonule and posteriorly is adjacent to the retina on its entire surface. The volume of the vitreous cavity is 4.5 ml. The vitreous is a transparent tissue and has properties of a gel. It is spherical in shape except for the anterior portion which has the impression of the lens. The vitreous body adjacent to the lens which produces a hollowed-out space is called the anterior hyaloid membrane. The vitreous body is attached to the entire retina by scattered collagenous filaments. There is a firm attachment to the ciliary body and ora serrata of the retina and to the margin of the optic nerve.

The vitreous body is divided into two parts:

1. The cortical portion adjacent to the retina.

2. A central gel which has a collagen-like fibrous network and a mucopolysaccharide (hyaluronic acid) in which is suspended a large amount of water (99%).

OPTIC NERVE

The optic nerve extends from the eye to the optic chiasm and consists of bundles of nerve fibers separated by septa that are continuous with the pial sheath and carry minute blood vessels to the nerve. There are approximately one million fibers within the nerve. The optic nerve has four portions.

A. The intraocular portion includes the optic disc and the part of the nerve within the posterior scleral forament.

B. The orbital portion has a S-shaped curve to allow movements of the eye and is 30 mm long. At the apex of the orbit, the nerve is surrounded by the ligament of Zinn which is the tendinous origin of the rectus muscles.

C. The intracanalicular portion is about ½ mm long and passes through the optic foramen. It acquires meningeal coverings of the pia mater, dura mater, and

arachnoid. The pia mater extends to the globe, while the dura mater divides within the orbit so that one portion is continuous with the orbital periostium and the other part continues to the globe as the dural sheath of the optic nerve.

D. The intracranial portion of the optic nerve is 10 mm long and is located above the diaphram of the sella turcica. Lateral to each optic nerve is the internal carotid artery.

ORBIT

The bony orbits are the cavities in which the eyes are suspended. The anterior two-thirds of the orbit is shaped like a four sided pyramid while the posterior third of the orbit assumes the shape of a three sided pyramid. The medial walls run parallel to each other and are formed mainly by the orbital plate of the ethmoid bone. This structure is so thin that it is called the lamina papyracea and is a frequent site of the transmission of ethmoidal pathology into the orbit. The lateral walls diverge from the medial walls at an angle of 45 degrees. The lateral walls anteriorly are formed from the zygoma and posteriorly from the greater wing of the sphenoid. The superior margin is formed from the frontal bone and the inferior border by the zygoma and body of the maxilla. The optic foramen is located at the apex of the orbit in the body of the spenoid bone. Through it passes the optic nerve, ophthalmic artery, and sympathetic nerves. Lateral to the optic foramen is the superior orbital fissure.

The orbital contents are held together by the orbital fascia. These connective tissues divide the orbit into clinically important spaces which define the localization of hemorrhage and infection.

EXTRINSIC MUSCLES

The extrinsic muscles of the eye are the four rectus muscles and the two oblique muscles. The four rectus muscles originate from the ligament of Zinn which encircles the optic foramen and the medial portion of the superior orbital fissure. The superior oblique muscle originates at the apex of the orbit from the periosteum in the body of the sphenoid medially and above the optic foramen. The inferior oblique muscle arises from the floor of the orbit at the anteromedial portion of the maxilla. The four rectus muscles insert into the sclera anterior to the equator and the two oblique muscles insert into the sclera posterior to the equator.

As the rectus muscles pass forward and diverge from the ligament of Zinn, they form the muscle cone of the orbit. Each muscle is about 40 mm long and 9 to 11 mm wide. The medial and lateral rectus muscles arise from the ligament of Zinn and pass medially and laterally respectively around the globe to insert into the anterior sclera. The superior rectus muscle passes forward and laterally from the apex forming an angle of 23 degrees with the sagittal diameter of the globe. The inferior rectus muscle passes forward and laterally also forming an angle of 23 degrees.

LACRIMAL APPARATUS

The lacrimal apparatus consists of a secretory and a collecting portion. The lacrimal gland is located in the anterior and lateral portion of the roof of the orbit in the lacrimal fossa. The collecting portion is made up of the canaliculi, lacrimal sac and nasolacrimal duct located at the nasal side of the orbit.

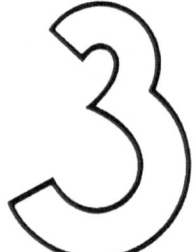

sonoanatomy

Routine application of the contact real-time scanning method is not optimal for displaying the anterior segment of the globe because the ultrasonic beam is out of focus for first 5 mm. However, special modifications such as using a water bath or a large amount of gel may visualize the anterior structures. A common method of examination is to hold the transducer against the closed lid. Consequently, the anterior pole anatomy is out of the examination field. The anterior segment can be studied clinically in the majority of cases by using a water bath system.

NORMAL PUPIL

The examination starts at a convenient position near the equator of the globe, and ultrasonic beam is directed toward the optic nerve. After visualization of the optic nerve, the probe should sweep anteriorly towards the iris lens complex in all quadrants. As the ultrasonic beam strikes the posterior aspect of the lens in the most extreme anterior position, a

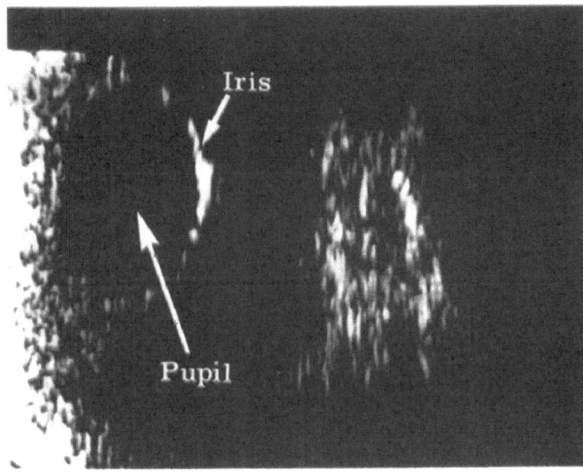

FIGURE 3.1a
Pupil open. The anterior segment of the eye is scanned obliquely. The ovoid echogenic boundary has an echo-free center. Note the thin and large outline with big echo-free central region with the fellow eye open.

constant artifact will be seen on the T.V. monitor which causes a typical scalloping of the orbital fat pattern. This scalloping tells the examiner that he has arrived at the anterior position, and the sonic beam location is traveling anteriorly. If the examiner continues to probe anteriorly, a cross sectional view of the iris and pupil will be seen on the display monitor especially well if the patient has a deep anterior chamber. After visualization of the pupil, its contractual response to light can be followed with the real-time scanner (Figure 3.1a and b).

The anterior globe may be studied by application of a thick column of viscous methylcellulose gel to elevate the transducer head away from the skin surface. The anterior and posterior lens capsule, anterior chamber, iris, and skin of the upper lid are clearly imaged (Figure 3.2a). The other method of anterior chamber scanning is to inject sterile saline solution or local anesthetic into the soft tissues of the lid. When sterile saline has been injected into the soft tissues of the upper lid there is an elevation of the anterior lid and the transducer head away from the anterior eye structures (Figure 3.2b). Novocaine may also be used and produces less pain than saline. When the sonic beam tangentially sections the lens (Figure 3.3) as mentioned, the anterior and posterior outline of the lens are usually imaged. The anterior segment of the eye can be scanned obliquely, and pupillary contraction from the light can be detected when the anterior segment of the eye is scanned obliquely. The ovid echogenic boundary of the iris has an echo-free center. In the absence of light stimuli (Figure 3.4a), there is a thin veil of tissue with a large echo-free central region outline with the fellow eye open.

In the presence of light stimuli, the pupil assumes a thicker boundary, with a small echo-free center as the iris responds with pupillary contraction from the light stimulus (Figure 3.4b).

The posterior segment from the posterior lens capsule to the posterior ocular wall is well visualized by the contact real-time scanner. In the hands of an experienced person, the posterior lens capsule and optic nerve can be imaged in the same plane and photographed. The vitreous is

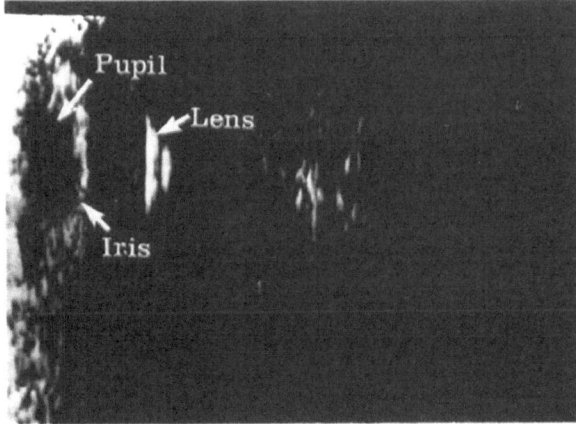

FIGURE 3.1b
Pupil closed. Thick and smaller outline with small echo-free center as light falls on the fellow eye. Iris with pupillary contraction from light stimulus.

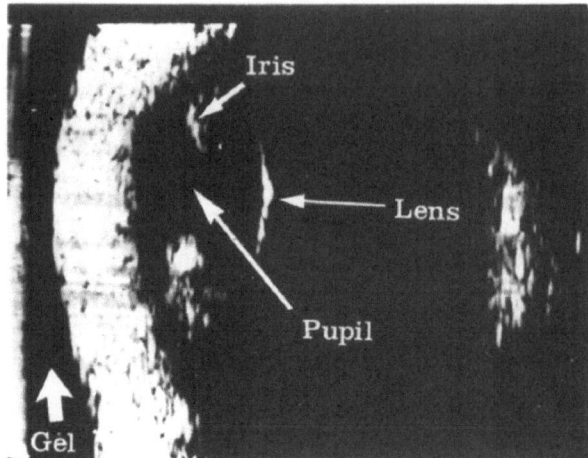

FIGURE 3.2a

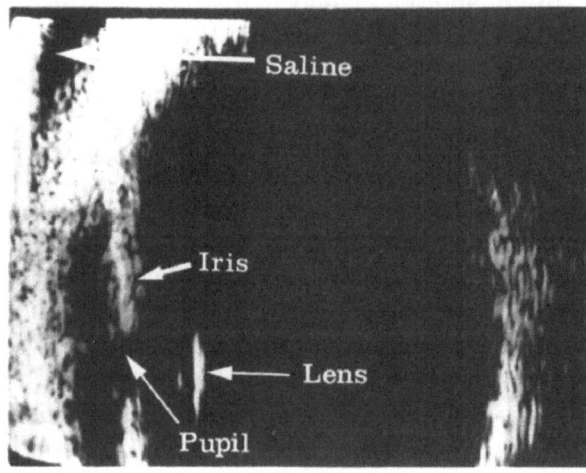

FIGURE 3.2b

FIGURE 3.2a
The anterior globe may be studied by application of a thick column of viscous methylcellulose gel to elevate the transducer head away from the skin surface. The anterior and posterior lens capsule, anterior chamber, iris, and skin of the upper lid are clearly imaged.

FIGURE 3.2b
Sterile saline has been injected into the soft tissue of the upper lid producing an elevation of the anterior lid and the transducer head away from the anterior eye structures. Novocaine may also be used and produces less pain than saline. Note that the anterior and posterior outline of the lens are imaged.

FIGURE 3.3
Tangential scanning of the lens produces a thin, echo-poor outline of the posterior lens capsule. Note internal echoes due to cataract.

FIGURE 3.4a
Thin and echo-poor outline of dilated iris is noted in the absence of light stimuli.

clear and appears as an echo-free structure (Figure 3.4c).

The optic nerve appears as a single structure. It may or may not have a few echoes inside it as a normal variant. The ciliary body can be detected from the opposite side of the eye with extreme downward or upward gaze. In displaying the sonoanatomy, optimal study is obtained with the real-time scanner when maximum effort is exerted to optimally visualize the anterior chamber, lens, pupil, vitreous cavity, and optic nerve. The optic nerve may have a wide variety of echo

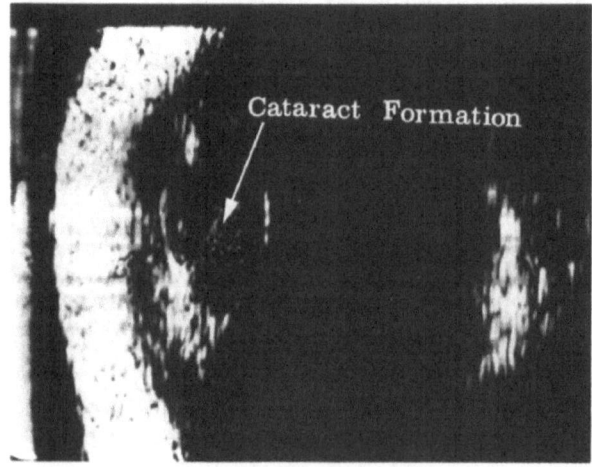

FIGURE 3.3

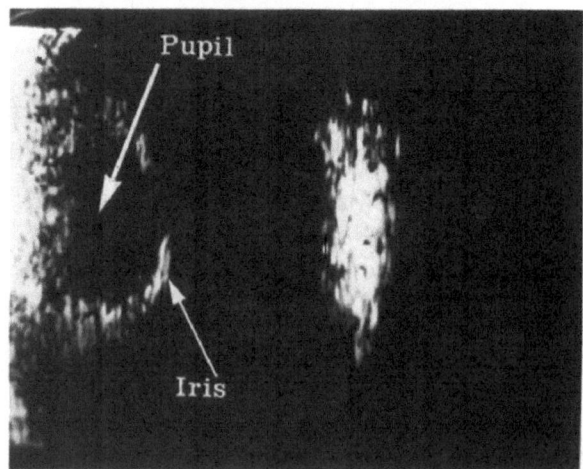

FIGURE 3.4a

34

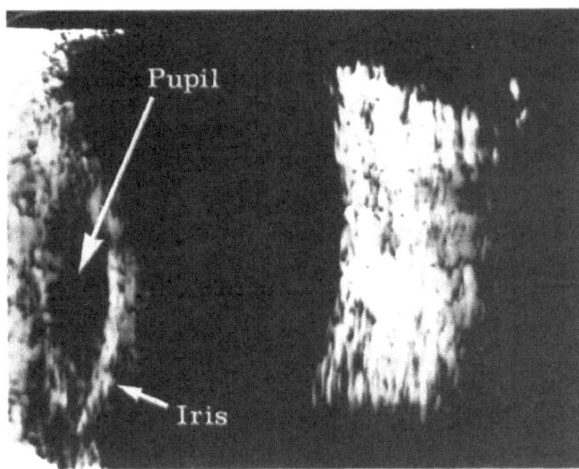

FIGURE 3.4b

FIGURE 3.4b
Light contracts the pupil now appearing as a small echo-free zone surrounded by a thick echogenic zone.

FIGURE 3.4c
The normal vitreous is acoustically homogeneous and appears echo-free.

FIGURE 3.5
Normal echogenic optic nerve.

FIGURE 3.6
Normal echo-poor optic nerve.

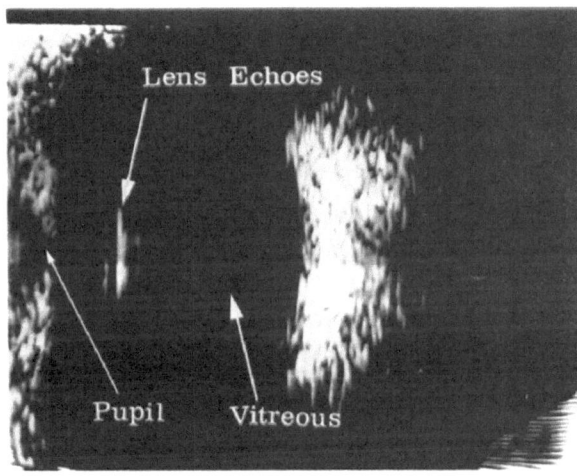

FIGURE 3.4c

patterns with which the examiner should be totally familiar.

Normally the real-time scanner shows the optic nerve inserting perpendicularly into the optic disc as it passes through the orbital fat echoes. A variety of optic nerve appearances are illustrated, which have been frequently demonstrated with real-time scanning.

A. Normal echogenic optic nerve (Figure 3.5).

B. Normal echo-poor optic nerve (Figure 3.6).

C. Partially septate echo-poor optic nerve (Figure 3.7).

D. Wide echogenic optic nerve (Figure 3.8).

E. Wide echo-poor optic nerve (Figure 3.9a and b).

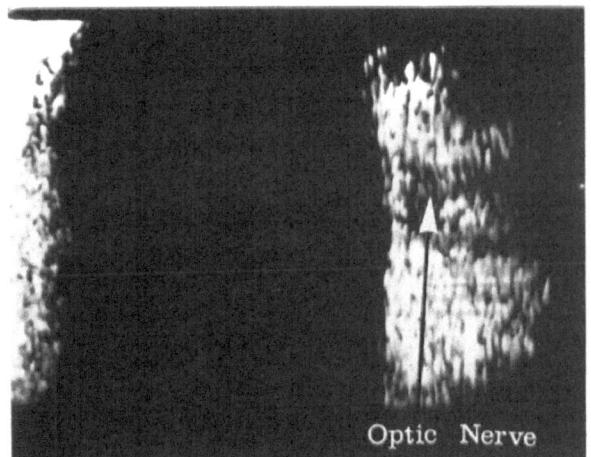

FIGURE 3.5

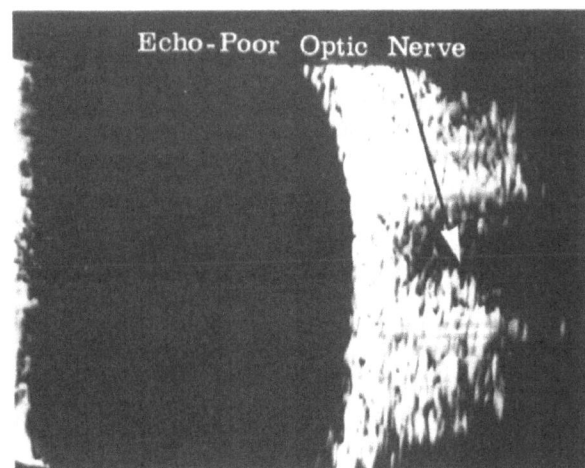

FIGURE 3.6

FIGURE 3.7
Partially septate echo-poor optic nerve.

FIGURE 3.8
Wide echogenic optic nerve.

FIGURE 3.9a
Wide echo-free optic nerve.

FIGURE 3.9a
Wide echo-free optic nerve.

FIGURE 3.10
Wide anteriorly echogenic optic nerve.

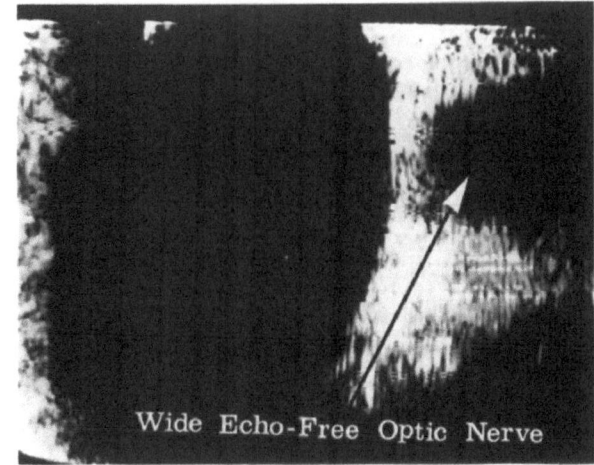

FIGURE 3.9a

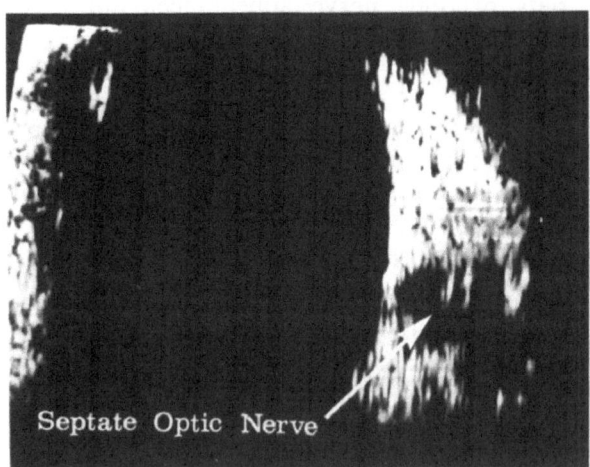

FIGURE 3.7

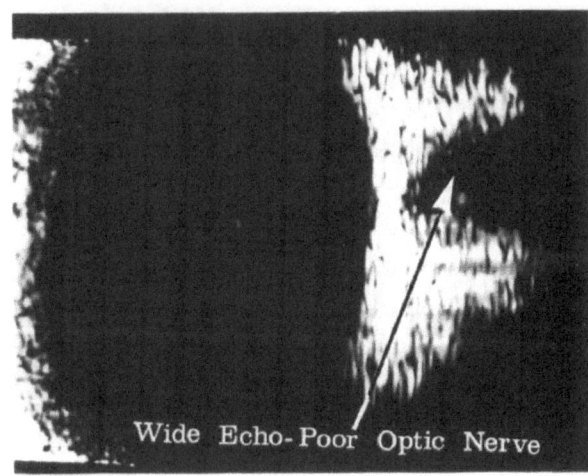

FIGURE 3.9b

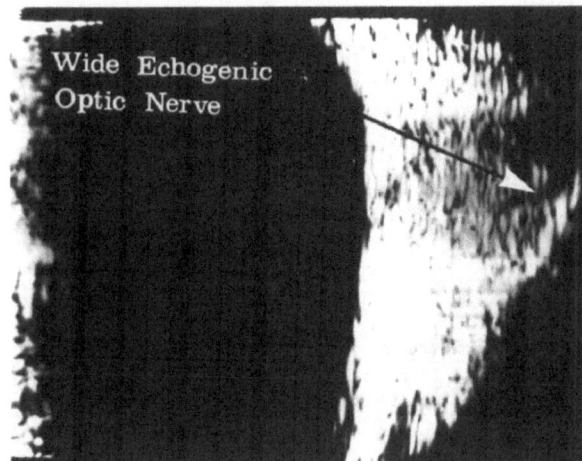

FIGURE 3.8

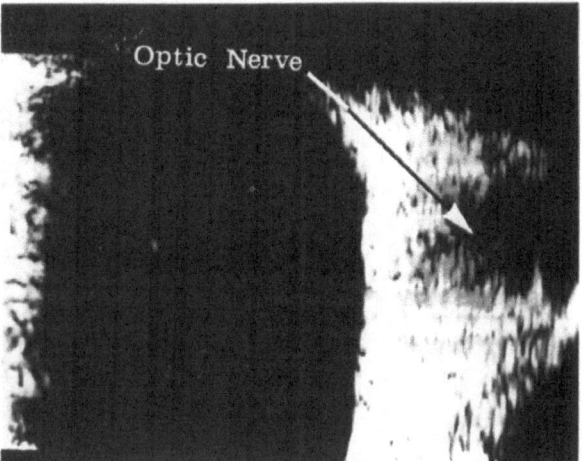

FIGURE 3.10

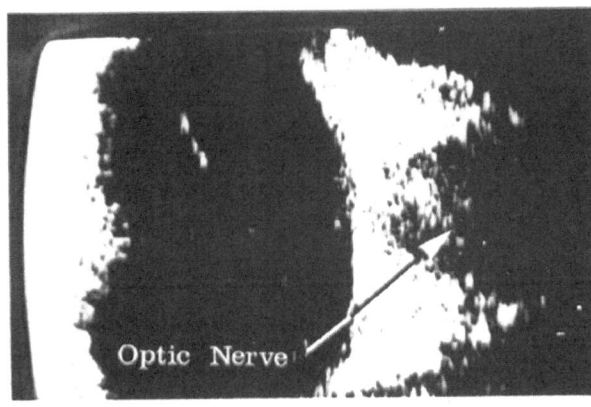

FIGURE 3.11

FIGURE 3.11
Very wide anteriorly echogenic optic nerve.

FIGURE 3.12a
Heavy centrally echogenic optic nerve.

FIGURE 3.12b
Light centrally echogenic optic nerve.

FIGURE 3.13
Very heavy centrally echogenic optic nerve.

FIGURE 3.14
Very wide echo-poor optic nerve. Incidentally noted is a retinal detachment.

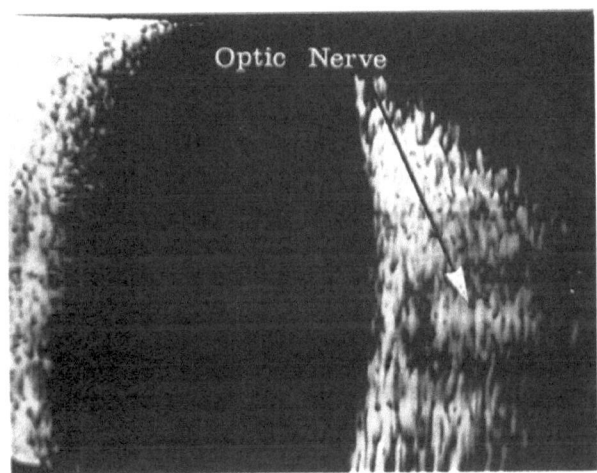

FIGURE 3.12a

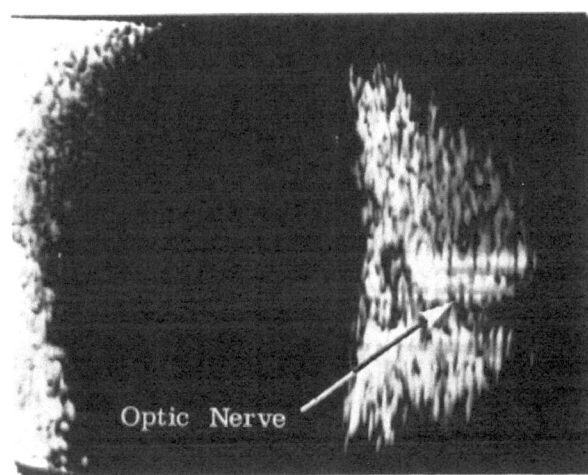

FIGURE 3.13

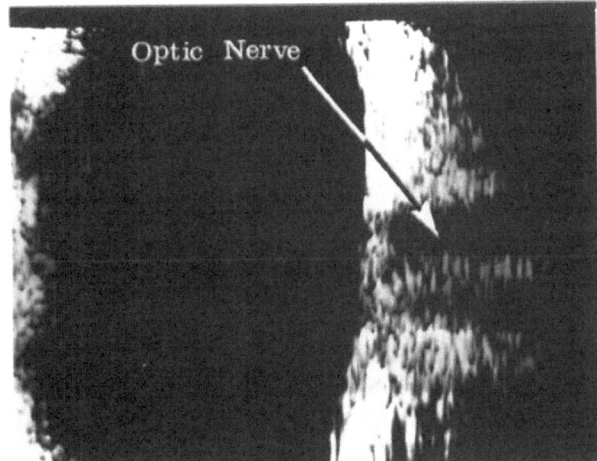

FIGURE 3.12b

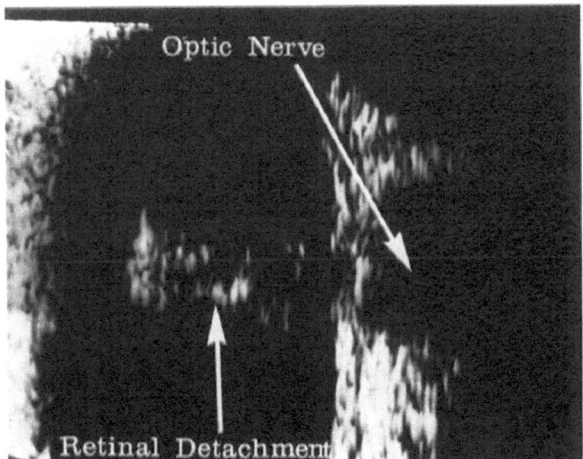

FIGURE 3.14

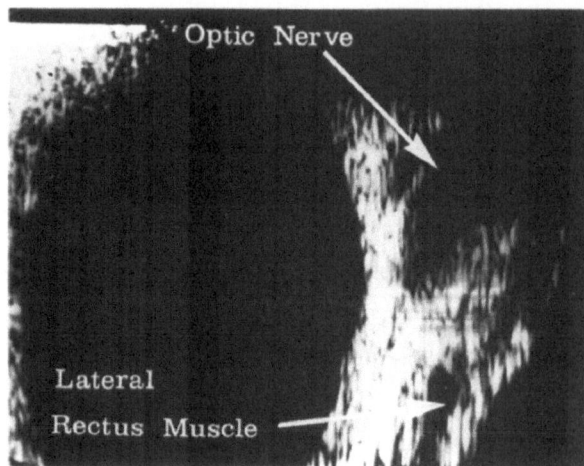

FIGURE 3.15

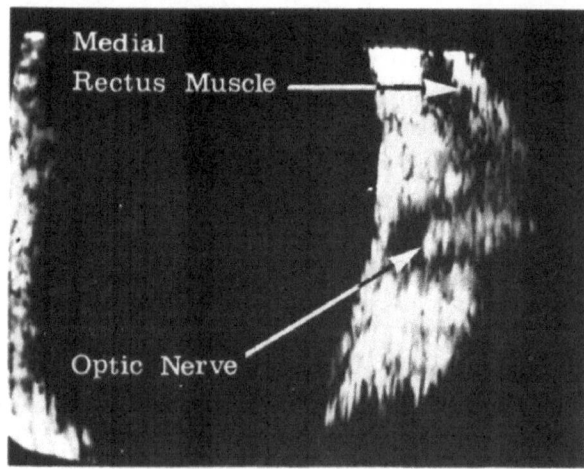

FIGURE 3.16

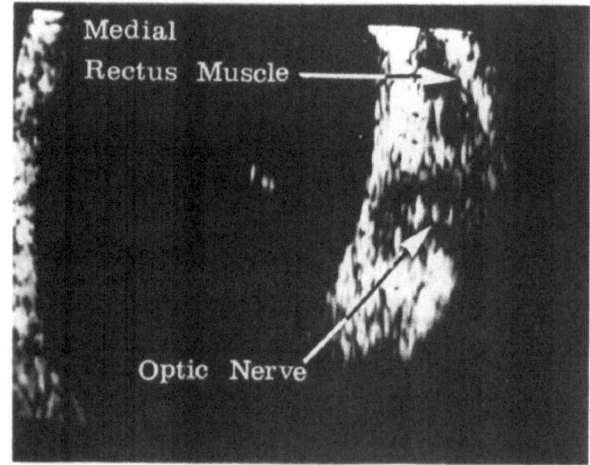

FIGURE 3.17

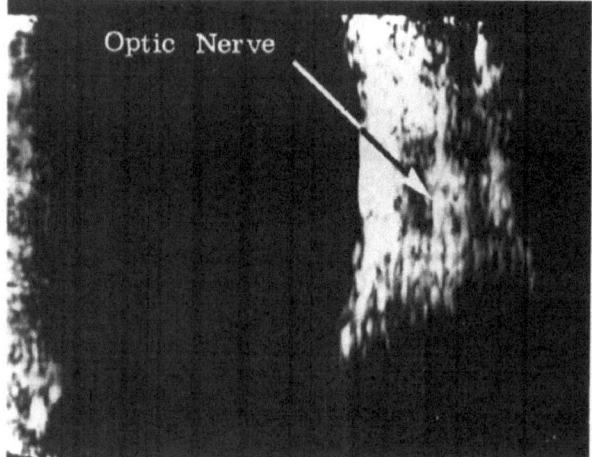

FIGURE 3.18a

FIGURE 3.15
Very wide optic nerve during medial gaze.

FIGURE 3.16
Merging of echogenic nerve with rectus muscle.

FIGURE 3.17
Merging of echo-poor optic nerve with rectus muscle.

FIGURE 3.18a
Cross section of optic nerve simulating very echogenic solid tumor.

F. Wide anteriorly echogenic optic nerve (Figure 3.10).

G. Very wide anteriorly echogenic optic nerve (Figure 3.11).

H. Centrally echogenic optic nerve (Figure 3.12a and b).

I. Centrally highly echogenic optic nerve (Figure 3.13).

J. Very wide echo-poor optic nerve (Figure 3.14).

K. Very wide obliquely inserting optic nerve (Figure 3.15).

L. Merging of echogenic optic nerve with rectus muscle (Figure 3.16).

M. Merging of echo-poor optic nerve with rectus muscle (Figure 3.17).

N. Cross section of optic nerve simulating solid tumor (Figure 3.18a and b).

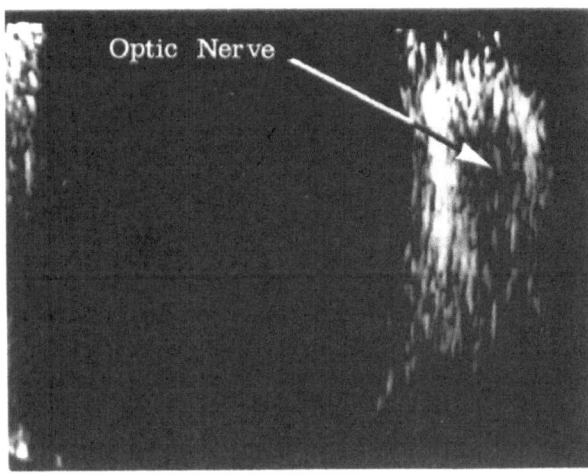

FIGURE 3.18b

FIGURE 3.18b
Cross section of optic nerve simulating poorly echogenic solid tumor.

FIGURE 3.19a
Cross section of optic nerve simulating regular cystic tumor.

FIGURE 3.19b
Cross section of optic nerve simulating irregular cystic tumor.

FIGURE 3.20
Cross section of optic nerve may simulate a cystic lesion next to echo-free rectus muscle.

FIGURE 3.21
Cross section of optic nerve which in medial gaze is parallel to the echo-poor lateral rectus muscle.

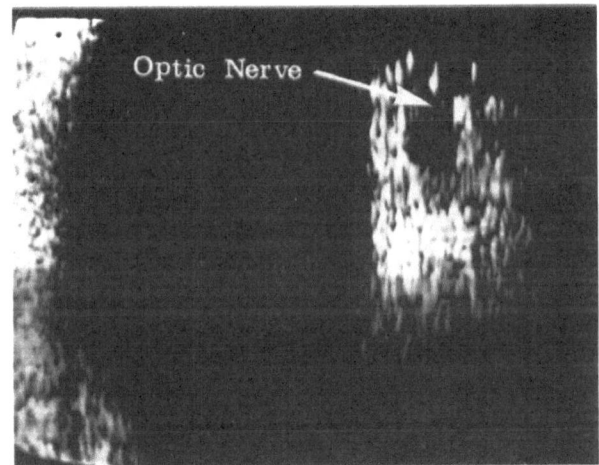

FIGURE 3.19a

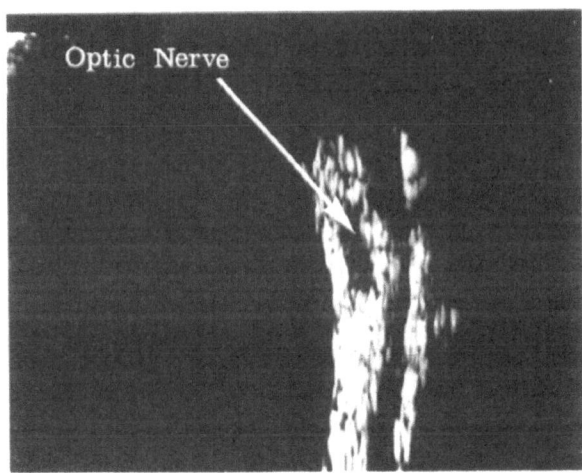

FIGURE 3.20

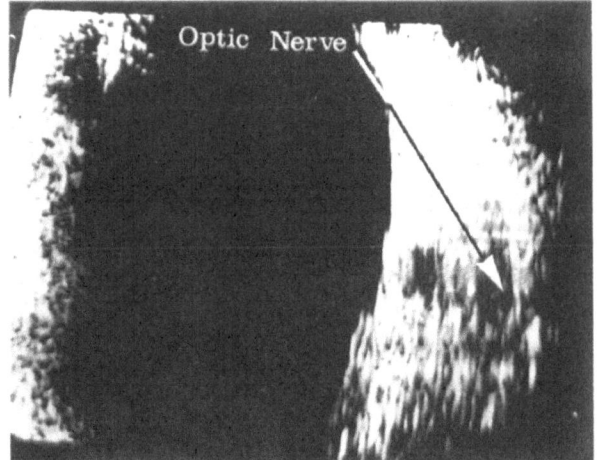

FIGURE 3.19b

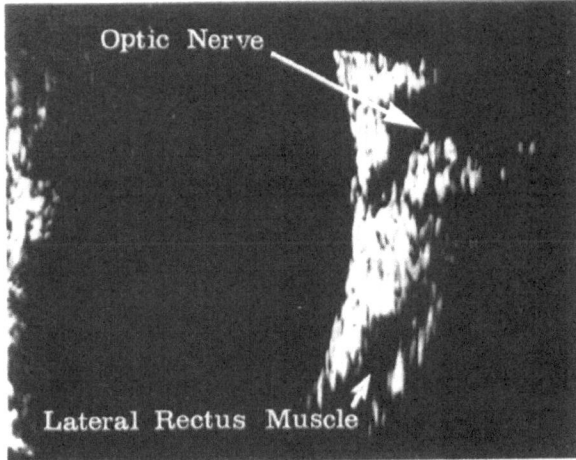

FIGURE 3.21

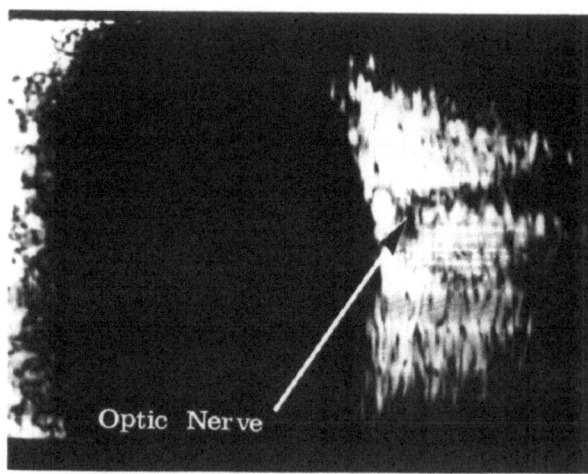

FIGURE 3.22

FIGURE 3.22
Strong echogenic areas of optic nerve head.

FIGURE 3.23
Variation of nerve with minimal gaze.

FIGURE 3.24
Variation of nerve with medium gaze.

FIGURE 3.25
Variation of optic nerve with maximal gaze.

FIGURE 3.26
There may be no definitive or clear imaging of the optic nerve in the normal eye. Incidentally note the disc.

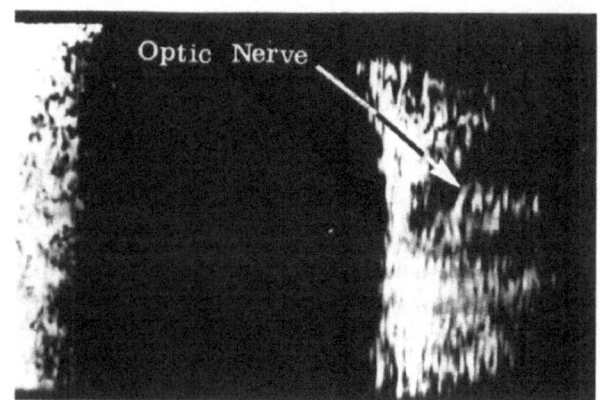

FIGURE 3.23

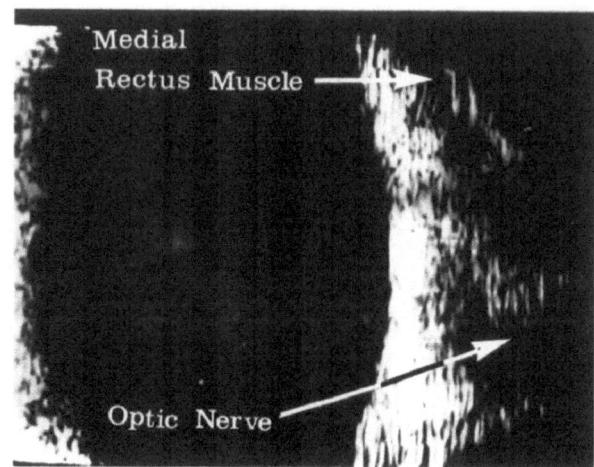

FIGURE 3.25

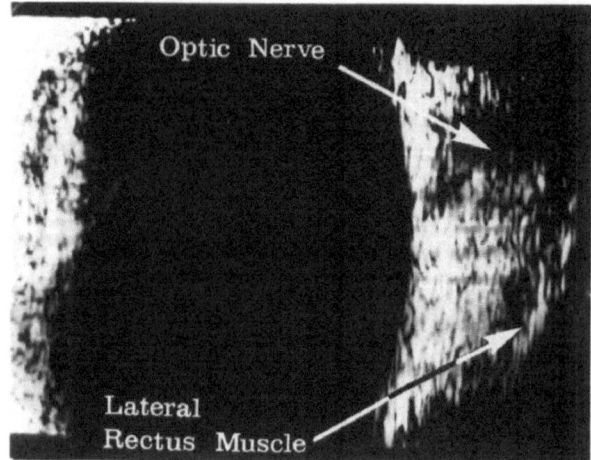

FIGURE 3.24

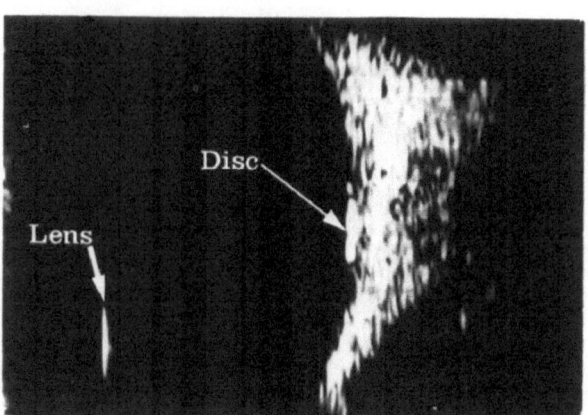

FIGURE 3.26

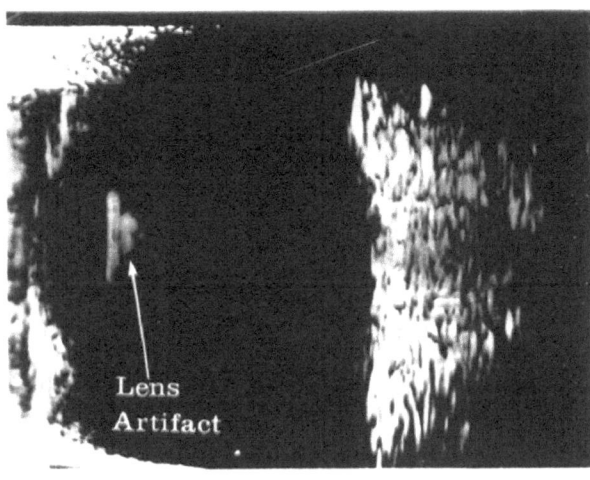

FIGURE 3.27
The lens artifact may produce an echo-poor area in the orbital fat echo pattern simulating the optic nerve head. To make sure this shadow is the optic nerve the eye should be evaluated in such a manner that the lens is out of the field of examination.

O. Cross section of optic nerve simulating cystic tumor (Figure 3.19a and b).

P. Cross section of optic nerve adjacent to echo-poor rectus muscle (Figure 3.20).

Q. Cross section of optic nerve paralleling echogenic rectus muscle (Figure 3.21).

R. Strongly echogenic areas of optic nerve head (Figure 3.22).

S. Variation of nerve with minimal gaze (Figure 3.23).

T. Variation of nerve with medium gaze (Figure 3.24).

U. Variation of nerve with maximal gaze (Figure 3.25).

V. There may be no definitive or clear imaging of the optic nerve in the normal eye in all planes (Figure 3.26).

In scanning the optic nerve, maximum effort should be used to avoid the lens artifact which obscures the details of the course of the optic nerve as the following case illustrates. The posterior wall of the lens is imaged anteriorly and produces a sonic shadow in the posterior orbital fat which simulates the image of the optic nerve. Scanning through the lens may produce multiple artifacts and the optic nerve is best evaluated when the scan beam is out of the plane of the lens (Figure 3.27).

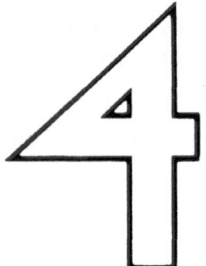

ultrasonic patient history

A detailed history of the patient's ocular disorder is essential to tailor the examination to meet the specific clinical problem. The lack of a point of information, such as previous surgery, can cause tbe sonographer endless frustration with the confusing scan picture. Symptoms referring to the anterior chamber of the eye will modify the scan with the addition of either a water bath system or a gel stand-off set up to produce better imaging of the anterior structures.

An ultrasonic history need not be totally comprehensive, but it must touch on all the pertinent material necessary to optimize performance and interpretation of the sonogram. Additionally, there will be a rapport established with the patient who feels the sonographer is interested in his problem. The patient will be much more cooperative with the sonographer's commands and maneuvers, making the scan simpler for both participants.

Initially, a chief complaint is obtained from the patient. The stated problem will bring to the sonographer's mind a number of possible diagnoses. The physician should then ask appropriate questions designed to confirm or exclude these tentative diagnoses. Although the history will narrow the diagnostic possibilities, the sonographer should have all the potential problems in mind as he is scanning the patient. The maxim that "one sees what one knows" is key to ophthalmic scanning. While the sonographer scans with a mental picture of the expected scan findings, during the course of the examination, unexpected echo patterns may be discovered. At this point, the examiner should think again of the likely etioloiges and question the patient further in his investigation of the new scan data.

SYMPTOMS

Clinicians engaged in eye scanning must be thoroughly aware of the limited but complicated spectrum of eye pathology and the symptoms produced by ocular disorders. The sonographer must have a thorough knowledge of systemic diseases simulating or aggravating ophthalmic problems. A patient may have suddenly lost vision in one eye. The blindness may be total, painless, and permanent. The infarcted retina may appear gray and the ultrasound picture of the eye will most likely be inconclusive at an early stage. Since the patient has the characteristic clinical picture of occlusion of the central retinal artery, the sonographer must be aware that this occlusion is usually due to occlusive carotid artery disease with small pieces of atherosclerotic plaque becoming loose and embolizing or to the areas of thrombosis in the left heart chambers which may shoot off small emboli. At this point the sonographer may solve the clinical problem by scanning the affected carotid artery and the cardiac chambers.

DECREASED VISION IN THE ELDERLY

Diminished vision in old age is very common and the gradual loss of sight is often accepted by the elderly as a natural accompaniment of old age. The normal eye is a tough organ and should be able to see clearly well into the geriatric years.

PRESBYOPIA

This is the inability to accommodate and affects all persons beyond middle age by the loss of near detail imaging. The decreased visual acuity of presbyopia is correctable with proper reading glasses.

CATARACT

The cataractous lens (Figure 4.1) is the most common disorder producing gradual, painless, visual loss and may occur often over a period of several years before it significantly affects the involved eye. Sensitivity to glare is an early symptom. This produces night blindness since the patient cannot see due to the brightness of the oncoming headlights. Surgery is indicated only for the mature cataract. Some elderly people are unfortunately not advised to visit the physician until they are handicapped by the loss of vision. This is tragic when the loss of vision is due to glaucoma, rather than a cataractous lens.

GLAUCOMA

Visual loss is irreparable in glaucoma. The symptomology is similar to that of cataracts. Tonometry affords early diagnosis of this disorder and may prevent blindness by proper treatment. Cupping of the optic disc is seen both clinically and in the hands of the experienced sonographer.

MACULAR DEGENERATION

The elderly patient may have a loss of central vision due to degenerative changes of the macula. Peripheral vision is spared as contrasted to the characteristic glaucomatous visual loss of peripheral vision.

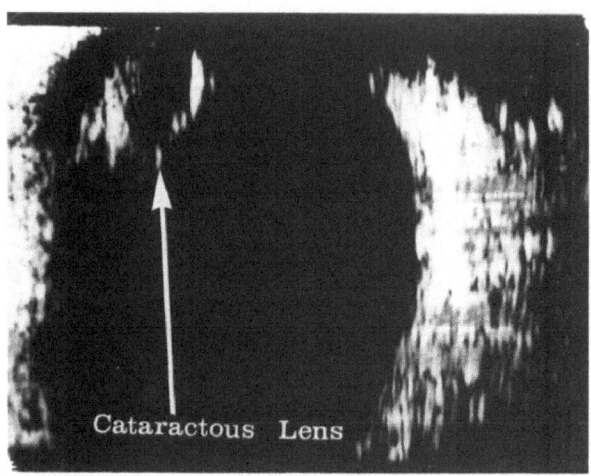

FIGURE 4.1
Cataractous lens. Early cortical cataract appears as an anterior irregularity in the normally smooth lens outline. The posterior lens is as yet unaffected. Moderate visual deterioration clinically.

RETINOPATHY

Diabetes and hypertension produce typical patterns of retinopathy (Figure 4.2) which may cause either a gradual or acute visual loss. Prognosis is poor with diabetic disorders, but newer methods of vitrectomy surgery offer great hope in this field. Hypertensive retinopathy may show dramatic improvement with systemic therapy.

OPTIC ATROPHY

This entity produces gradual and painless visual loss. This may be caused by irreparable degenerative diseases or by curable entities such as early neurosyphilis and small brain tumors. Pallor of the optic disc is the fundoscopic finding.

ACUTE VISUAL LOSS

Often, sudden loss of vision is the end stage of a slowly progressive gradual blindness which the patient has not previously noted. However, there are many instances of sudden loss of sight. Occlusion of the central retinal artery causes painless and total blindness. Embolic closure of the lumen of the artery is the usual etiology of the untreatable disorder. Occlusion of the central retinal vein decreases the visual acuity over a period of weeks. Retrobulbar neuritis may produce a large scotoma, or visual loss in the visual field, within a day. Multiple sclerosis is the most frequent demyelinating disease causing this process. Macular hemorrhage from diabetes, blood dyscrasia, macular degeneration, chorioretinitis, or hypertension, will obscure vision in the area of hemorrhage. Vitreous hemorrhage (Figure 4.3) is associated with the above conditions as well as with trauma and may block the entire visual field. Acute macular chorioretinitis may wipe out the central visual field within a few day's time, producing a central scotoma. Central corneal edema will produce blurred vision. This is seen with bacterial corneal ulcers, herpes simplex ulceration, acute glaucoma, or corneal abra-

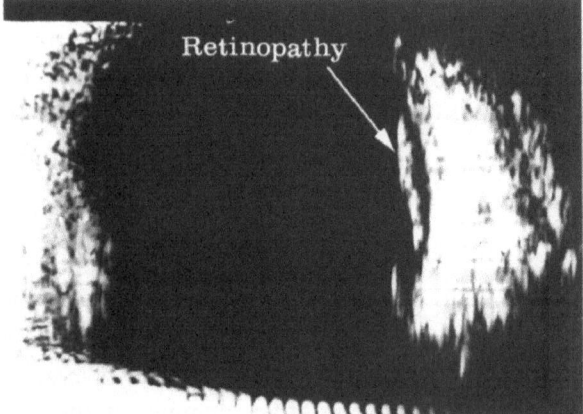

FIGURE 4.2
Diabetic retinopathy. Retinopathy may be due to various etiologies and often shows sheet like echoes emanating from the surface of the retina with limited mobility.

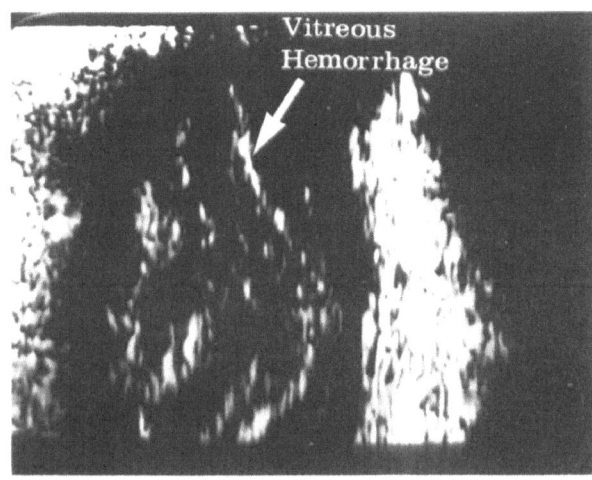

FIGURE 4.3
Vitreous hemorrhage. Typical low amplitude echo pattern of multiple linear membranes with good mobility in this example of traumatic vitreous hemorrhage of the liquid and formed vitreous.

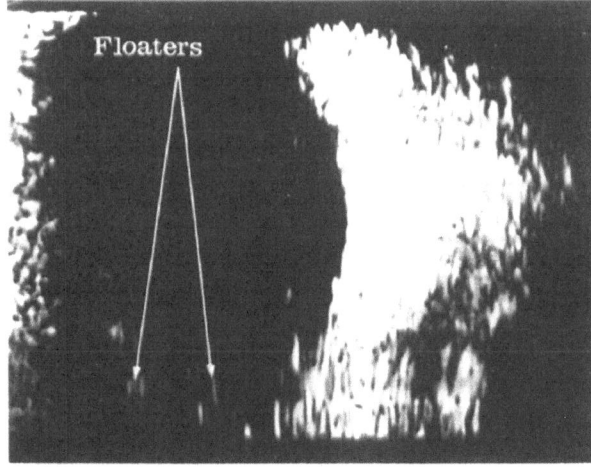

FIGURE 4.4
Vitreous floaters. Low amplitude echoes within the vitreous are often innocuous in nature. However, their sudden appearance in the visual field may signify the onset of a retinal detachment.

sion. Trauma to the eye, especially when a miniscule foreign body has entered the eye without the patient's notice and produced a vitreal hemorrhage, or corneal edema, must always be considered. Methyl alcohol (wood alcohol) poisoning may cause total blindness within several days of ingestion.

FLOATERS

Small moving specks in the visual field are common and are called floaters (Figure 4.4). Many floaters are benign or not treatable. However, the onset of floaters may indicate a serious disorder. Developmental remnants may be due to incomplete disappearance of intravitreal hyaloid arteries. These hyaloid strands are nonprogressive and are often discovered accidentally and dramatically. Vitreous hemorrhage may produce large or small floaters, depending on the magnitude of the intravitreal hemorrhage. The patient may notice a reddish discoloration of the vision. Sonography may show the cause of the bleeding as well as the geographic localization of the hemorrhage which is of paramount importance in planning therapy. Intraocular hemorrhage may be secondary to trauma or spontaneous in the systemic disorders such as diabetes, increased intracranial pressure, hypertension, and blood dyscrasias. Inflammation of the retina or uveal tract produces inflammatory debris which may enter the vitreous and produce the complaint of floaters. This may form a network of opacities within the vitreous which may seriously affect vision. Degenerative changes may be hereditary, traumatic, or post-inflammatory. The most important degenerative condition resulting in floater production is retinal detachment (Figure 4.5). As the retina tears, a shower of cells is thrown into the vitreous producing a burst of floaters. Emergency surgery is necessary to correct retinal detachment as a cause of vitreous floaters. Detachment of the vitreous occurs in the elderly with some frequency. The separation of the vitreous from the retina may cause cellular material to cling to the posterior vitreous surface and cast floating shadows.

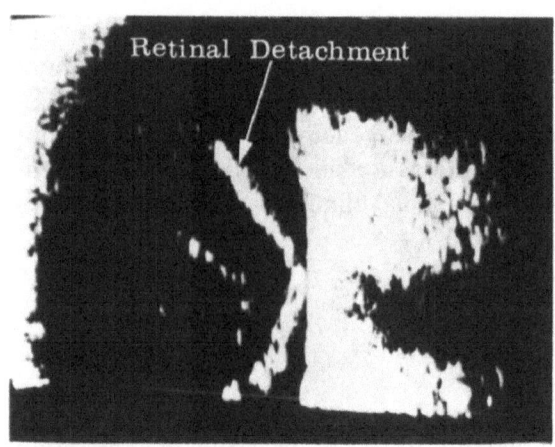

FIGURE 4.5
Retinal detachment. Retinal detachment has a high incidence in aphakik (without lens) and highly myopic eyes. This patient had cataract surgery one year previously.

VISUAL FIELD DISORDERS

Floaters usually produce small defects in the visual field. Scotomata and sector defects are due to lesions in the retina or the visual pathways. Causes of this type of visual field loss include senile macular degeneration, injury, chorioretinitis, and vascular occlusion. The patient will often give a history of blurred vision when in fact there is a focal and geographic loss of the visual field. Metamorphopsia is a distortion of the shape of an object and is due to a lesion of the central retina. Inflammatory conditions usually produce this disorder, but this may also be noted in neoplasm or retinal detachment. Diplopia is double vision due to the eyes not properly oriented in space. This is often due to weakness or paralysis of the extraocular muscles and the sonographer must search for orbital pathology, central nervous system disease, and myasthenia gravis. Errors of refraction may produce eye strain, headache, or blurred vision.

PAIN

Ophthalmic pain may be varied in location, such as the orbit, frontal, temporal, or occipital areas. The ache may be dull as in the pain from refractive error, or intense and excruciating as that associated with acute glaucoma. Unilateral serious eye disease may produce local pain of acute onset. Refractive headaches are characteristically made worse with the use of the eyes. Burning and irritation may be due to chronic lid infection, allergy, and smoke or dust exposure, and excessive use of the eyes to the point of fatigue. Photophobia is non-specific and may accompany many types of ocular irritation and inflammation.

Iritis is a cause of significant photophobia of acute onset. Epiphoria or watering of the eye is usually due to excessive secretion. This may be produced by foreign body irritation, local ocular inflammation, or allergy. Blockage of the nasolacrimal duct is a less common cause of tearing. Foreign body sensation may be produced either by an actual foreign body or by a corneal epithelial abrasion. Corneal ulcers and the early stages of acute conjunctivitis may cause mild foreign body sensation.

EYE EXAMINATION

After an appropriate history is taken, the eye is routinely examined prior to ultrasonography. Correlation of the history and physical examination guide the hand of the sonographer towards the optimal study of the globe and orbit. The physical examination is divided into an external examination and a fundoscopic study.

The external physical exam begins with routine visual acuity testing to evaluate the presence and degree of impaired vision. This is customarily performed with a letter chart at 20 feet. When vision is diminished severely, counting fingers is used as a gross acuity test. In the most advanced cases of poor vision, the ability to detect light perception as a flash light is shined directly into the eye is used as a crude evaluation. Color vision may be tested since this may be impaired in disorders of the optic nerve occuring in retrobulbar neuritis where there is a transmission impairment of the nerve. This exam is not routinely performed prior to sonography. The lids are checked briefly to assure that they close adequately to cover the eyes. Lid edema or ptosis should be noted. The lacrimal apparatus is visually examined and palpated only when clinically indicated. The bulbar conjuctiva is noted and the palpebral conjunctiva is studied when necessary. Dilatation of the conjunctival vessels produces a red eye and may point to various disease processes.

A transparent and smooth cornea is a requirement for good vision. Abrasions and opacities are searched for with indirect illumination from a small flash light. A look at the anterior chamber will show if this zone is abnormally shallow, which may possibly contraindicate the use of dilating drops. Corneal sensitivity testing is performed only when pathology of the fifth nerve is suspected.

The pupil is next examined and compared with the opposite side (Figure 4.6) for roundness, size and equality, and constriction to light stimulation. Consensual pupillary reaction where the opposite pupil constricts is checked as this physiologic stimulus is often used during the ocular sonographic procedure for identification of certain echo patterns. The swinging flash light test is done to show a paradoxical dilatation of the pupil on which the light shines. The so-called Marcus Gunn pupil signifies a severe receptor or nerve transmission defect such as that occurring with a retinal detachment. This type of reflex is not noted with a cataract. Anisocoria or a discernable difference in pupil size occurs in approximately 5% of normal persons. Mydriasis or an enlarged pupil may be caused by recent or old ocular injury, acute glaucoma, or local dilating drops. Miosis or constriction of the pupil may herald iris inflammation, glaucoma patients treated with pilocarpine, or drug effect such as morphine. Irregularity of the pupil contour occurs in iritis, central nervous· system syphilis, trauma, and congenital defects.

Intraocular pressure is checked grossly by finger tension although a tonometer may be used if the history, physical, or ultrasonic exam warrant a finer test of intraocular pressure alterations.

The extraocular muscles are checked first by finding a symmetrically located light reflex in the two pupils. If there is an asymetric light reflex or orbital pathology is suspected, the eye is rotated to the six cardinal positions of gaze that test the function of each muscle.

The orbit is evaluated by noting the position of the globe in the bony socket. This may be displaced forward, termed exophthalmos, by tumors, trauma, inflammation, and thyroid disease. Backward displacement occurs with developmental defects and post traumatic and chronic inflammatory conditions and is called enophthalmos.

Visual fields are checked when abnormality of the visual pathways associated with neuro-ophthalmological diseases is suspected. It is not part of the routine pre-sonographic examination.

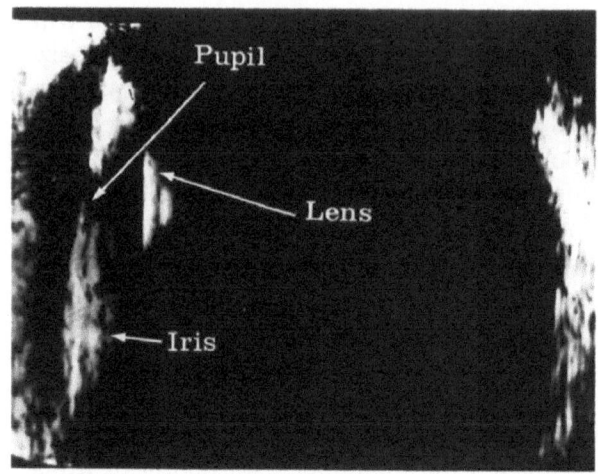

FIGURE 4.6
Pupil. Real-time ultrasonography of the iris pupil complex is best accomplished by the use of a water bath. The echoes of the iris are interrupted at the location of the pupil which is located immediately anterior to the lens.

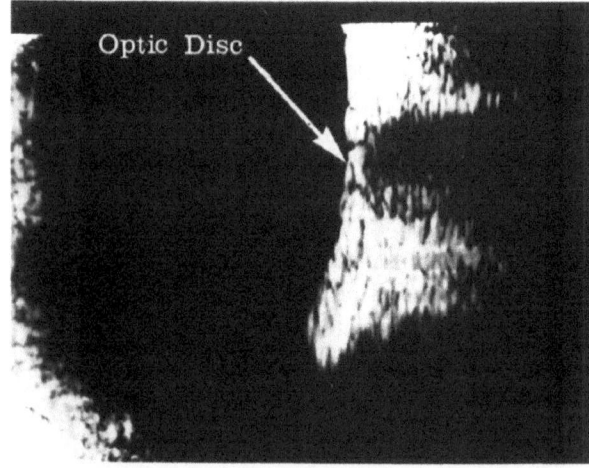

FIGURE 4.7
Optic disc. The optic disc is the most visible fundoscopic and ultrasonic landmark. This is usually 1.5 mm in diameter when visualized at the posterior pole with the ophthalmoscope.

The second part of the examination of the eye prior to sonography is the ophthalmoscopic study of the fundus or posterior part of the eye. The procedure not only shows findings related to ocular and orbital disease, but often provides helpful clues to serious systemic diseases, and may direct the sonographer to study other parts of the body following ophthalmic sonography.

The fundoscopic examination may be performed either with a standard direct ophthalmoscope or the binocular indirect ophthalmoscope. Direct ophthalmoscopy must be performed at a close distance to the patient, so that the examiner almost touches the patient's head with his forehead. The indirect scope study may be performed at a distance with a hand-held lens close to the patient's eye. Although the indirect ophthalmoscope affords a stereoscopic view of the fundus with bright light, the image seen through the convex lens is inverted and the interpretation of this test is best in the hands of the physician skilled in the use of this sophisticated instrument.

In the examination of the ocular fundus, a specific routine is followed. The optic disc is the most obvious landmark and is studied first. The size of the optic disc is noted and is usually 1.5 mm in diameter (Figure 4.7), although this appears many times magnified through the ophthalmoscope. The disc diameter is important since other areas on the posterior ocular wall are measured with respect to their number of disc diameters from the optic disc. Generally the macula, an important target in sonography, is 2 DD temporal (disc diameters) from the optic disc. The normal round or oval shape is noted and the pink color is due to the rich capillary network. A small cup is generally noted slightly temporal of the center of the disc and is a physiologic depression called the cup. The margins of the disc are regular and often pigmented areas overlie the borders of the optic disc.

Next the central retinal artery and vein and their branches are studied. The arteries are narrower than the veins and have a characteristic arteriolar light reflex in the center of the artery. The macula is an area about 1 DD in diameter and located 2 DD temporal to the disc. This area is normally avascular. The periphery of the fundus is finally examined with the patient's help in directing his eye in various gaze positions.

Although the history and physical examination are vitally important in arriving at the correct diagnosis, the correlation between the ophthalmoscopic findings and the ultrasonic pathophysiologic picture is key to the interpretation of the gross pathologic changes in the eye. Indeed, it is essential for the beginning ocular sonographer to scan those eyes into which he can clearly image visually so that he may gain experience and confidence in diagnosing routine vitreous and retinal disorders when the media is opaque or the lens is cataractous. Only when the sonographer has a thorough understanding of ocular pathology as seen through the fundoscope, can he go on to piece together the complex picture of sheets, strands, and amorphous echoes appearing on the sonogram into a meaningful diagnostic interpretation. A clear uniform red reflex seen with the ophthalmoscope rules out serious eye pathology in the axial parts of the cornea, aqueous, lens, and vitreous. Any defect in these regions will produce a dark shadow within the red reflex. Indeed, vitreous hemorrhage and dense cataract formation will completely destroy the red reflex.

The disc is a common site of pathologic changes. The appearance of an excessively large disc usually means that there is a pathologic area adjacent of the disc, which may simulate an enlarged disc to the observer. A myopic crescent is a form of slow atrophy on the one side of the disc. Circumpapillary chorioretinal atrophy completely or partially surrounds the disc like a doughnut and may be due to aging or post inflammatory changes and is often an incidental finding. A coloboma is a congenital absence of the retinal and choroid layer and in the disc appears as a large inferior elongation of the disc which is pale and has a distorted arterial distribution. A pale disc suggests optic atrophy. A red or hyperemic disc indicates papilledema or optic neuritis. Irregular margins of the disc may be seen in normal patients, with localized optic nerve head drusen, disc edema, or local scar tissue. True edema of the disc is seen with trauma, inflammation, ischemia, or papilledema (Figure 4.8).

The vessels of the retina provide much clinical information due to changes in their caliber, color, distribution, and pulsation. Neovascularization produces great distortion of the retinal vessel pattern. The new vessels are tortuous and irregular. This occurs in diabetic retinopathy, venous occlusion, and some types of chorioretinitis. Diabetic changes are much worse in the region of the macula although they are diffuse in distribution. Chronic chorioretinitis produces peripheral and focal areas of neovascularization. Branch venous occlusion is usually confined to the geographic distribution of the occluded branch vein. Microaneurysms are common near regions of neovascularization and are indicative of diabetic retinopathy. The retinal vessels may be elevated in the conditions of retinal detachment, choroidal melanoma, and metastatic tumors which are usually located in the vascular choroid layer. The retinal detachment looks like a clear gray curtain behind which is a dark fluid. Choroidal metastases and malignant malanoma appear as a fleshy solid elevation. Retinitis proliferans may cause large vessels to grow forward into the vitreous.

The caliber of the vessels may increase in hypercirculatory states, such as polycythemia, papilledema, central retinal vein occlusion, and carotid cavernous fistula. Smaller vessel diameter is seen in hypertension, eclampsia, retinitis pigmentosa, and occlusion of the central retinal artery. The retinal arteries may collapse during diastole indicating that the intraocular pressure exceeds diastolic pressure and is found in glaucoma and aortic insufficiency with a wide pulse pressure. The light reflex of the arteriole will increase in size and become wider as arteriolar sclerosis develops.

The macula is the visual zone of highest acuity. For this reason, a small lesion in this area may handicap the patient while a large lesion in the periphery may go unnoticed. The macula must be studied carefully both ophthalmoscopically

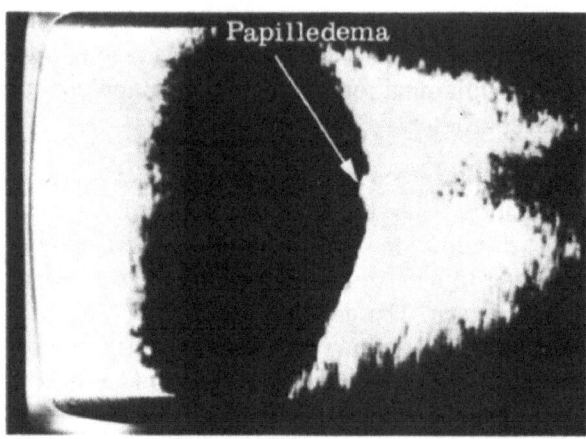

FIGURE 4.8

Papilledema. Elevation of the optic nerve head was due to increased intracranial pressure in this patient with a brain tumor. The raised portion of the optic nerve head is moderately echogenic.

and sonographically. The rich blood supply of the macula predisposes it to certain diseases related to an abundance of blood flow. Metastatic tumors and infectious chorioretinitis occur frequently in this area. Certain degenerative disorders prefer the posterior pole of the eye.

The periphery of the fundus may be affected by many processes that may be imaged both by ophthalmic and ultrasonic imaging. Edema of the retina thickens the membrane and changes the appearance from transparent to gray in color. Edema indicates recent or active pathology. Peripheral retinal edema is diffusely present in conditions such as ocular contusion, active chorioretinitis, hypertensive retinopathy, and occlusion of the central retinal artery. Hemorrhage produces red patches in the retina. Deep retinal hemorrhages are rounded, while bleeding into the more anterior nerve fiber layer of the retina appears flame shaped. The larger retinal vessels lie in this anterior layer so that hypertensive retinal hemorrhage is characteristically flame shaped. The space between the anterior retina and the vitreous face is called the preretinal space. The nature of this region permits blood to pool in large rounded pockets. The intact vitreous face prevents blood from entering the vitreous cavity. Large preretinal hemorrhage may be noted in acute hemorrhagic disorders. When the hemorrhage breaks through the vitreous face, the blood scatters diffusely throughout the vitreous. Blood in the vitreous often obscures the details of the fundus and may destroy the red reflex. Fresh blood may not show up on all ultrasonic examinations. The vitreous may be blood filled and the sonogram will appear absolutely normal. Vitreous hemorrhages are often produced by trauma and by the retinal tears that precede retinal detachment, although they may occur in a wide variety of ocular and systemic disorders. Gravity affects the shape and consistency of the hemorrhage which alters the ophthalmic and ultrasonic appearance. The plasma rises superiorly while the red cells settle inferiorly. These two layers are thus separated by a horizontal line or interface. Blood is more echogenic than plasma and echoes may be greater in number in the dependent portion of the anterior chamber and the preretinal space.

Exudates indicate fundal disease. Since they occur in all types of degenerative and inflammatory disorders, they are nonspecific, and are found in many systemic diseases such as diabetes, hypertension, and collagen disorders. Hard exudates are the name given to discrete areas while soft exudates are fuzzier and slightly larger. Hard exudates represent intraretinal lipoid deposits occurring with chronic disease. Soft exudates are areas of microinfarctions in the retina and occur more rapidly than hard exudates. Drusen may be mistaken for hard exudates. Drusen are benign hyaline degenerative deposits on the elastic membrane between the retina and choroid. They appear as whitish translucent areas, often in both eyes. Drusen are often an incidental finding: however, they may simulate papilledema when located at the optic nerve head or areas of hard exudates in other portions of the retina. The experienced ophthalmologist can differentiate drusen from ocular disease. The sonographer may easily differentiate drusen by their highly echogenic nature, often persisting down to 40 dB during ultrasonic scanning.

Chorioretinitis is acute focal inflammation of the choroid and retina which produces a picture similar to a soft exudate with associated retinal edema and hemorrhage in or adjacent to the focus of chorioretinitis. Pigmentary changes are associated with many disorders of the choroid and outer retina and are nonspecific, since they may occur following trauma, degeneration, or inflammation. The most common pigmentary alterion of the choroid is the benign nevus, which occurs in approximately 1% of the population. They may vary in size from $\frac{1}{3}$ DD to more than 3 DD and are usually gray in color and often have overlying drusen. Nevi present the problem of a tumor in the eye possibly being a malignant melanoma. The presence of associated drusen indicates the chronicity of the lesion, although other clinical tests are necessary for further confirmation. Nevi are generally not elevated and do not induce neovascularity, exudates, edema, or hemorrhage.

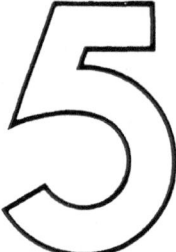

oculosonotomography

In order to obtain maximum information through ophthalmic sonography by the real-time scanner, we utilize the following procedure:

PATIENT PREPARATION

The patient should be reassured that the examination is simple and painless except for minimal pressure over the eye. The patient is instructed that the lid will be wet by methylcellulose and that this may penetrate into the eye but is completely harmless, since this liquid is used in eye drops. If the patient is cooperative or if conditions permit during the examination, the opposite eye should be opened. The purpose is to direct the patient's gaze at the examinaer's finger in order that the position of the eye under examination can be determined by the direction of the fellow eye being used as a visual reference point. This is difficult in the geriatric patient and often impossible in pediatric subjects. In patients with injured eyes or dense cataracts, this manuver cannot be executed.

AXIAL LENGTH MEASUREMENT

Historically many researchers and investigators have been interested in the axial length measurement of the eye for different purposes. Some researchers are basically interested in biometrics and they measured axial length with accuracy in the vicinity of 0.1 mm. This work was used for studies of myopia, lens changes, and accommodation. This is also of great interest for ophthalmologists inserting intraocular lenses as a means of deciding the strength of the intraocular lens. Other researchers' techniques have produced high accuracy measurements, but these are unsatisfactory for routine clinical application. Their measurement lies in the vicinity of 1 mm accuracy. By these measurements, microphthalmia, myopia, and early phthysis bulbi can be evaluated.

The contact B-scanner can be used to grossly measure the axial length since its accuracy is within 1 mm. With this unit the intraocular lens strength or quantification of myopia cannot be judged, due to limited axial resolution and pressure exerted upon the globe during scanning. By placing the probe in the center of the eye, we try to visualize the posterior lens capsule. In this view, the optic nerve usually can be seen. A photo is taken for axial measurement with the overlay grid.

The axial length of the globe may be calculated from the polaroid photographs. This is accomplished by using the overlay grid which is supplied by the manufacturer. The vertical lines of this chart are placed side by side with the border of the polaroid. If the posterior lens capsule is seen on the photo and the deepest part of the posterior wall of the eye is displaced upward or downward on the photo, the grid may be adjusted vertically to correspond to the proper dimension. The portion of the overlay marked 1.5–4.5 cm depth can be used similarly when the depth control is adjusted.

The normal eye has an average axial length of approximately 24 mm, by the contact real-time scanner. As mentioned earlier, the posterior lens capsule and optic nerve definitely should be in

the polaroid film before using the overlay grid. The photo can be taken at 80 dB, however, 70 dB gives a clearer view for overlay grid application.

We use a large amount of methylcellulose to avoid any indentation or pressure over the eye. Staphyloma (Figure 5.1), myopia (Figure 5.2), and microphthalmia (Figure 5.3) may be studied further by the ultrasonic appearance and by the use of axial length measurement.

SONOFLUOROSCOPY OF THE GLOBE AND ORBIT

By moving the probe throughout the entire area of the globe and orbit, both eyes may be scanned. If any abnormality is noted, the identification system which will be described later should be used for evaluation of the pathology. It is essential to examine the unaffected eye first, because not only may an unsuspected lesion be found, but it is extremely helpful for comparison. In the study of the normal eye the pupillary response to light stimuli can be detected. Usually a section taken from the most posterior portion of the globe with the beam directed vertically shows that the pupil appears as a round echo free structure anteriorly. As light is flashed into the open opposite eye, the pupillary zone becomes smaller in the eye being scanned (Figure 5.4a and b). The position of transducer is extremely important. In the majority of cases, by directing the transducer in the anteroposterior plane, the iris appears anterior to the posterior lens capsule echo as a break in the irregular moderately echogenic band of approximately 4 mm. Light shined in the contralateral eye causes closure of the scanned pupil as a narrowing of the discontinuous echoes of the iris (Figure 5.5a, b, and c).

SENSITIVITY SETTING FOR TISSUE CHARACTERISTICS

If any abnormal echo pattern is encountered, it should be investigated with different sensitivity settings. For example, to differentiate vitreous

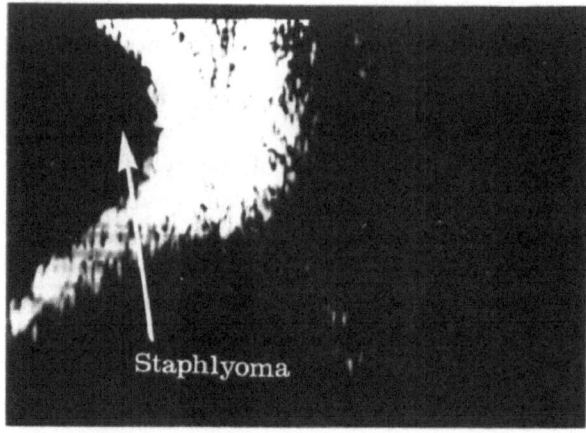

FIGURE 5.1

FIGURE 5.1
Staphyloma. There is a bulge to the posterior ocular pole which distorts the normally smoothly concave outline of the vitreoretinal interface. Scan at 1.5–4.5 cm depth.

FIGURE 5.2
Myopia. There is markedly increased axial length of the eye which produces myopic errors in focusing. This type of globe is prone to retinal detachment.

FIGURE 5.3
Microphthalmos. Congenital rubella has produced this disorganized small eye with disruption of the normal posterior ocular structures and small vitreous cavity.

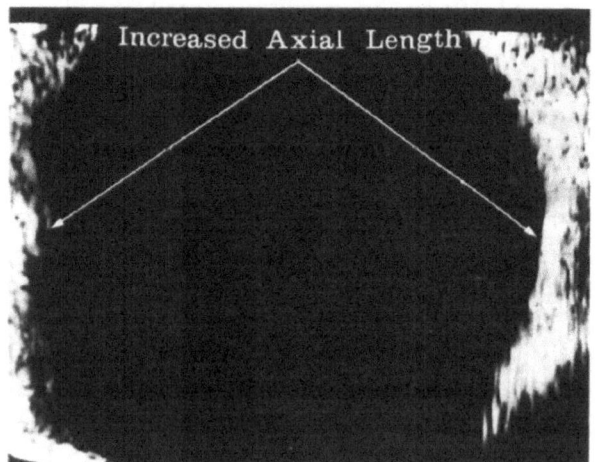

FIGURE 5.2

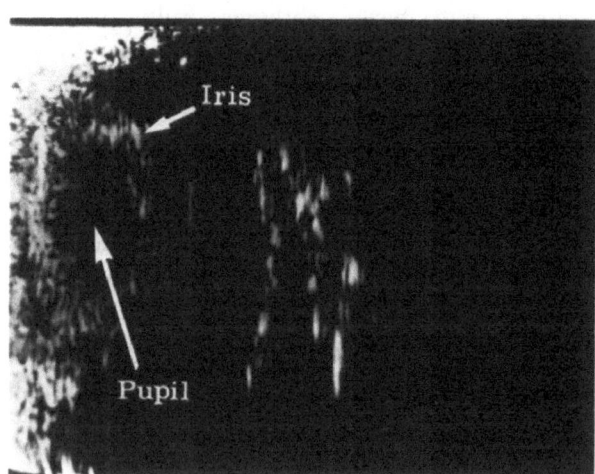

FIGURE 5.4a

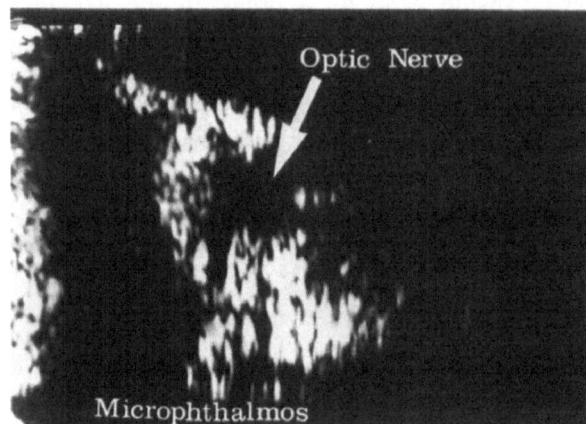

FIGURE 5.3

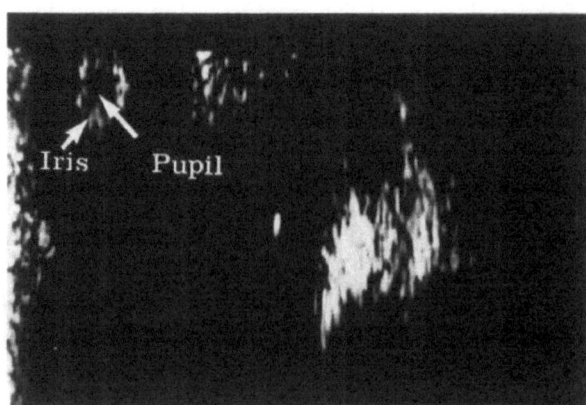

FIGURE 5.4b

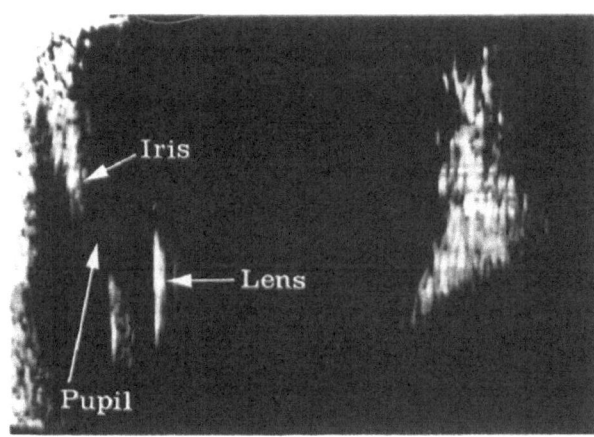

FIGURE 5.5a

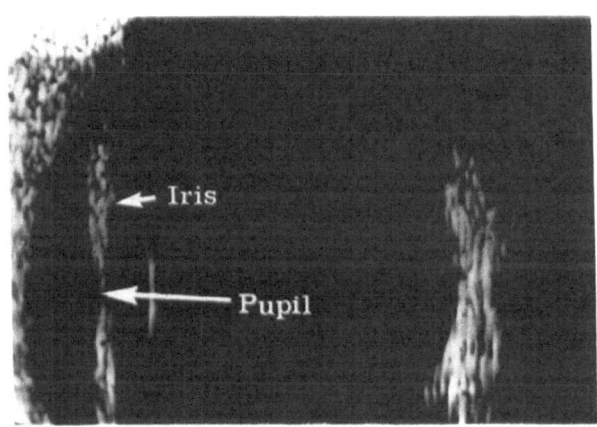

FIGURE 5.5b

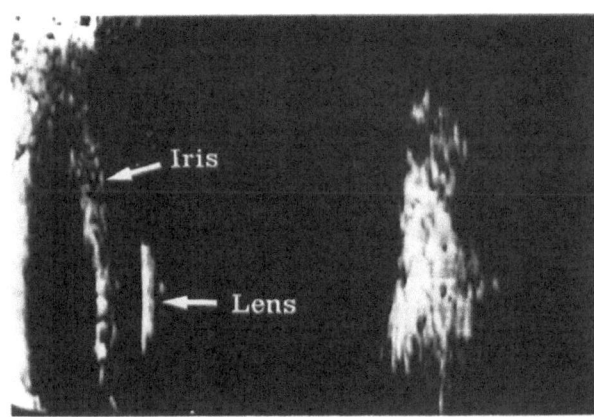

FIGURE 5.5c

FIGURE 5.4a
Pupillary response to light stimuli. The pupil appears as a round echo-free structure anteriorly. As light is flashed into the open opposite eye, the pupillary zone becomes smaller in the eye being scanned.

FIGURE 5.4b
Pupillary response to light. Light shined in the contralateral eye shows closure of the scanned pupil as a narrowing of the discontinuous echoes of the iris.

FIGURE 5.5a
Iris and pupil. Frontal scan through the iris-lens complex in a dark room demonstrates the linear echoes of the iris as a membrane interrupted over the region of the lens. The posterior lens echo is well delineated.

FIGURE 5.5b
Pupil. Light illumination on the eye is increased and the iris mechanism has closed down partially narrowing the aperture of the pupil and closing the gap in the echo pattern of the iris as compared to the dilated iris.

FIGURE 5.5c
Maximal closure of pupil. The previously interrupted echo pattern of the iris cannot be resolved by the transducer since the margins of the structure are very closely approximated and appear as a sheet-like echo.

hemorrhage from asteroid hyalosis we note that at 60 dB the echoes of the hemorrhage completely disappear from the screen while some of the echoes of the asteroid hyalosis will persist (Figure 5.6a and b).

DYNAMIC STUDY

By dymanic study further information can be gained in specific conditions. In the case of vitreous hemorrhage, the mobility of the hemorrhage can be easily analyzed by having the patient look rapidly from side to side and suddenly stop the eye motion. The aftermovements of the hemorrhage are seen as a characteristic jelly-like flutter. Aftermovements of an organized retinal detachment show limited motion of the leaves (Figure 5.7a,b,c,d, and e). If an anterior echogenic area is noted in the substance of vitreous and there is any doubt whether the pupil projects inside the vitreous, the study of the pupil can be completed by light examination of the pupil of the opposite side to evaluate the consensual light reflex. This condition occurs among very un-

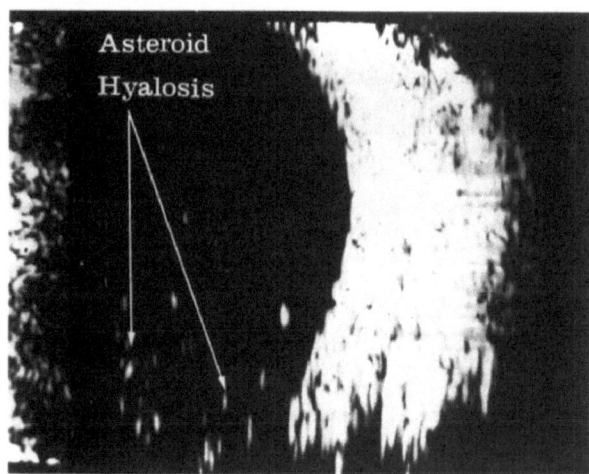

FIGURE 5.6a
Asteroid hyalosis. At 80 dB there are multiple strong reflectors in the midvitreous having a characteristic aftermovement. Diagnosis of this condition rests on the appearance of the ultrasonic picture at different sensitivity settings.

cooperative patients or patients with certain anomalies. As mentioned earlier, frontal scan usually through the lens and optic nerve reveals the posterior lens wall flanked on either side by linear high amplitude echoes of the iris which directly can be seen on the T.V. monitor.

The echo free space in the center of the iris is the pupil. The pupil narrows as light is directed on the opposite open eye confirming that this is the iris mechanism.

COMPRESSION TECHNIQUE

While observing the lesion on the T.V. monitor, the globe is compressed by moving the scanning head inward. For example, in certain lesions such as hemangioma or varix, compression of the eye by the probe may be of extreme help by showing alteration of the echo pattern or decrease in size of the lesion.

EXAMINATION OF THE TRAUMATIZED EYE

In examination of the injured globe, physical examination should be carried out with extreme

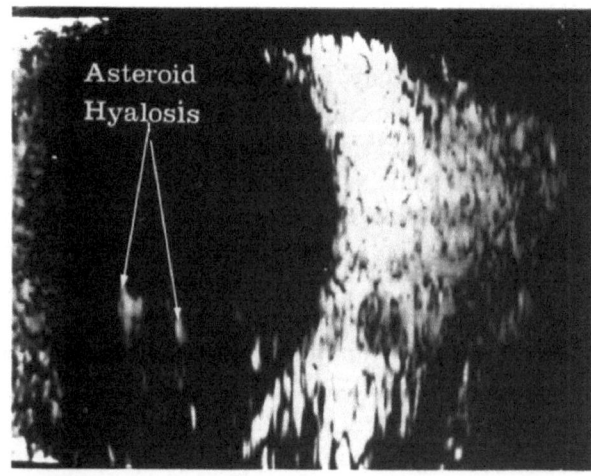

FIGURE 5.6b
Sensitivity study. Asteroid hyalosis. At 70 dB there has been a notable decrease in the number of reflecting surfaces in the midvitreous as compared with the scan at 80 dB which is typical of this disorder.

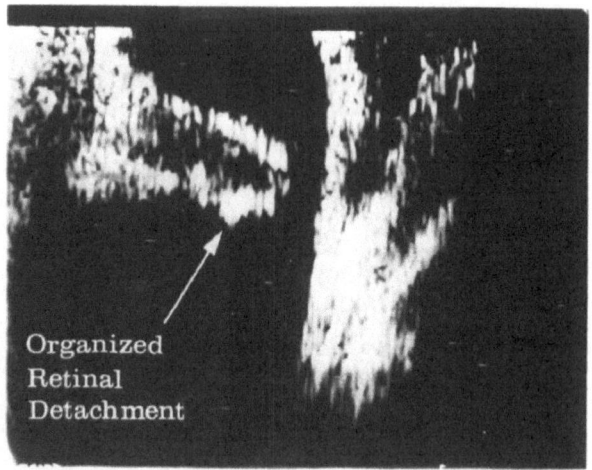

FIGURE 5.7a
Dynamic Study. Scan is in the plane of the lateral rectus muscle with the echogenic leaves of the retinal detachment pointing superiorly on the monitor. Note the oblique insertion of the optic nerve.

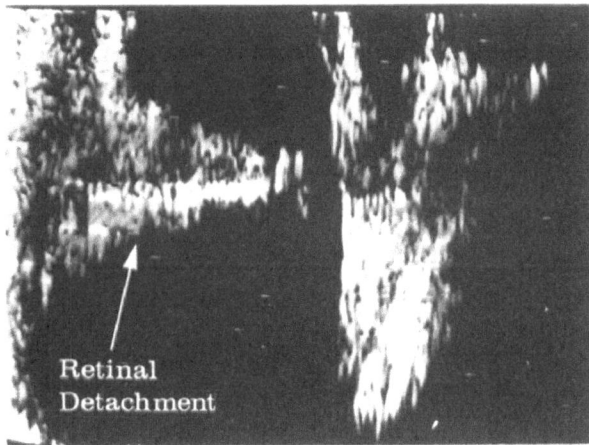

Retinal
Detachment

FIGURE 5.7b

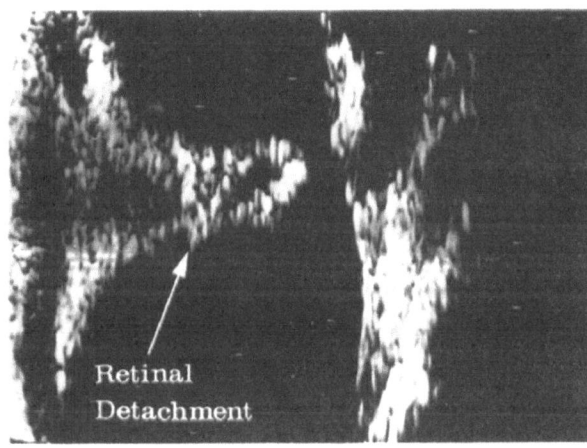

Retinal
Detachment

FIGURE 5.7c

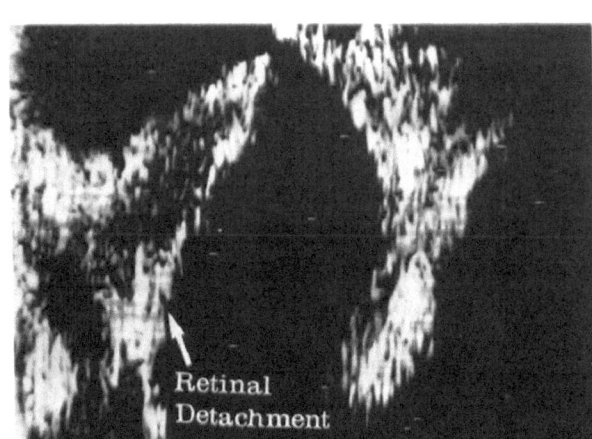

Retinal
Detachment

FIGURE 5.7d

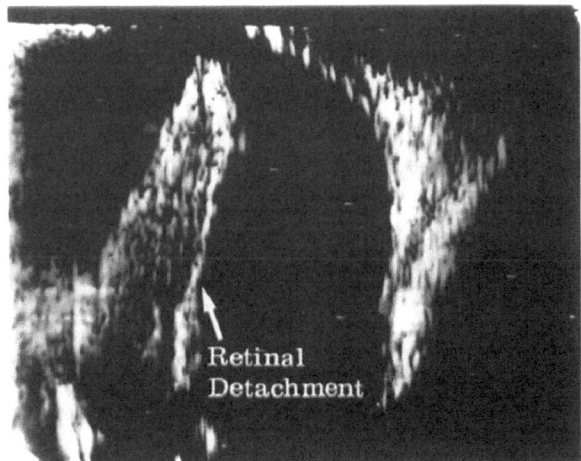

Retinal
Detachment

FIGURE 5.7e

FIGURE 5.7b
Motion of the globe upon command shows shifting of the detachment of the retina to a position parallel to the scan beam.

FIGURE 5.7c
As the retinal detachment begins to point inferiorly on the monitor, the leaves do not show any significant change in size, shape, or position.

FIGURE 5.7d
The echoes of the lateral rectus muscle become more echogenic as the gaze becomes more extreme.

FIGURE 5.7e
Maximal gaze shows essentially the same shape and echo pattern as the initial scan plane for this old and organized retinal detachment. This is of prognostic value in consideration of retinal surgery.

rior laceration is essential. In searching the laceration site in the anterior chamber, it should be kept in mind that a posterior laceration may accompany a laceration of the anterior segment. In performing sonography, after local application of generous amounts of sterile methylcellulose, the weight of the probe is buffered to avoid any unnecessary pressure on the globe.

The degree of lid edema is important, since it may directly affect the attenuated returning echoes. In marked edema, the energy of the distal echoes may be markedly reduced due to the greater distance over which the sound beam travels, and as a result, evaluation of the distal part of eye may become extremely difficult. Minimal pressure may be of help, because it may

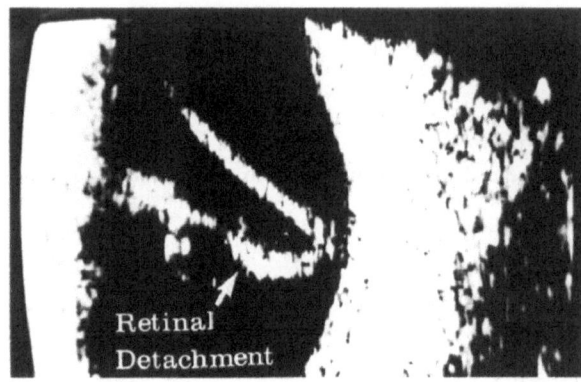

FIGURE 5.8a
Retinal detachment. Funnel shaped retinal detachment diverges from the region of the optic nerve head. A retinal cyst is noted projecting from the inferior leaf.

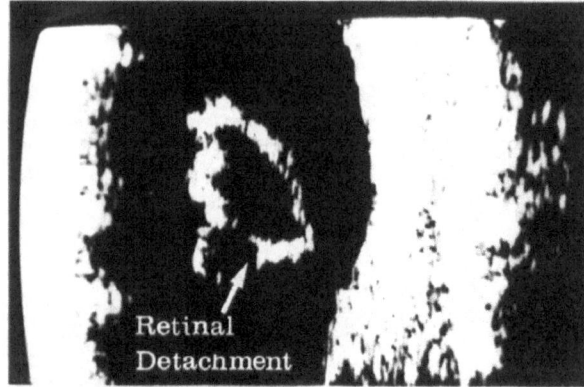

FIGURE 5.8b
Cross section of retinal detachment. Perpendicular section taken through the level of the retinal cyst which appears at the lower portion of the circular echogenic structure. The three-dimensional build up verifies the funnel shape of the detachment and the circular shape of the retinal cyst.

displace some edema and shorten the scan path. This may be dangerous if there has been significant injury to the globe.

THREE-DIMENSIONAL BUILD-UP

In sonography the examination of the organ is performed in various specific planes, usually cross-sectionally and sagittally. However, the area of pathology must always be confirmed in two planes. The shape, location, and configuration of the lesion should be evaluated by right angle scanning studies, to produce a three-dimensional representation of the pathological region. In order to accomplish mental integration of the scan data, the examiner should concentrate continually on visualizing in his mind the picture imaged on the T.V. monitor as a three-dimensional construct.

As the scan information appears on the monitor, the examiner builds up a three-dimensional object which is the summation of the two-dimensional scan planes. For example, a retinal detachment with folds could be seen easily in one direction with its attachment, but with rotating the transducer it could be displayed on the T.V. monitor in a manner that only two unconnected layers or a circular echogenic region in the vitreous may be seen (Figure 5.8a and b).

Similarly, when scanning the globe in an oblique plane, the leaves of a funnel-shaped retinal detachment will appear on the T.V. monitor as membranes with an arc shaped pattern. As the oblique scan plane approximates the perpendicular plane, the detached retina may mimic an ovid cystic lesion in the vitreous (Figure 5.9a and b). This latter appearance is quite common in the condition of bulbous retinal detachment, but the diagnosis is made with certainty as the membrane is followed to its insertion into the optic nerve head (Figure 5.10a and b). Although oblique scan planes are useful to evaluate difficult pathologic lesions, the inexperienced sonographer should attempt to obtain maximum information from the routine axial and perpendicular scan positions.

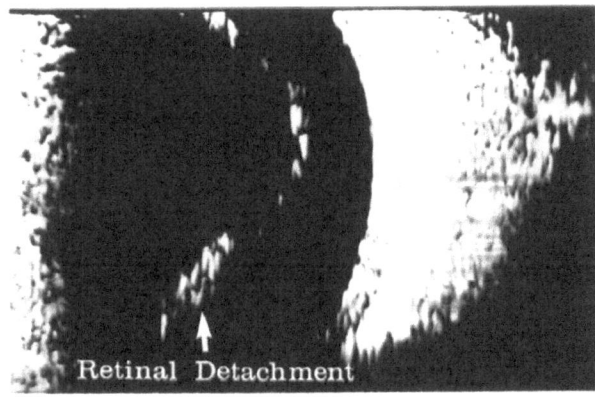

FIGURE 5.9a

FIGURE 5.9a
Oblique scan of retinal detachment. Several disc diameters away from the plane of the optic nerve the converging leaves of the retinal detachment bow gracefully towards the posterior ocular wall. Further angulation is necessary to demonstrate the insertion of the retina into the disc.

FIGURE 5.9b
Retinal detachment. Cross section scan through a cone shaped retinal detachment appears ovoid in nature. The optic nerve head cannot be imaged in this plane.

FIGURE 5.10a
Retinal detachment. The retina assumes a cylindrical form as the leaves of the retina lie parallel as it courses through the distal vitreous due to localized adhesions.

FIGURE 5.10b
Frontal section of retinal detachment. Scan taken near the posterior ocular interface demonstrates the leaves of the echogenic retinal detachment to insert into the optic disc.

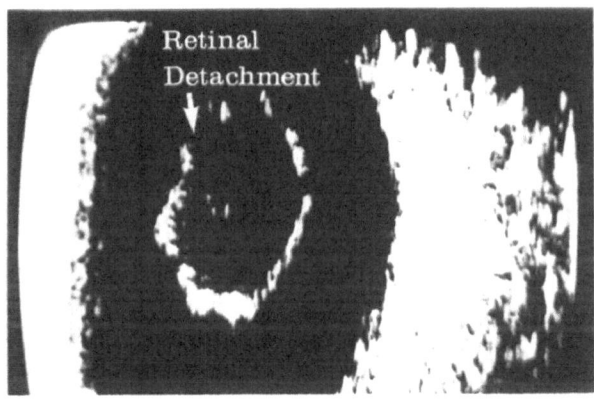

FIGURE 5.9b

The three-dimensional concept is most fascinating and helpful when applied to choroidal detachments. Although this lesion produces a choroidal effusion which circumferentially pushes the choroid medially, the choroid is anchored to the sclera at the insertion of echo of the four vortex veins near the equator of the globe. The typical biconcave appearance often called kissing choroidals is readily imaged. The sonographer should appempt to demonstrate the tent-like configuration of the choroid attached by the vortex vein to the sclera in two scan planes if possible (Figure 5.11a and b).

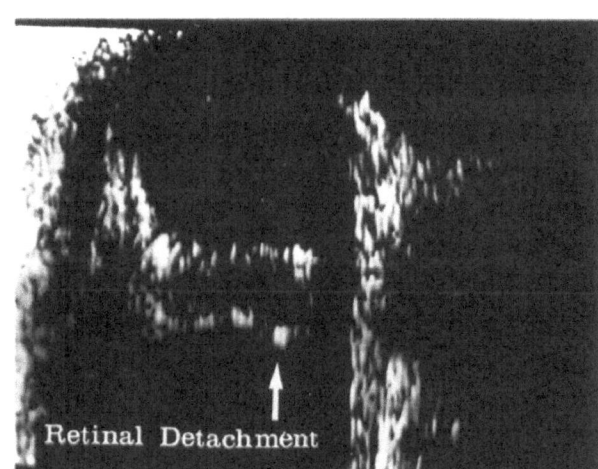

FIGURE 5.10a

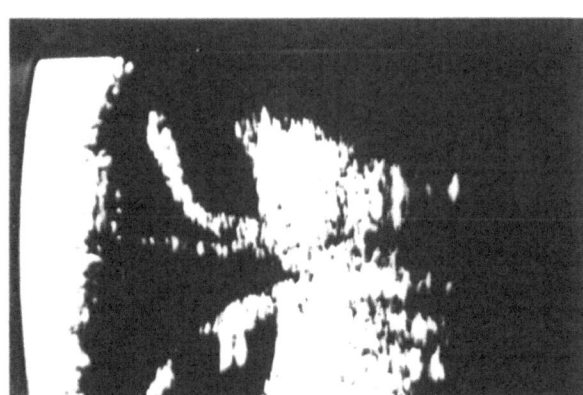

FIGURE 5.10b

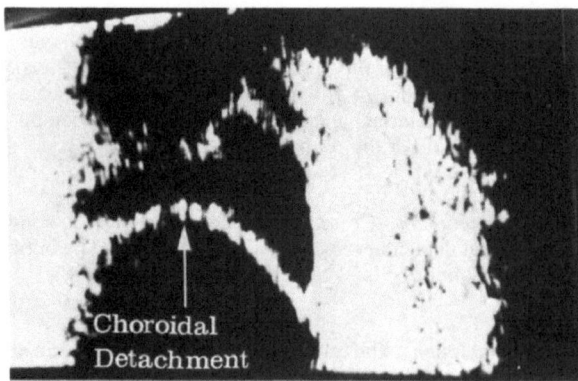

FIGURE 5.11a

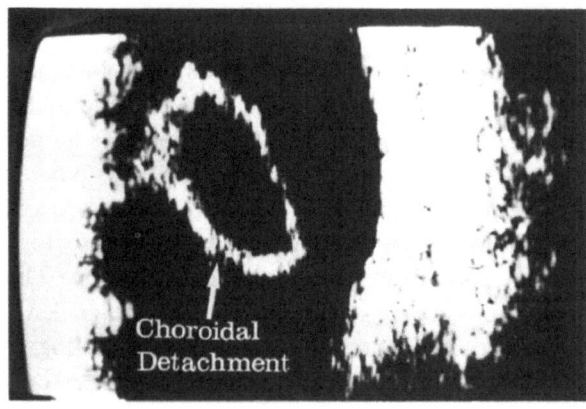

FIGURE 5.11b

FIGURE 5.11a
Choroidal detachment. The effusion of the choroid circumferentially pushes the choroid medially producing the typical biconcave appearance. The superior leaf is pulled towards the sclera by the vortex vein insertion.

FIGURE 5.11b
Scan through the vortex vein insertion. A circular array of echoes is noted since the choroid is tented superiorly by the vortex veins piercing the sclera and fixing the choroid at this level.

FIGURE 5.12a
Sensitivity controls. At 80 dB this posteriorly dislocated lens appears totally echogenic with a strong sonic shadow demonstrated.

FIGURE 5.12b
Sensitivity change. As the sensitivity control is decreased to the 70 dB setting, the previously highly echogenic central substance of the lens becomes totally echo-free.

The dynamic range of the real-time contact scanner is limited. For this reason, although one may make rough estimates of the echo strength of a given structure, the sensitivity control is of critical importance in accurately quantifying the reflectivity of an echgenic region. Typically, vitreous hemorrhage appears echogenic at 80 dB and often is totally absent at the 70 dB setting. In a similar manner, solid lesions at 80 dB may appear with an echo-free center as the sensitivity control is decreased to the 70 dB range (Figure 5.12a and b).

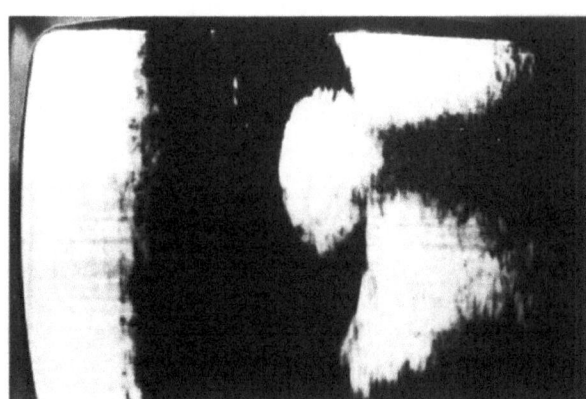

FIGURE 5.12a

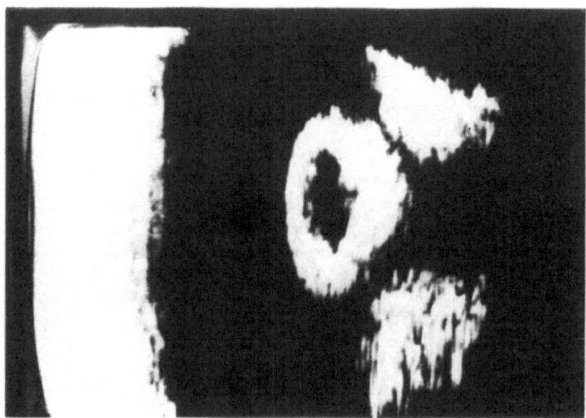

FIGURE 5.12b

IDENTIFICATION SYSTEM

Ultrasonic energy is markedly attenuated by the orbital fat. As a result, the apex of the orbit is not as clearly imaged by ultrasonography as the tissues of the globe.

The orbital contents are markedly echogenic. This echogenicity is produced by the many fine interlacing tissue interfaces. For this reason, it is highly unlikely that these echoes arise from a pure fatty substance. At high sensitivity setting (80 dB) the fatty tissues appear on the monitor as a solid pattern with gray white color. The gray-scale display helps tremendously in the recognition and the documentation of tissue signatures. However, this feature is limited in the orbit because the normal orbital fat echo pattern produces an unsharp view of this area. Most orbital pathology is echo-poor and appears as a homogeneous area. The pathological area shows if it has an echo pattern different from the normal echogenic orbital pattern. An irregular, echo-poor area within the orbital echogenic tissue may have numerous shapes and represent many pathological conditions or may be the product of an improper examination with incorrect transducer maneuvers. This is the reason that technically the examination of the orbit is simple, but ultrasonic interpretation is very difficult. Even in the hands of experienced examiners, false positives and false negatives may be produced by various scan maneuvers. The geographic orientation of the lesion is extremely important. After localization of the pathological area, (the shape must be reproducible) its size, position, and tissue signature are described. One point should be kept in mind that interpreting shades of gray on the echogenic background is extremely difficult. On the other hand, the diagnosis of the pathological echoes (white or gray) in the echo-free region of the globe is simple.

Even though there are numerous structures in the orbit only the optic nerve and larger ocular muscles are visible. Sonographically, the systematic examination of the orbit is similar to the globe.

1) Each eye is examined and scanned and the axial length measurement is photographed on the polaroid film.

2) The display setting control is changed from the 0–3 cm range to the 1.5–4.5 cm setting, in order to shift the entire picture on the screen towards the left. As a result, the posterior ocular wall and orbital tissue can be seen more easily. This time gating control allows the sonographer to examine various segments of the eye in greater detail. The optic nerve appears as an echo-free V-shape and is used as a reference point.

3) The position of the filling cap on the probe head should always be either superior, towards patient's head or medially, towards patient's nose for simple orientation. If the filling cap on the probe head is located nasally, the top of the T.V. monitor represents the nasal orbit and the bottom of the display monitor represents the temporal aspect.

It should be emphasized that using the contact B-scanner for the ophthalmic examination is a relatively simple technique. However, a system of identification is essential for proper interpretation and documentation of the ultrasonic findings. Excellent diagnostic information may be obtained if the study is carefully carried out. If the examination is not performed in a logical and systematic manner, regions of pathological changes may be completely missed.

Since the ultrasonic beam is not transmitted through air, a coupling agent is necessary for sonic conduction. Methylcellulose solution is generally used for this purpose. Methylcellulose is sterile, and, in cases of penetrating injury of eyes, there is no danger of infection. The agent may be placed directly on the transducer head or spread over the eyelid.

The patient usually lies in the supine position. The scanning head of the transducer may be placed against the closed eyelid or directly in contact with the cornea. We generally apply the scanning head over the closed eyelid to which a large amount of methylcellulose has been applied. This method of examination is both convenient for the examiner and comfortable for the patient. Indeed, this may be the only acceptable means to study the pediatric or geriatric patient. When studying post-operative or post-traumatic patients, a generous amount of highly viscous methylcellulose is applied to form a very thick layer over the eyelid. This is done to minimize pressure on the globe due to the weight of the metallic transducer probe. This jelly-bath may also be used to image the anterior segments of the eye. Alternatively, subcutaneous injections of a gasless, sterile solution such as saline or lidocaine into the loose skin of the eyelid will separate the transducer head from the anterior segment of the eye.

The scanning procedure is started with the patient looking down and the transducer positioned over the upper lid. As soon as the patient realizes that the procedure is painless, a systematic investigation is performed. The following definitions are used:

right eye = o.d.
left eye = o.s.

With the patient's eyes closed, and the transducer in place horizontally in such a manner that the housing cap points medially in the transverse position or superiorly in sagittal section, we have the TOD (transverse right eye) and TOS (transverse left eye) positions.

While the closed eye is being examined the patient is asked to open the opposite eye and look at the finger tip of the examiner. When the patient follows the finger movement, the eye is rotated into any desired direction. In the majority of patients it is difficult to open the opposite eye. During the examination, the patient is instructed to look right, left, superior, and inferior according to the examiner's required plane of study.

The longitudinal scanning planes are obtained by changing the transducer from a horizontal to a vertical direction. The LOD and LOS scan planes are obtained and, as in the above manner, the eye is studied in any desired plane.

The transducer is aimed through the center of the cornea at the optic nerve (either in the T or L planes which is TOD or TOS) and an axial length measurement is obtained and recorded photographically. Polaroid films are usually taken for documentation of the various scans of each eye. The main consideration in the dynamic study of the eye is to manually shift the transducer forward, backward, medially, and laterally to examine all areas of the globe. This is similar to the fluoroscopic part of a G.I. series.

Specific areas of pathology should be confirmed with sufficient polaroid pictures in various planes and localized with respect to the anatomic landmarks of the globe.

Some examiners consider two practical points on the globe for identification of the scan planes. The center of the cornea is the zero (0) point and the most posterior part of the globe is the four (4) point. Other examiners have used a system from 0–4. However, we have found reproducibility of these intermediate settings difficult in the clinical setting.

Another useful anatomic site is the o'clock position of the globe. The extreme cephalic position of the globe is called 12 o'clock directions. The extreme inferior aspect of the globe is at the 6 o'clock position.

To these directional markings, the sensitivity setting of the machine should be recorded on the polaroid film for a complete listing of the variable factors.

In the 0/0/80 position, the scan is performed through the center of the cornea with maximal gain setting. The scan done at 4/12/60 has the probe at the extreme superior aspect of the globe with the eye gazing at the twelve o'clock position and utilizes an intermediate sensitivity setting. A polaroid marked with 4/6/40 has the eye gazing up with the minimal gain of the unit and the probe inferiorly.

We use the following identification system for both orbit and globe for greater practicality and better localization of eye pathology. Once more it should be emphasized that proper evaluation of the orbit requires identification of the landmarks within this bony structure. The optic nerve is easily observed in its proximal aspect within the orbital fat echoes. At the junction of the optic nerve with the apex of the muscle cone the attenuated sonic beam portrays this conglomerate of structures as a vaguely defined echo-poor region.

Of greatest value to the sonographer in the optimal study of orbital disease are the muscles forming the muscle cone. These may be serially and simply identified with the following localization system. On the other hand, by identifying the muscles and optic nerve we have more reference points for localization of pathology in the globe. In our system the scan head is always positioned with the cap facing either superiorly or nasally with respect to each eye. As the first step in scanning the orbit or globe we hold the transducer head either in the transverse or longitudinal position. In the study of the orbit for the localization of each muscle and space occupying lesions we use an identification system based on five years of practical experience. In this system the recti muscles stand as landmarks. The right eye, as mentioned earlier, is called OD and if the sector scan is used transversely, it is called TOD. The sector scan used longitudinally is called LOD. (TOD = transverse scan of right eye) (LOD = longitudinal scan of right eye).

Similar terminology is used for the left eye (TOS = transverse scan of left eye) (LOS = longitudinal scan of left eye).

To identify each muscle we designated the letter M for medial rectus, L for lateral rectus, S for superior rectus, and I for inferior rectus muscle. As a result, when each specific letter is used in accordance with the above identification system it is concluded that a scan in the plane of the specific muscle of the interest has been studied. The optimal position in scanning the medial rectus muscle is in the temporal gaze. The transducer should be held transversely at the temporal side. Since the metallic cap of the transducer housing corresponds to the superior

portion of the T.V. monitor, the medial rectus muscle appears as a linear band passing along the upper aspect of the T.V. monitor and finally will be registered on the top of the polaroid film (Figure 5.13).

Scanning of the lateral rectus muscle is best accomplished with the eye in extreme nasal gaze while holding the transducer medially with the cap towards the nasal area. The lateral rectus muscle will be displayed on the lower aspect of the T.V. monitor and finally registered in the lower portion of the polaroid film (Figure 5.14). Similarly, the superior rectus muscle of the eye is best imaged in the maximum inferior gaze while transducer is held in the most inferior portion of the orbital rim. This muscle appears as a sonolucent area in the upper aspect of the T.V. monitor (Figure 5.15). The inferior rectus muscle is better imaged in the superior gaze as the transducer is held on the superior portion of the orbital rim. This muscle appears on the inferior portion of the T.V. monitor (Figure 5.16). The superior and inferior rectus muscles usually are scanned longitudinally, but it may be done transversely to identify each muscle. In the transverse sector scanning plane with the sound beam transversing a nasotemporal path, in the medial gaze the structure appearing as an echo-poor (echo-free at 70 dB) linear band extending inferiorly along the screen as it courses posteriorly will be the lateral rectus muscle. The polaroid picture is taken when the muscle is maximally imaged and the assistant is instructed to label the film TOS-L (L for lateral rectus). Each muscle can be studied in maximal gaze for extreme stretch or in neutral position, or it can be studied cross-sectional. It depends on the clinical aspect and presentation of pathology.

Similarly, as the probe scans in the transverse plane from temporal to nasal, an echo poor image will appear extending from the top of the screen inferiorly as it progresses posteriorly. This is the medial rectus muscle and the picture is labelled TOS-M. In the longitudinal scan plane, again with the cap pointing upward, the muscle identified along the infero-anterior orbit is the inferior rectus muscle. Since the superior

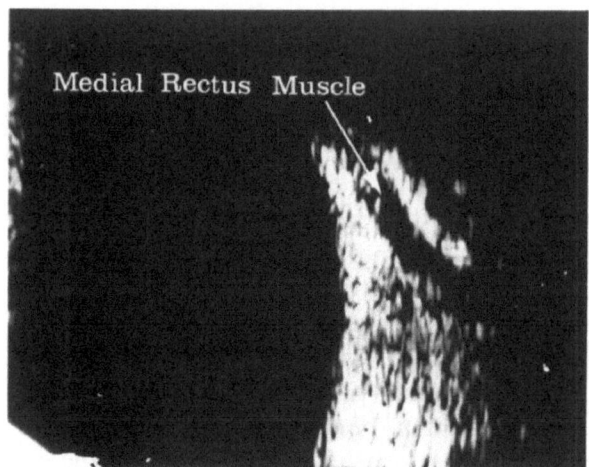

FIGURE 5.13

FIGURE 5.13
The medial rectus muscle appears as a linear band at the top of the screen and is an important landmark.

FIGURE 5.14
The lateral rectus muscle lies at the inferior aspect of the monitor. The screen cap of the unit points nasally.

FIGURE 5.15
The superior rectus muscle lies at the top of the screen with the transducer cap pointing superiorly.

FIGURE 5.16
The inferior rectus muscle appears as a mirror image to the superior rectus muscle and is at the bottom of the screen.

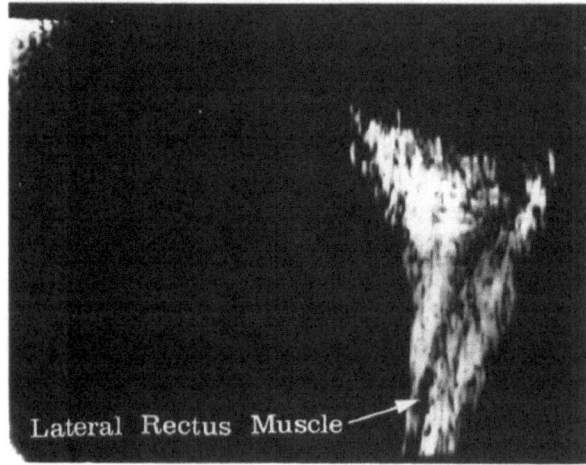

FIGURE 5.14

and inferior rectus muscles run at a lateral angle to the sagittal plane of the orbit, special care must be taken to optimally image these muscles. The inexperienced sonographer may confuse the more proximally situated inferior rectus muscle with the more distal inferior oblique muscle. Similarly, appearing as a mirror image to the inferior rectus will be the superior rectus muscle. Again, care must be taken not to confuse the more proximal usperior oblique muscle with the more distal superior rectus muscle. The scans obtained on the superior and inferior rectus muscles are labelled as LOS-S and LOS-I. This manner of sequential rectus muscle imaging and immediately labelling each polaroid has proven of enormous value in the geographic localization of lesions of the orbit and muscle cone.

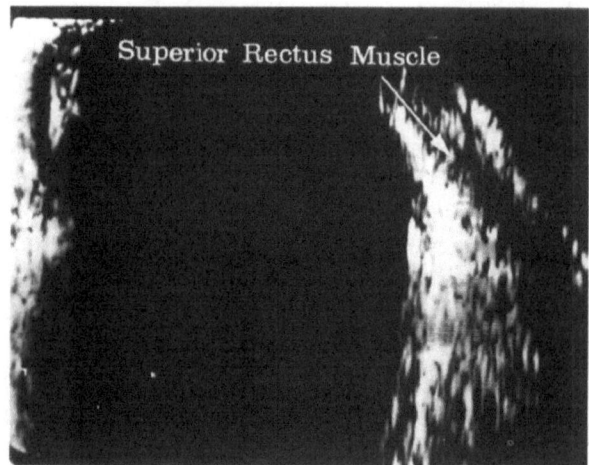

FIGURE 5.15

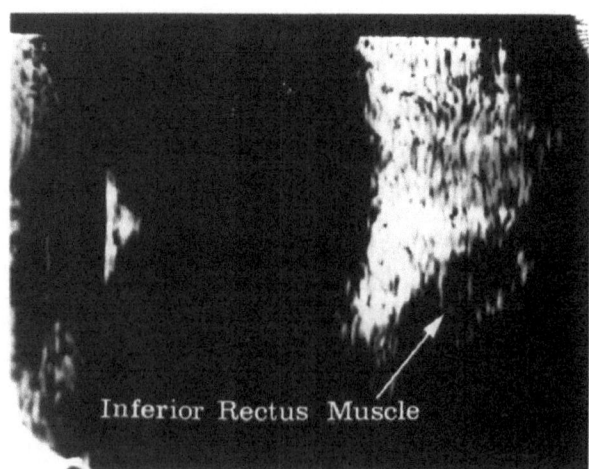

FIGURE 5.16

In order to avoid any mistakes, for example, an echo-free area in an echogenic substance of the orbit may be due to a tumor or cross-section of one of the hypertrophic recti muscles. To best visualize the medial recti muscles along their long axis, the probe is held against the lateral canthal area parallel with the closed palpebral fissure, and the eye is rotated laterally. This motion causes that muscle to extend along the medial orbital wall in total abduction. Again, the filling cap pointing towards the nasal area signifies that the top of the screen is the anterior orbit and the bottom is the posterior orbit. As a result, the medial recti muscle is seen as a relatively sonolucent stripe with light internal echoes surrounded by the normal orbital fat. From the insertion of the ocular wall the muscle extends posteriorly into the orbital fat at an oblique angle. After identifying the recti muscles, the area of the disc and macula can be evaluated grossly.

During the study, the sensitivity must be adjusted so that the globe and regions of pathology are analyzed at the range of sensitivities from the strongest to the weakest. Asteroid hyalosis and vitreous hemorrhage appear the same at the 80 dB gain setting. To obtain the characteristic tissue signature of the lesion for differential diagnosis, the sensitivity is lowered in 10 dB steps until the echoes disappear. The echoes of asteroid hyalosis are stronger than vitreous hemorrhage and will disappear at lower gain settings than the hemorrhage. At the end of the examination, the depth control is varied. The globe is best scanned in the 0–3 cm range. For complete study, the tissues of the orbit are best imaged in the 1.5–4.5 cm range. In dealing with a large space occupying lesion, it may be necessary to switch to the 3–6 cm range, although this is unusual in routine practice. Changing to a higher range setting shifts the posterior wall of the eye towards the left side of the screen.

MARKING OF THE POLAROID PICTURES

Total information is obtained when each polaroid picture is marked with the following information: direction of transducer, name of eye, globe location, gaze, and sensitivity setting.

The name, date, and age may appear on the back of the polaroid. It is good practice to string these pictures in order on a strip of marking tape for a serial review of the scanning procedure. The use of polaroid is easier than video tape since it can be developed immediately and illustrative scans may be sent to the referring physician for orientation. We find the new 667 film is far superior to the 107 type of polaroid film. In our camera we use f/11 at 1/8 second exposure. Some of the information displayed on the T.V. screen cannot be captured by the relatively less sensitive polaroid film and is lost during the exposure. However, in spite of this small information loss, we find that polaroid is still the most convenient method of documentation of the examination findings.

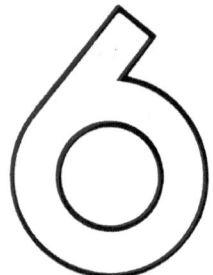

sonography of the injured eye

GENERAL INTRODUCTION

The patient with an eye injury usually seeks immediate attention when he is aware of the traumatic incident. Certain penetrating wounds may be painless. This occurs especially with small high speed particles such as stone or metallic slivers incidental to construction or machinery work. Thus, eye trauma must be suspected in patients with a suggestive work history, but no recall of the actual traumatic moment. The cardinal symptoms of eye damage include reduced vision and persistent discomfort. Visual acuity must be routinely measured when evaluating the potentially injured eye. Continuing discomfort following eye trauma indicates a certain degree of injury.

It must be emphasized here that the injured eye must be manipulated or examined with extreme care and gentleness. The eye is a delicate organ and rough handling may convert a salvageable eye into a useless organ. In certain instances the sonographer may be asked to provide essential data on the status of the globe, especially when fundoscopic examination

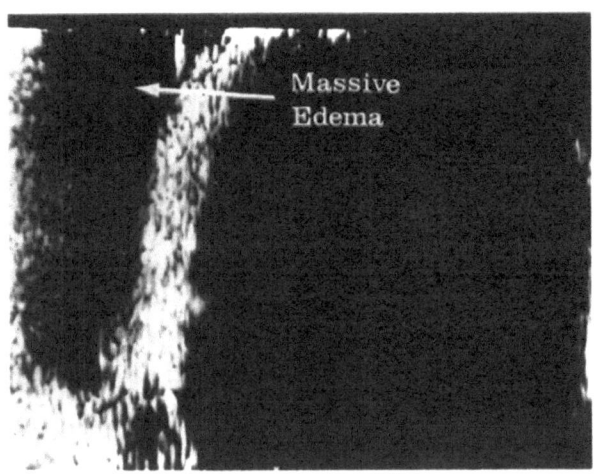

FIGURE 6.1
Edema of lid. Patient with eye lid contusion shows marked edema of the superior lid which produces an echo poor space between the outer surface of the eyelid and the sclera.

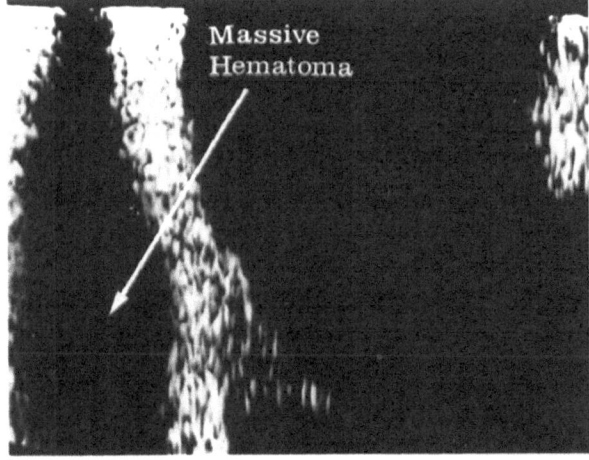

FIGURE 6.2
Hematoma of lid. Echo free zone is visible between the corneoscleral limbus and the exterior lid tissues. The space in between is filled with blood from recent trauma and produces a water bath effect. Anterior displacement of the probe results in poor imaging of the orbital fat.

is not practical due to the nature and extent of the injury. Great caution should be exercised in the ultrasonic study. Pressure over the globe should be avoided by the use of a very thick layer of viscous methycellulose gel. The sonographer must also be aware that immersion water bath techniques are contraindicated in the severely injured eye.

To properly study the injured eye, a variety of examinations may be performed. The eye must first be inspected. Then the lids should be separated without exerting pressure on the eyeball. Oblique illumination will satisfactorily examine the anterior transparent structures. The use of pressure on the injured globe may permanently ruin the vision. The sonographer is urged to look for the following objective signs of injury: lid abrasions, ecchymoses, and lid edema.

Edema of the eyelid due to a contusion shows marked swelling of the superior lid which produces an echo-poor space between the outer surface of the eyelid and the sclera (Figure 6.1). When there is injury to the eyelid the point of significant damage should be investigated.

Hematoma may follow a wound of the eyelid. An echo-free zone may occur between the corneoscleral limbus and the exterior lid tissues. The space in between is filled with blood from recent trauma and produces a water bath effect (Figure 6.2). Anterior displacement of the probe results in poor imaging of the orbital fat at the 0–3 cm setting. Since the eyelids are very thin, a laceration that is slightly deeper will involve the eyeball. Conjunctival hemorrhages and lacerations may mask a penetrating wound. Superficial corneal abrasions and foreign bodies are readily observed. Fluorescein stain will easily highlight corneal damage, but should not be attempted until a penetrating injury has been ruled out.

The anterior epithelium of the cornea is remarkably self healing and generally leaves no scar. The deeper cornea is protected by the tough Bowman's membrane. Injury to this layer or of the deeper corneal tissue will leave a permanent scar. Penetrating injuries of the cornea or sclera may show a protruding transparent jelly representing loss of vitreous or lens. A gray ring of

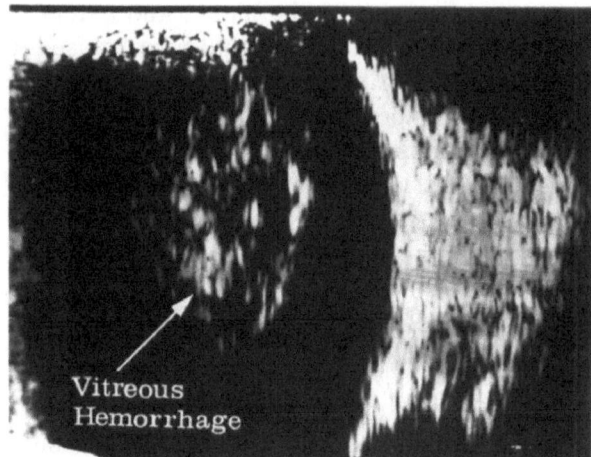

FIGURE 6.3

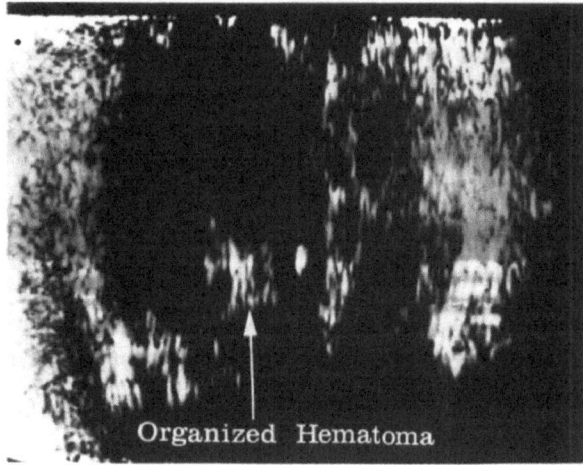

FIGURE 6.4

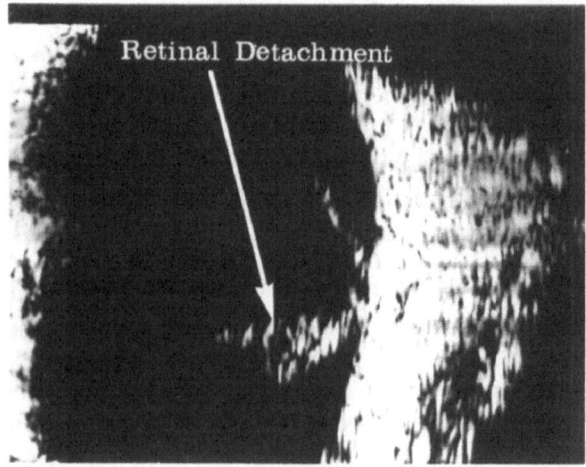

FIGURE 6.5

edema surrrounds corneal perforations and collapse of the anterior chamber may be noted. Displacement of the iris suggests prolapse of this structure toward the side of penetrating injury. Holes in the iris or notches are indicative of penetrating trauma. Intraocular bleeding results from either penetrating injury or ocular contusion. Recent blunt trauma may show focal areas of low amplitude, very mobile echoes due to acute vitreous hemorrhage (Figure 6.3). Long standing blood may produce multiple irregular internal echoes with a poorly marginated posterior retinal interface. Motility is severely limited (Figure 6.4). Vitreous hemorrhage may be quickly suspected from absence of the expected red reflex of the eye with the ophthalmoscope. Ophthalmoscopy will often show retinal edema, retinal tears, and foreign bodies if the vitreous hemorrhage does not obscure the retina. Retinal edema is most pronounced in the macula and appears as a gray discoloration. The foreign body will appear greatly magnified unless it has been obscured by the exudative reaction of the vitreous. Retinal detachment may occur (Figure 6.5). Trauma may produce either enophthalmos or exophthalmos. Enophthalmos or backward displacement of the eye is common to blow-out fracture of the orbit with herniation of the orbital contents into the maxillary sinus. Temporary exophthalmos results from orbital hemorrhage and edema. This may compromise the circulation to the optic nerve resulting in blindness. Crepitus of the lids is itself innocuous but indicates a fracture into the sinuses, usually the thin ethmoidal air cells. Appropriate measures should be taken to prevent orbital cellulitis. The

FIGURE 6.3
Recent vitreous hemorrhage. A midvitreous collection of low amplitude, mobile echoes due to recent vitreous hemorrhage.

FIGURE 6.4
Old vitreous hemorrhage. Multiple irregular internal echoes with a poorly marginated posterior retinal interface. Motility was severely limited. Organized vitreous hemorrhage.

FIGURE 6.5
Retinal detachment. Diverging leaves of a traumatic detachment extend from the posterior ocular wall.

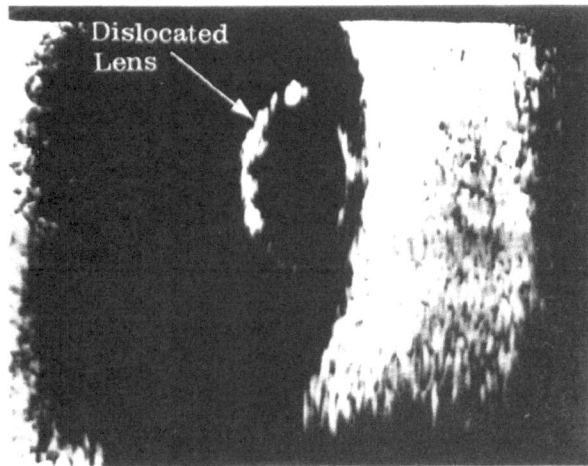

FIGURE 6.6a

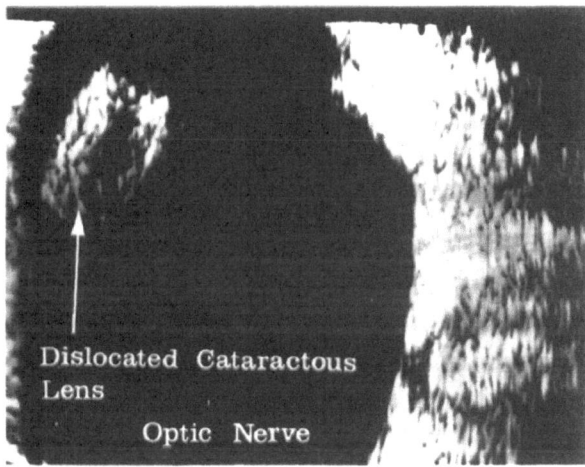

FIGURE 6.6b

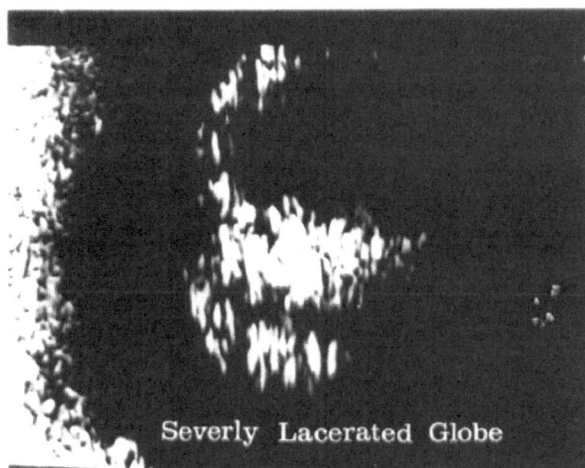

FIGURE 6.7

lens may dislocate as a result of trauma (Figure 6.6a and b) and acute glaucoma may follow anterior dislocation of the lens.

SONOGRAPHY OF THE INJURED EYE

In a severely traumatized eye, there is shortening of the axial length as vitreous is lost (Figure 6.7). The normal posterior ocular structures are not visualized and the orbital fat echoes are grossly irregular. Through transmission is impaired. When there is a history of burns, extreme caution should be exercised to prevent further damage.

Lid edema from a flash burn produces eyelids that are very edematous and may not be opened. The swelling of the lids (Figure 6.8) allows us to image the anterior chamber of the eye and also check for vitreous damage and retinal detachment.

Another post-traumatic condition that may occur is hyphema. Here, a water bath may be a great help. When there is a traumatic hyphema, a water bath scan is optimal as the following case with the water bath delay demonstrates (Figure 6.9). The anterior echo-free area in the scan represents the water bath. The upper lid appears triangular and echogenic. The lower lid is swollen and less echogenic due to more localized bleeding. Between the open lids is the anterior chamber with echoes noted in the inferior (dependent portion) aspect. Distal to this is the echo-free lens with its artifact. In some traumatized eyes, phythisis bulbi will occur. In the pre-

FIGURE 6.6a
Dislocated lens. Biconvex structure lies against the posterior ocular wall.

FIGURE 6.6b
Dislocated lens. Lens is filled with echoes due to cataractous changes.

FIGURE 6.7
Lacerated eye. Severely traumatized eye. There is shortening of the axial length. Normal posterior ocular structures are not visualized and the orbital fat echoes are grossly irregular. Through-transmission is impaired.

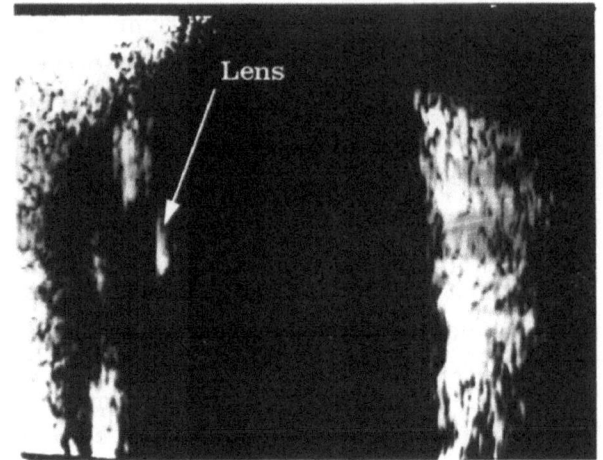

FIGURE 6.8

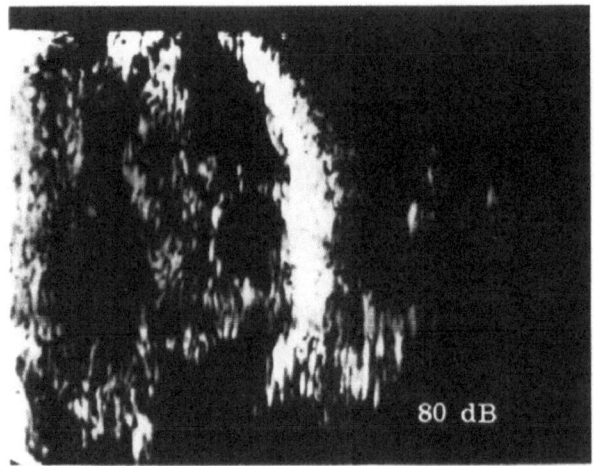

FIGURE 6.10b

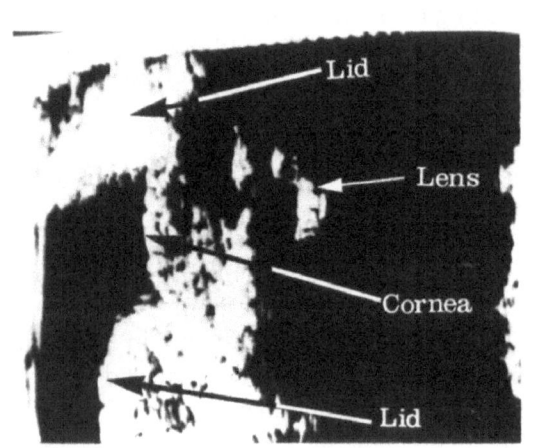

FIGURE 6.9

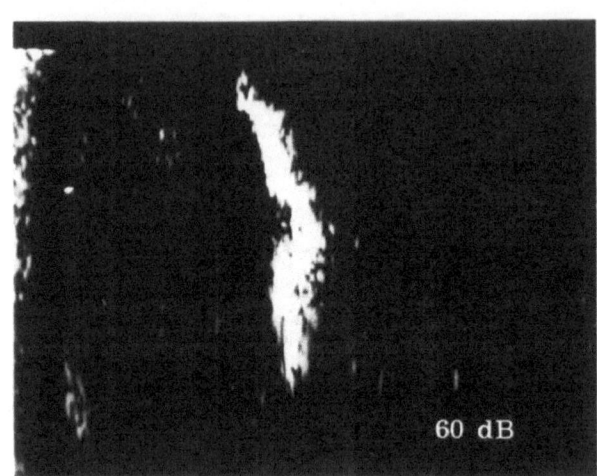

FIGURE 6.10c

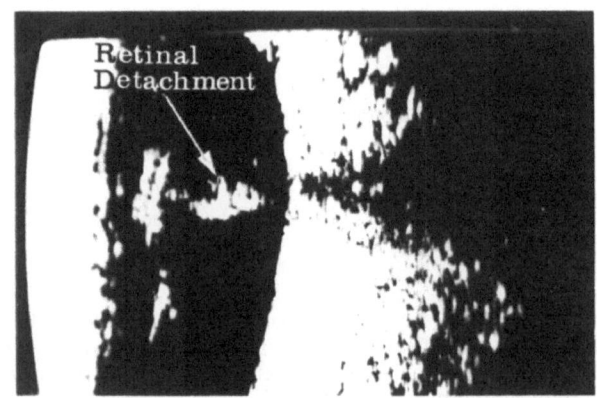

FIGURE 6.10a

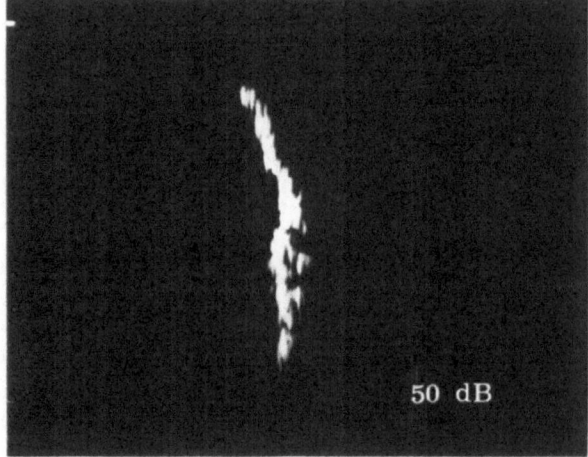

FIGURE 6.10d

FIGURE 6.8
Lid edema from burn. The eyelids were very edematous and could not be opened. The swelling of the lids allows us to image the anterior chamber of the eye and also check for vitreous damage and retinal detachment. There has been neither retinal detachment nor vitreous hemorrhage.

FIGURE 6.9
Traumatic hyphema. Water bath scan. Echo-free anterior space represents the water bath. Upper lid appears triangular and echogenic. Lower lid is swollen and less echogenic due to lesser bleeding. Between the open lids is the anterior chamber with echoes noted in the inferior (dependent portion) aspect. Distal to this is the echo-free lens with its artifact.

FIGURE 6.10a
Pre-phthisical globe. There is shortening of the axial length with a decrease in the intraocular pressure. A strong set of echoes projects and diverges into the vitreous from the optic nerve head which is the associated retinal detachment.

FIGURE 6.10b
At 80 dB, this pre-phthysical eye shows irregular vitreal echoes.

FIGURE 6.10c
At 60 dB, marked scleral thickening is noted.

FIGURE 6.10d
At 50 dB, only the irregular scleral outline appears.

FIGURE 6.11
Part of the choroidal detachment is noted in the vitreous. Choroidal thickening often accompanies the lowered intraocular pressure.

FIGURE 6.12
Abnormal echo pattern to the posterior portion of the globe. Disorganization due to rupture of the globe. Note shortened axial length.

phthisical stage (Figure 6.10a,b,c, and d), there is shortening of the axial length with a decrease in the intraocular pressure. Retinal detachment at this stage is usually a common occurrence and appears as a strong set of echoes projects and diverges into the vitreous from the optic nerve head. The pre-phthisical condition (Figure 6.11), may show an isolated part of the retinal detachment noted in the vitreous which may be associated with vitreous hemorrhage. Choroidal thickening accompanies the lowered intraocular pressure. Disorganization due to rupture of the globe shortens the axial length and produces an abnormal echo pattern in the posterior portion of the globe (Figure 6.12). In other traumatic conditions such as hyphema, when there is no associated rupture of the globe, the contact scanner can be applied directly to the lid without separating the transducer head from the lid by the subcutaneous injection of saline or thick gel layer if a water bath is not available. Hyphema presents as focal strong echoes which are demonstrated antero-inferior to the lens, indicative of clotted blood in the anterior chamber. As mentioned earlier in the case of edema of the eyelid (Figure 6.13), a frontal sonogram through the lens shows both posterior and anterior borders of the lens including parts of the iris. Edema fluid increases the distance from the transducer head to the anterior chamber of the eye and the near field dead zone does not distort the image of the

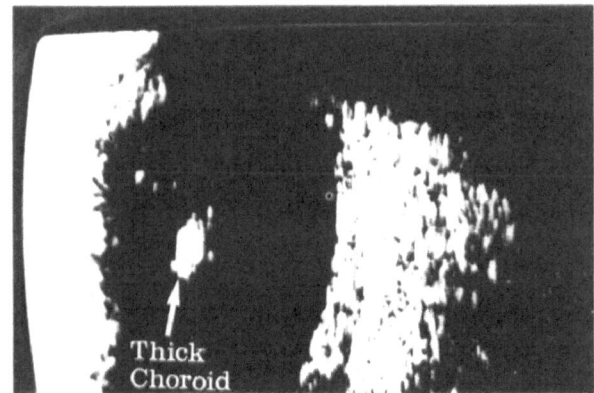

FIGURE 6.11

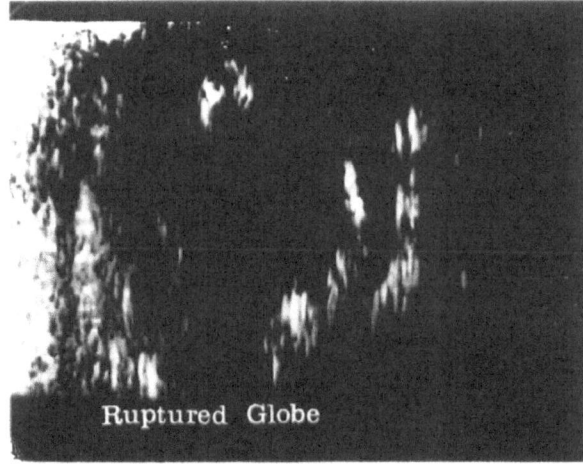

FIGURE 6.12

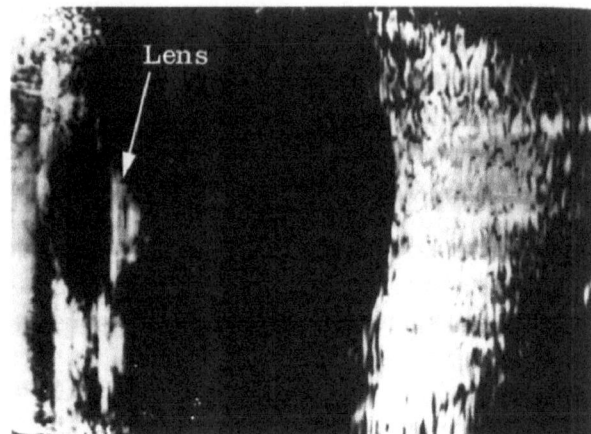

FIGURE 6.13

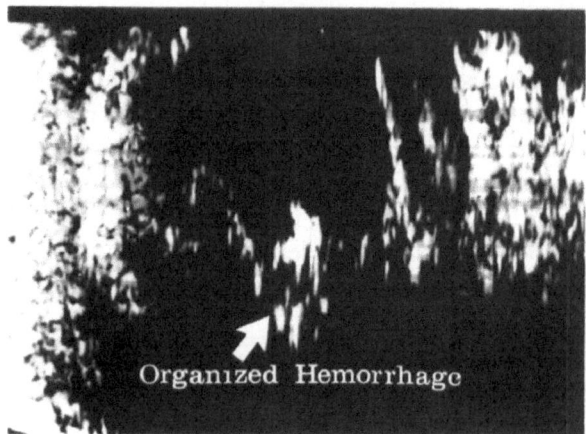

FIGURE 6.14a

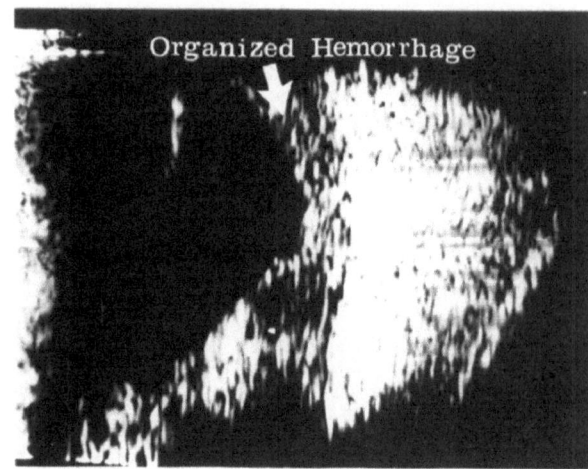

FIGURE 6.14b

anterior ocular structures permitting a scanning of the entire lens. Organized hemorrhage may cause a thick band of echoes which persist down to 50 dB. This situation is best imaged in a scan at 60 dB which demonstrates an irregular flattened area against the posterior ocular wall (Figure 6.14a and b), and simulates thickened choroid. Weak aftermovements noted show that the diagnosis is old post-traumatic vitreous hemorrhage.

The normal structures of the globe are not imaged in the enucleated eye which reveals the region of the globe filled with amorphous echoes. Sound transmission is usually poor (Figure 6.15a). Usually at 80 dB there is progressive attenuation of the echo pattern and at 60 dB scattered irregular echoes are noted which is the typical ultrasonic appearance of the orbit with the eye enucleated (Figure 6.15b). When artificial eye is placed (Figure 6.15c), the prosthetic device beneath the closed eyelid completely attenuates the sonic beam, producing a total sonic shadow distal to the anterior echo complex (Figure 6.15c).

FIGURE 6.13
Edema of the eyelid. Frontal sonogram through the lens shows both the posterior and anterior borders of the lens including parts of the iris. Traumatic edema has increased the distance from the transducer head to the anterior chamber of the eye. The near field dead zone does not distort the image of the anterior ocular structures permitting scanning of the entire lens.

FIGURE 6.14a
Organized hemorrhage. Disorganized internal echoes with medium and high amplitudes show poor mobility.

FIGURE 6.14b
Scan of vitreous blood clot at 70 dB with inhomogeneous echoes which move slowly following eye motion.

FIGURE 6.15a
Enucleated eye. The normal structures of the eye are not imaged. The region of the globe is filled with amorphous echoes and sound transmission is poor. At 80 dB there is progressive attenuation of the echo pattern.

FIGURE 6.15b
The same case of 6.15a demonstrated and changing the sensitivity to 60 dB scattered irregular echoes are seen. Ultrasonic appearance of the orbit with the eye enucleated.

FIGURE 6.15c
Artificial eye with total attenuation of the sound beam.

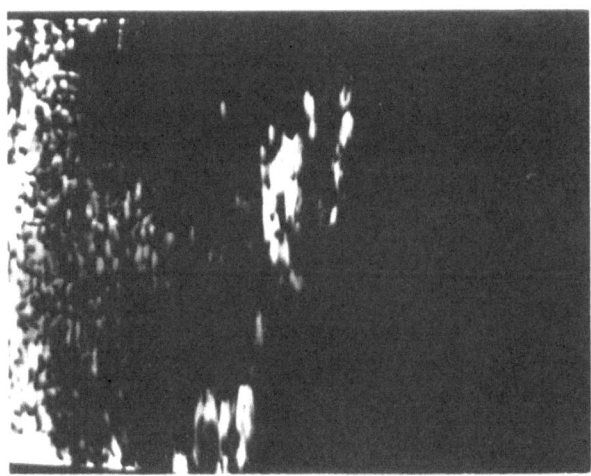

FIGURE 6.15a

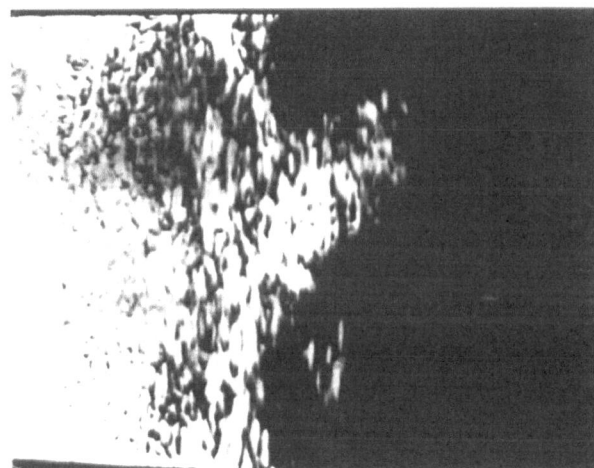

FIGURE 6.15b

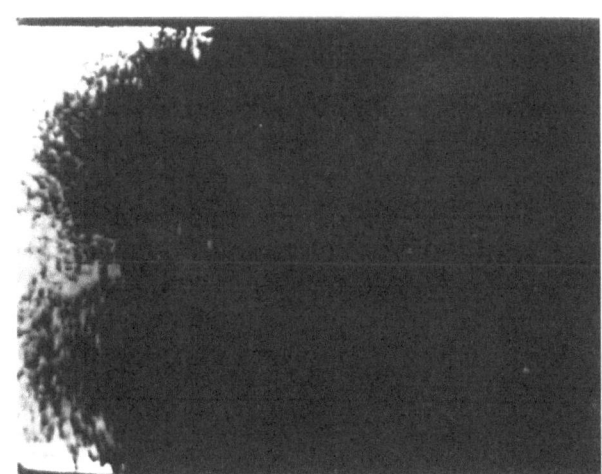

FIGURE 6.15c

INTRAOCULAR FOREIGN BODY

Most of the ocular foreign bodies are radiopaque and best demonstrated by radiographic localization techniques. This method is not precise since it assumes an average size of the eyeball of 24 mm. The normal globe varies from 22–27 mm in axial length and discrepancies from the normal result in errors in localization. By using sonography, the foreign body is demonstrated together with the ocular and orbital structure, without distortion or magnification. In well trained hands, more accurate localization can be achieved. Both A-scan and B-scan should be applied if at all possible. Foreign bodies are demonstrated in the vitreous with high accuracy, if of sufficient size and geometry to reflect back the ultrasonic wave. A foreign body within the globe and orbital cavity may be diagnosed with 70% accuracy. By sonography, the magnetic foreign body can be monitored as it moves under influence of the probe. As mentioned earlier by sonography, the foreign body can be located and its relation to the wall of the eye can be accurately assessed.

The associated damage with foreign bodies can also be evaluated. This investigation is important for surgery. Ultrasonography is another complement to the x-ray examination, slit lamp ophthalmoscopy, and the metal locator.

SONOGRAPHY OF FOREIGN BODIES

If the foreign body is free and lying in the vitreous it can be detected readily because of the high accoustical impedance between the foreign body and the vitreous. Foreign bodies are strong reflectors, and for this reason, their detection and localization are usually not too difficult. After localization, by using the overlay grid, it is possible to tell the distance between the posterior wall of the eye and the foreign body. The size and shape of the foreign body is better determined by x-ray.

If the foreign body is located on or near the posterior wall it may be very difficult to detect. In this area, the sensitivity changes are of ex-

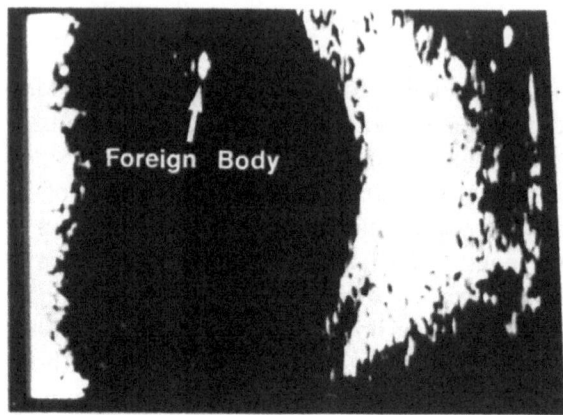

FIGURE 6.16
Foreign body. Scan at 80 dB. Metallic mid-vitreous foreign body casts a focal sonic shadow at 70 dB. At 80 dB there is no shadowing noted. The amount of shadowing depends upon the nature of the foreign body at its angulation with respect to the interrogating beam. At 60 dB a strong shadow was noted. It is imperative to vary the sensitivity settings while scanning for foreign bodies.

treme help. As the sensitivity setting is changed from 80dB to 50 dB, the stronger sonic reflection from the foreign body can be seen in contrast to the weaker echo pattern of the posterior wall. Metallic mid-vitreous foreign bodies cast a focal sonic shadow at 70 dB, although at 80 dB no shadowing may be noted (Figure 6.16). The amount of shadowing depends upon the nature of the foreign body and its angulation with respect to the interrogating beam. At 60 dB a strong shadow is expected. It is imperative to vary the sensitivity setting while scanning for foreign bodies. It is very difficult to locate a small foreign body in the retina. If a foreign body is not perpendicular to the beam axis or a few reflected echoes are detected due to its angulation, the eye should be examined from several different directions. A foreign body having weak reflections at 6 o'clock may have strong reflections at 12 o'clock.

A water bath is needed for localization of a foreign body in the anterior chamber. Even with generous usage of methylcellulose, the proper examination by real-time scanning may fail to localize a foreign body. There are a number of pathological conditions such as drusen of the optic nerve head which may simulate a foreign body. In essence, the presence or absence of a foreign body in all cases can not be unequivocably decided by sonography. In metallic foreign bodies, we use the sonic shadow sign as an extremely helpful guide along with changing the sensitivity setting to make foreign bodies more easily detectable. An irregular echogenic projection may be noted on the screen at 80 dB (Figure 6.17a), and at 70dB a hollowing or echo-poor area occurs about the metallic foreign body which represents the local tissue edema (Figure 6.17b). At 60 dB a small zone of sonic shadowing appears distal to the foreign body (Figure 6.17c). Radiographic localization may not be certain if a foreign body is in or out of the globe.

The localization of a large foreign body is simple, but special care should be taken when it is located in the posterior region. Sonic shadow may obscure part of the retina and the reflected echoes of a foreign body. For example, if a foreign body has also dislocated the lens, which

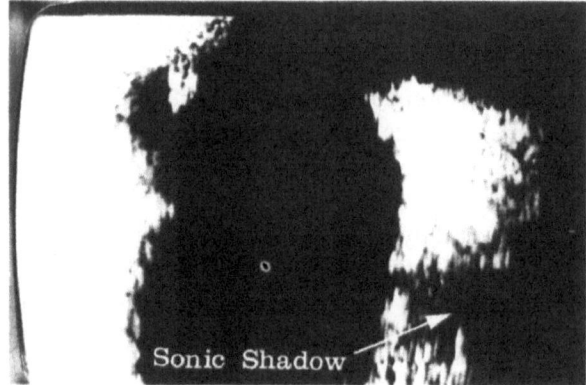

FIGURE 6.17a
Foreign body. Optic nerve head is at lower area of screen. An irregular echogenic projection is noted at top portion of screen at 80 dB.

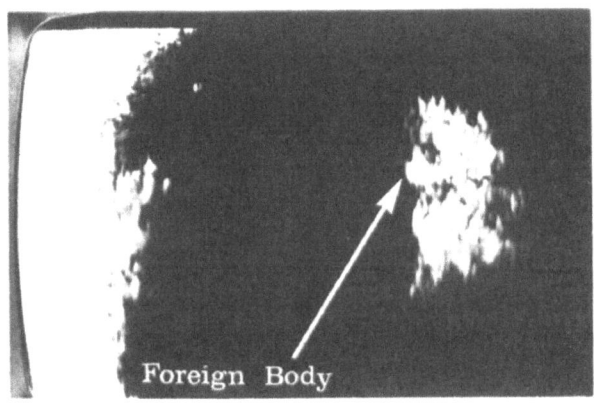

FIGURE 6.17b
At 70 dB a hollowing or echo-poor area is noted about the metallic foreign body which represents local edema.

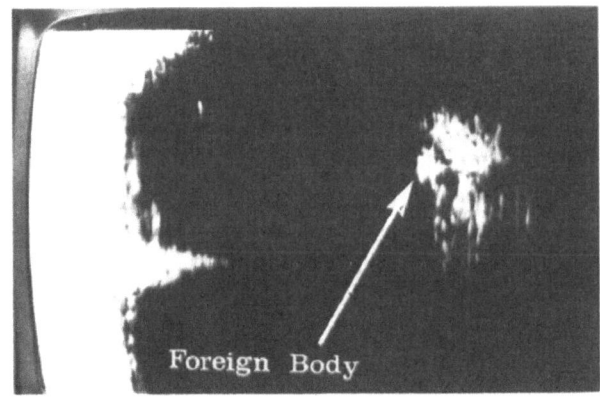

FIGURE 6.17c
At 60 dB sonic shadowing is noted distal to the foreign body. Radiographic localization was not sure if this was in or out of the globe.

has become cataractous, the sonic shadow produced may hide the foreign body if it lies directly in the path of the sonic shadow. Multiple scan planes must then be used.

The evaluation of foreign bodies in the orbital region is very difficult, and in many cases it is impossible. The anterior foreign body in the orbit may be lost in the fatty tissue and those which are located in the apex cannot be seen often.

All maneuvers, especially sensitivity setting adjustment, are important to detect, localize, and evaluate a foreign body.

ASSOCIATED DAMAGE FROM FOREIGN BODY

Hemorrhage and cataract formation may result from a foreign body in the eye. By ultrasound, the extent of the damage and location of the foreign body can be detected in order to extract the foreign body from the lacerated region or to decide that extra action is practically impossible. Again sensitivity setting changing from 80 dB to 50 dB is of extreme importance. A foreign body which may not be detectable at 80 dB (Figure 6.18a) will stand out at 70 dB (Figure 6.18b) and be optimally imaged at 60 dB (Figure 6.18c). The foreign body track also can be visualized through ultrasonography. A track of low amplitude echoes through the vitreous usually points to the location of the foreign body.

By the magnet test, the nature of the foreign body, and whether it is free or movable, can be determined.

Localization of a foreign body by sonography and x-ray study should be combined and other necessary examinations should be performed for optimal results.

PRE-PHTHISIS BULBI

The pre-phthisical eye can be serially followed with ultrasonic examinations and its previously inexorable course to a useless and sightless appendage may now be reversed with certain mod-

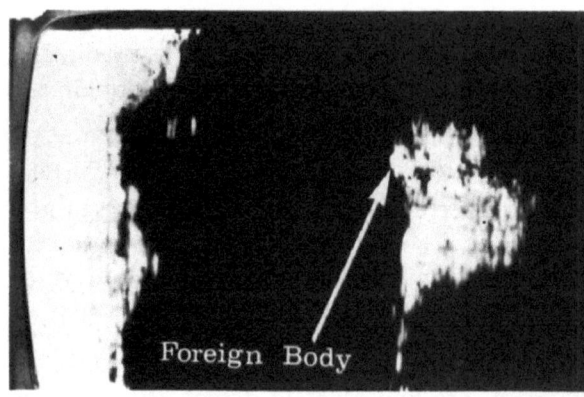

FIGURE 6.18a

FIGURE 6.18a
Foreign body. Roughening of the ocular wall noted at 80 dB.

FIGURE 6.18b
Separate high amplitude echoes appear at 70 dB.

FIGURE 6.18c
At 60 dB, scan shows well defined echo complex of foreign body.

FIGURE 6.19a
Axial length shortening. The most common finding is decrease in the antero-posterior diameter of the eye which is usually accompanied by a variety of other signs. Incidentally noted is an area of vitreous hemorrhage.

FIGURE 6.19b
Prephthisical eye. Axial length shortening is noted along with linear but irregular and thick membranes of vitreous hemorrhage.

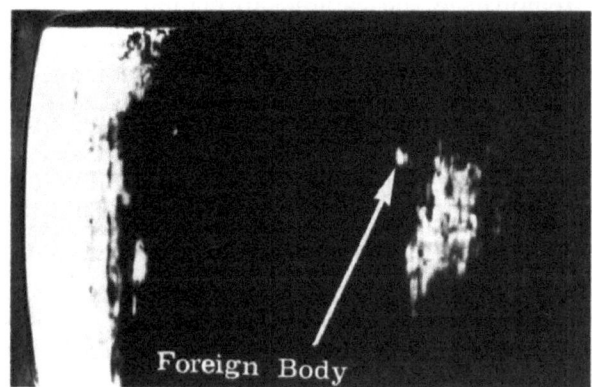

FIGURE 6.18b

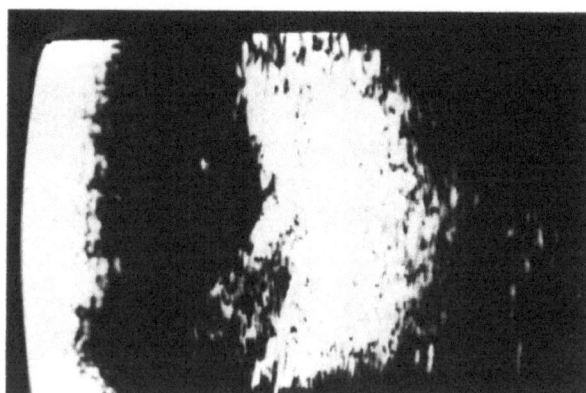

FIGURE 6.19a

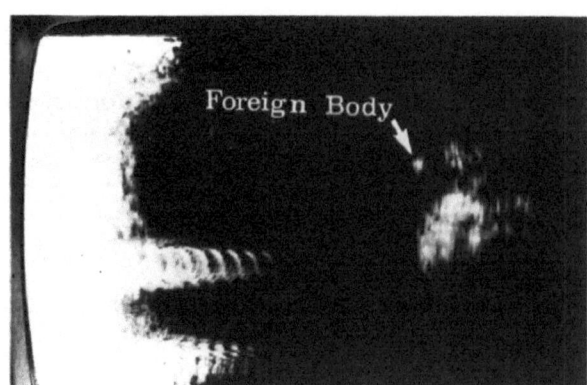

FIGURE 6.18c

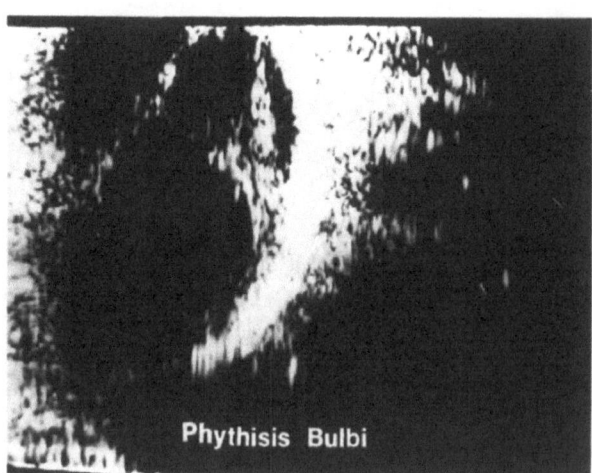

FIGURE 6.19b

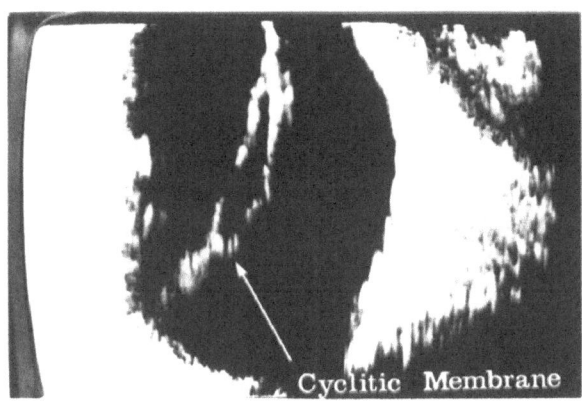

FIGURE 6.20

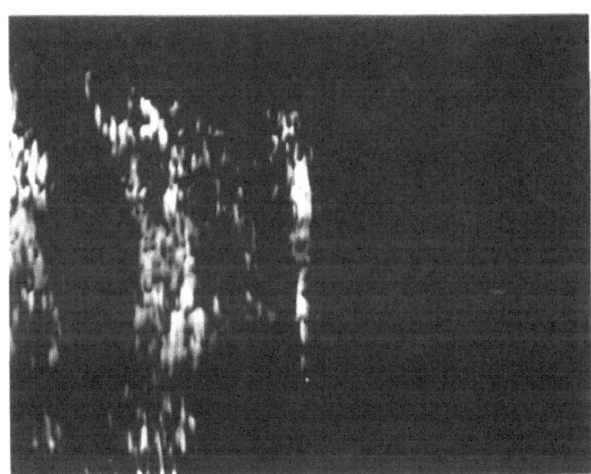

FIGURE 6.21

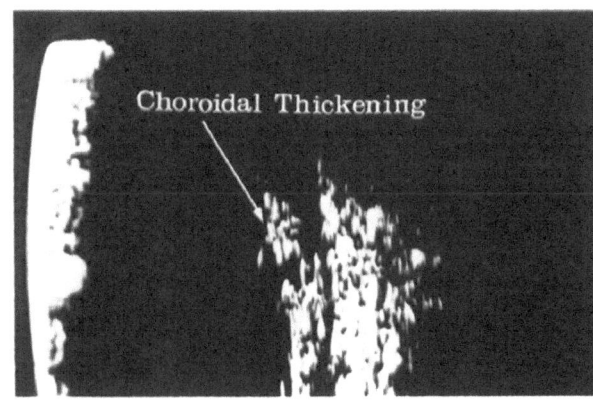

FIGURE 6.22

FIGURE 6.20
Cyclitic membrane. This linear band between the ciliary bodies may be irregularly thickened and folded in the pre-phthisical eye.

FIGURE 6.21
A thickened sclera is demonstrated by an irregularly enlarged scleral outline with decreased through transmission.

FIGURE 6.22
Choroidal thickening. Elevation of the choroid layer is associated with decreased intraocular pressure and may produce elevation of the ciliary body.

ern surgical techniques. There are a number of objective sonographic findings which allow the surgeon to determine which early phthisical eyes are potentially salvageable. These sonographic signs depend upon the severity of the degenerative changes.

The four most common ultrasonic findings are axial length shortening (Figure 6.19a and b), cyclitic membrane (Figure 6.20), thickening of the scleral layer (Figure 6.21), and thickening of the choroid with accompanying elevation of the ciliary body due to hypotony of the globe (Figure 6.22). If the above signs are present, the degen-

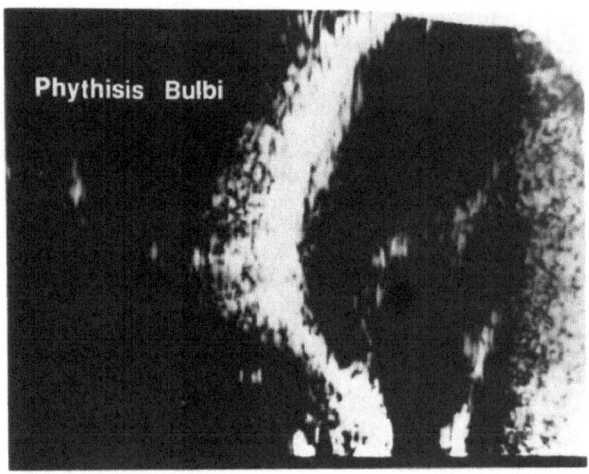

FIGURE 6.23

FIGURE 6.23
Phthisis bulbi. Marked shortening of the axial length with the presence of thick moderately echogenic membrane in the midvitreous with good mobility which disappear at 60 dB. A retinal detachment is not present. Phthisis bulbi with vitreous hemorrhage.

FIGURE 6.24a
Retinal detachment. Retinal detachment shows the diverging sheet-like echoes associated with significant decreased axial length in this phthisical globe.

FIGURE 6.24b
Oblique scan shows sheet-like linear membrane.

FIGURE 6.25
Choroidal detachment. Choroidal effusion is anchored at top by vortex vein.

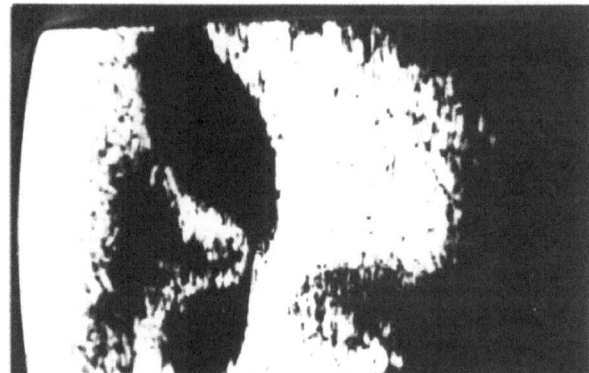

FIGURE 6.24a

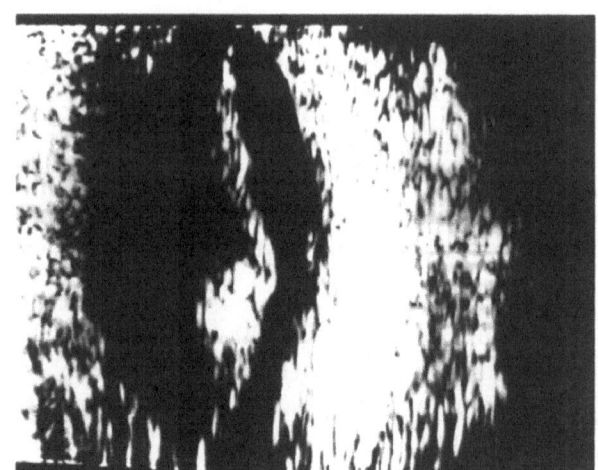

FIGURE 6.24b

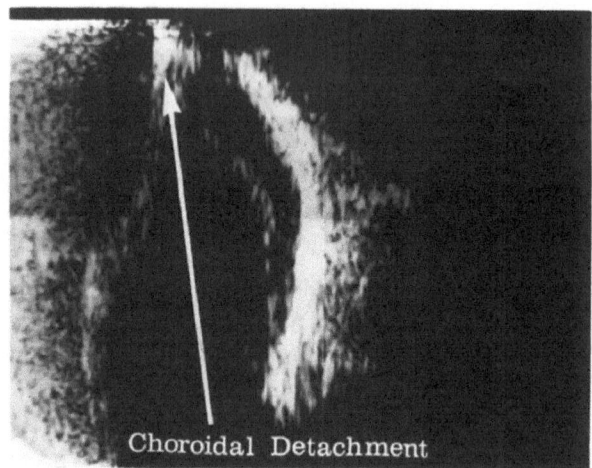

FIGURE 6.25

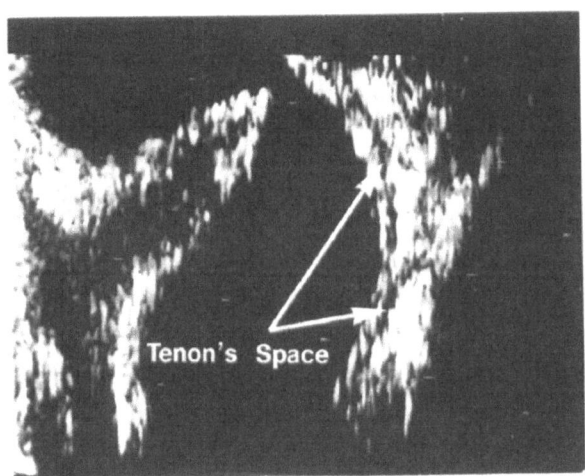

FIGURE 6.26a
Tenon's Space. Edema of tenon space occures in the pre-phthysical eye and appears as an echo-free curvilinear space paralleling the sclera in the immediate episcleral region.

erating globe may exhibit further findings. Other changes that may be present include vitreous hemorrhage (Figure 6.23), retinal detachment (Figure 6.24a and b), choroidal effusion with choroidal detachment (Figure 6.25), and episcleritis with edema of Tenon's capsule (Figure 6.26a).

The signs described above may be present in any combination and without specific pattern. Without proper correction, the early phthisical eye will progress to irreparable phthisis bulbi (Figure 6.26b).

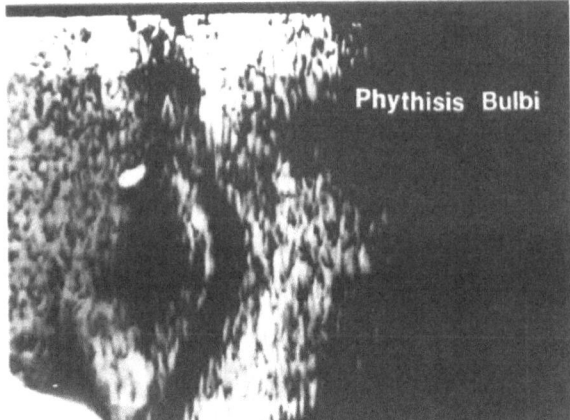

FIGURE 6.26b
Prephthisical eye. Slight axial length shortening is noted along with a total retinal detachment and scattered vitreous hemorrhage. At 80 dB the choroid cannot be well evaluated for thickening.

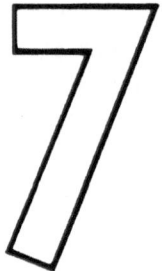

sonography of the lens

GENERAL INTRODUCTION

The lens is the gateway to the sensory retina. As the lens opacifies, the visual impression of the outside world becomes cloudy and eventually the patient becomes visually handicapped. A totally opaque lens locks the hands of the ophthalmologist since he can no longer image the vital structures of the posterior pole. Will a cataract removal restore vision to a patient with severe retinitis proliferans or an old retinal detachment? These questions may be answered after careful ultrasonography of the vitreoretinal structures. Indeed, a dislocated lens may be discovered floating in the vitreous and cataractous changes in the normally situated lens may be studied.

CATARACT

A developmental or degenerative opacity of the lens is called a cataract. Development may occur during early life as

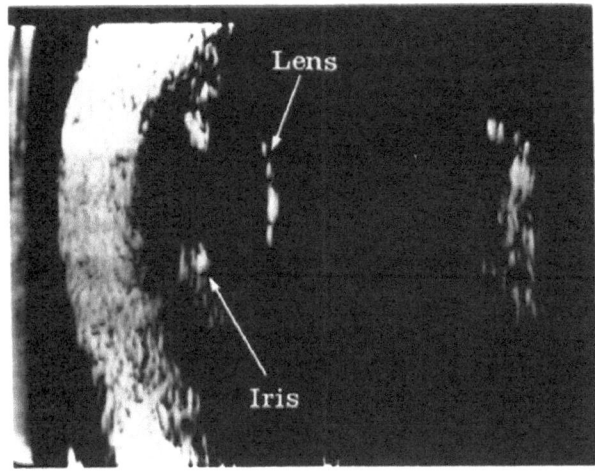

FIGURE 7.1
Normal lens. The echo-free lens is noted between the echogenic iris diaphragm with a sharply outlined anteriorly concave strongly reflecting posterior interface.

a result of heredity, or nutritional or inflammatory disturbances. Degenerative cataracts are characterized by a gradual loss of transparency in the normally developed lens.

CAUSES OF CATARACTS

There are many causes of cataractous lenses, although the most common is the so called senile cataract. Cataracts are stated to be a common cause of blindness; however, this type of visual impairment is surgically correctable. Senile cataracts are genetically determined opacities of the normally transparent crystalline lens occurring commonly at all ages past 40 years. Visual loss is gradual and progressive and is frequently bilateral. The cataract may be examined either by an ophthalmoscope or the slit lamp, to observe the common nuclear, cortical, and subcapsular cataracts. Nuclear cataracts are centrally located within the lens producing a central dense opacity. Cortical or soft cataracts are more peripheral and give rise to spoke-like clefts. Progression of these wedge shaped opacities gradually involves the central area. Subcapsular cataracts are posteriorly located and produce early visual loss. Surgical removal of the cataract is optimal when the visual acuity of the patient no longer permits the usual functioning. Congenital cataracts are hereditary and bilateral. Anomalous biologic condition will produce opaque fibers in the developing lens. Other congenital anomalies may coexist with the congenital cataract. Developmental cataracts occur when the rings of growing lens fibers do not remain clear. Minor developmental opacities are present in most lenses and many do not produce visual loss. Penetrating injury or blunt trauma causes the traumatic cataract. This may occur within days or gradually progress over a period of years. The lens is very sensitive to radiation exposure which results in a cataractous lens if a large dose is absorbed by the organ. Cataractous changes that accompany diabetes mellitus and hypoparathyroidism are called endocrine cataracts.

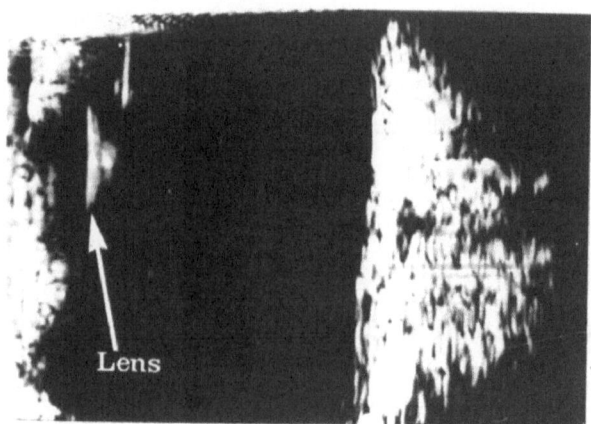

FIGURE 7.2

SONOPATHOLOGY OF CATARACT

When the process is clinically obvious, there is no need for sonography. In earlier cataracts, the lens is more echogenic than normal. However, the examiner should be familiar with ultrasonic appearance of the normal lens (Figure 7.1). When the cataract develops the degree of echogenicity of the lens increases. The cataractous lens may have many ultrasonic appearances:

A. Normal lens showing anechoic substance with strongly echogenic posterior capsule with one thick reverberation echo (Figure 7.2).

B. Normal lens with two thin reverberation echoes (Figure 7.3).

C. Early cataract with thickening of posterior lens capsule (Figure 7.4).

FIGURE 7.2
Normal lens showing anechoic substance with strongly echogenic posterior capsule with one thick reverberation echo.

FIGURE 7.3
Normal lens with two thin reverberation echoes noted distal to the posterior lens capsule.

FIGURE 7.4
Early cataract with thickening of posterior lens capsule.

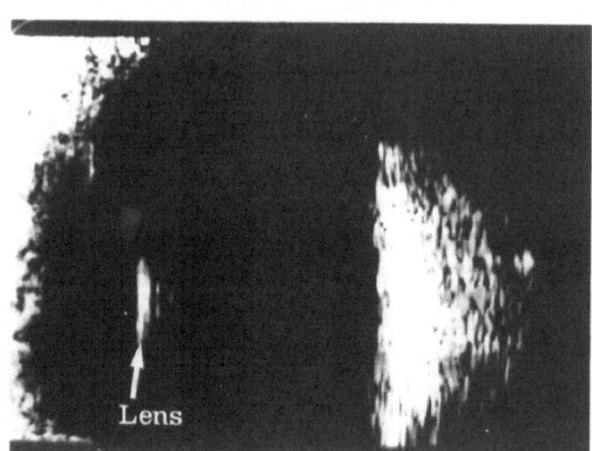

FIGURE 7.3

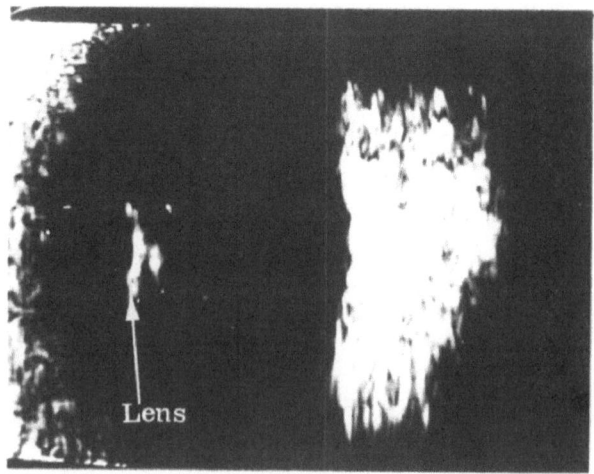

FIGURE 7.4

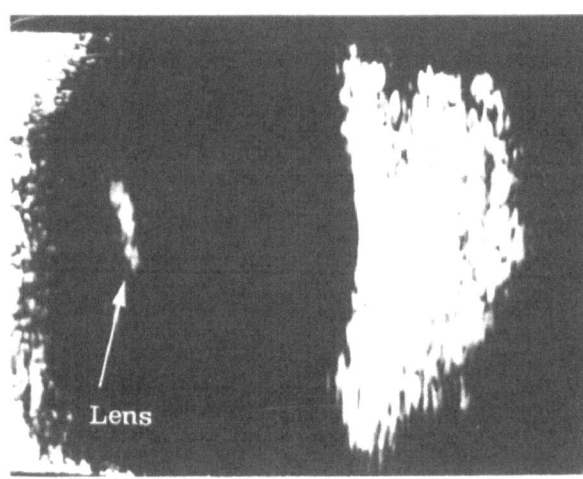

FIGURE 7.5

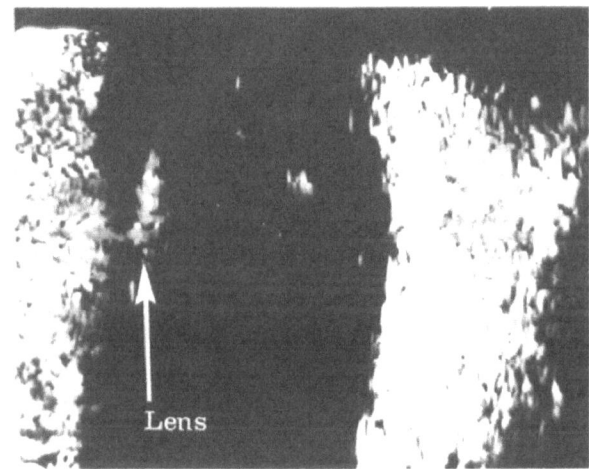

FIGURE 7.6

D. More severe cataract with roughening of the posterior lens capsule and low amplitude posterior lens echoes (Figure 7.5).

E. Moderate thickening of the posterior lens capsule (Figure 7.6).

F. Roughening of the posterior capsule with low amplitude echoes along anterior edges of the lens (Figure 7.7).

G. At 70 dB parts of the irregular posterior capsule no longer generate echoes. (Figure 7.8).

H. Markedly distorted lens with low amplitude internal echoes and retinal detachment (Figure 7.9).

I. Anterior and posterior lens capsule imaged due to traumatic edema of the

FIGURE 7.5
More severe cataract with roughening of the posterior lens capsule and low amplitude posterior lens echoes.

FIGURE 7.6
Moderate thickening of posterior lens capsule.

FIGURE 7.7
Roughening of posterior capsule with low amplitude echoes along the anterior edge of the lens.

FIGURE 7.8
At 70 dB parts of the irregular posterior capsule no longer generate echoes.

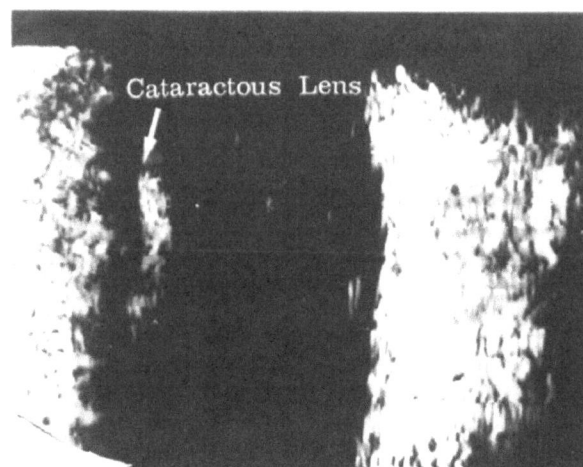

FIGURE 7.7

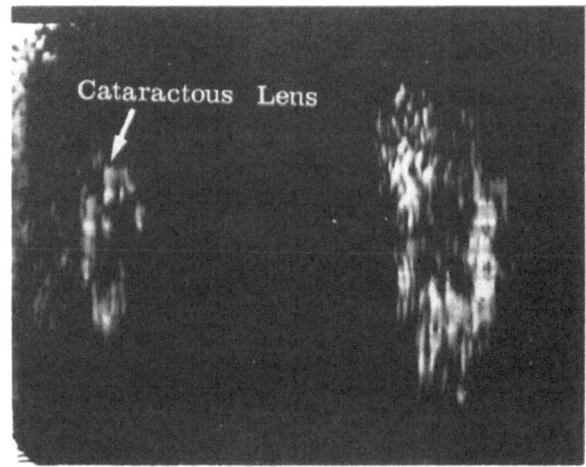

FIGURE 7.8

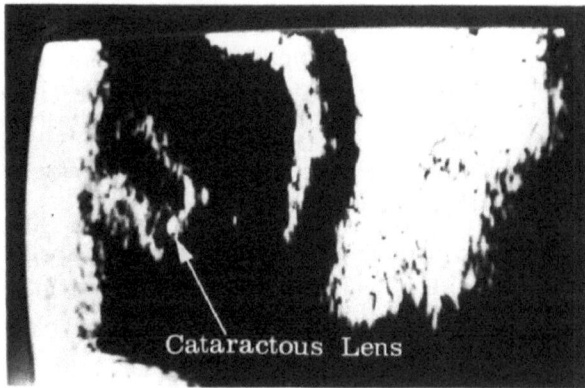

FIGURE 7.9

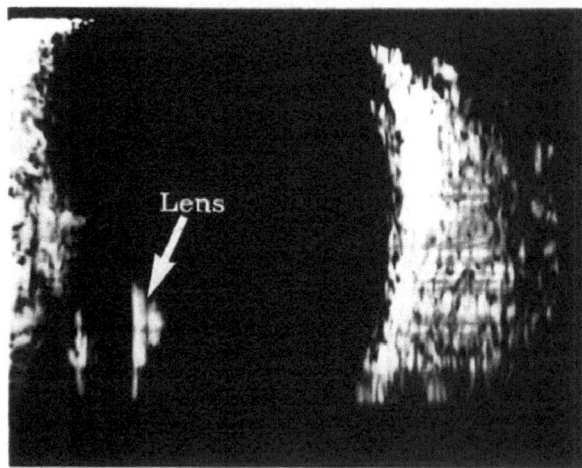

FIGURE 7.10

eyelids. Incidentally noted is an echogenic area of hyphema anteriorly (Figure 7.10).

J. Minimal dislocation of cataractous lens with a sonic shadowing (Figure 7.11).

K. Minimal dislocation with strongly reflecting anterior lens echoes producing echo-poor distal lens image (Figure 7.12).

L. Small dislocation with strongly diffracting lens presenting as echo-poor anterior lens tissue (Figure 7.13).

M. Mid-vitreous dislocation with lens artifact and minimal shadowing (Figure 7.14).

FIGURE 7.9
Markedly distorted lens with low amplitude internal echoes and retinal detachment.

FIGURE 7.10
Anterior and posterior lens capsule imaged due to traumatic edema of eyelids. Incidentally noted is echogenic area of hyphema anteriorly.

FIGURE 7.11
Slight dislocation of cataractous lens with sonic shadow.

FIGURE 7.12
Minimal posterior dislocation with strongly reflecting anterior lens echoes producing echo-poor distal lens image.

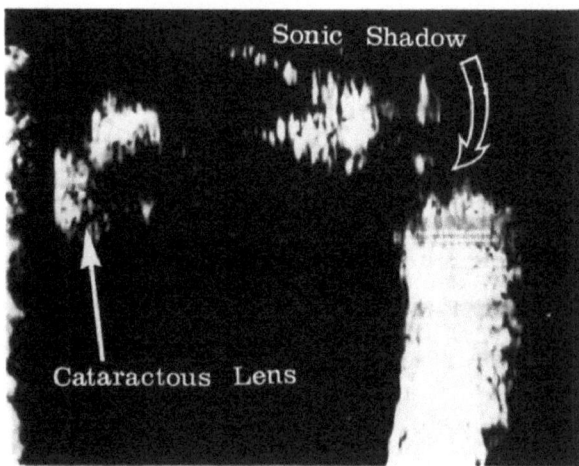

FIGURE 7.11

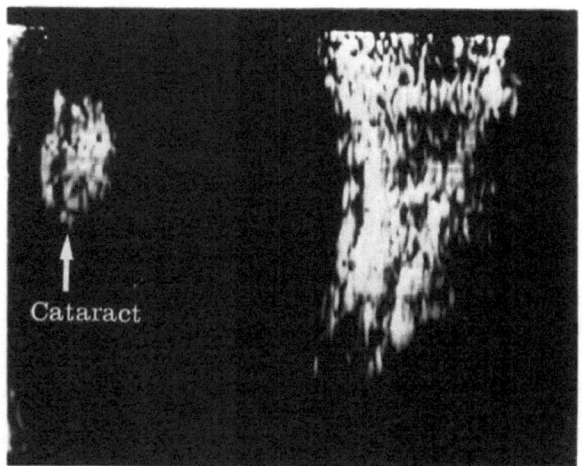

FIGURE 7.12

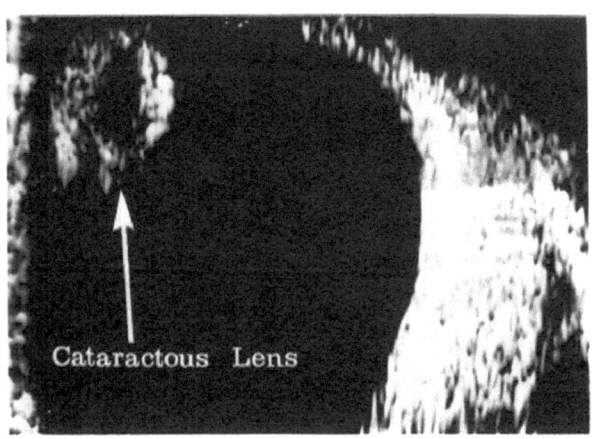

FIGURE 7.13

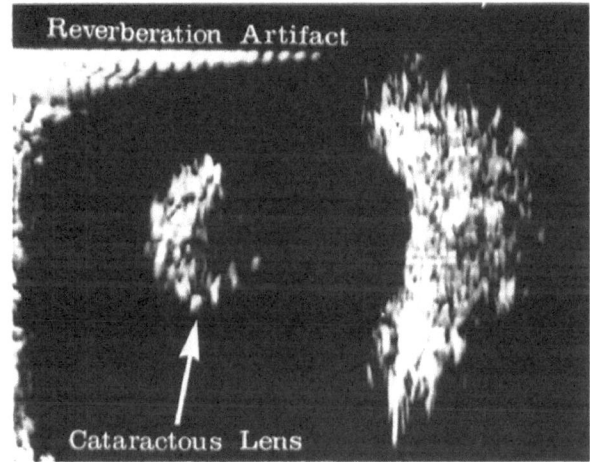

FIGURE 7.14

N. Circular echoes of cataract simulating retinal detachment (Figure 7.15).

O. Amorphous echoes of cataract simulating vitreous hemorrhage (Figure 7.16).

P. Posterior dislocation of normal lens with no shadowing (Figure 7.17).

Q. Posterior dislocation of cataractous lens with no shadowing (Figure 7.18).

R. Anterior border of dislocated lens simulating sheet-like band (Figure 7.19).

S. Posterior lens simulating collar-button type of malignant melanoma (Figure 7.20).

The cataractous lens should be differentiated from a calcified hematoma or malignant melanoma. Both conditions appear within the posterior vitreous as an ovoid shaped echogenic struc-

FIGURE 7.13
Slight posterior dislocation with strongly diffracting lens presenting as echo-poor anterior lens tissue.

FIGURE 7.14
Mid-vitreous dislocation with lens artifact and minimal shadowing.

FIGURE 7.15
Circular echoes of cataract simulating retinal detachment.

FIGURE 7.16
Amorphous echoes of cataract simulating vitreous hemorrhage.

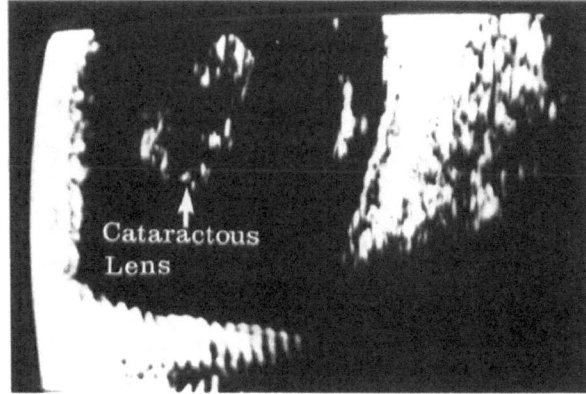

FIGURE 7.15

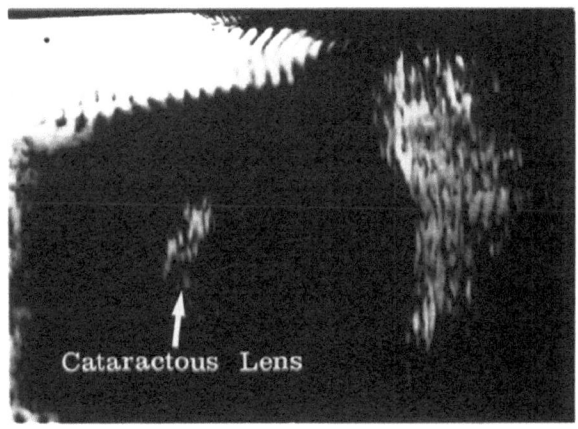

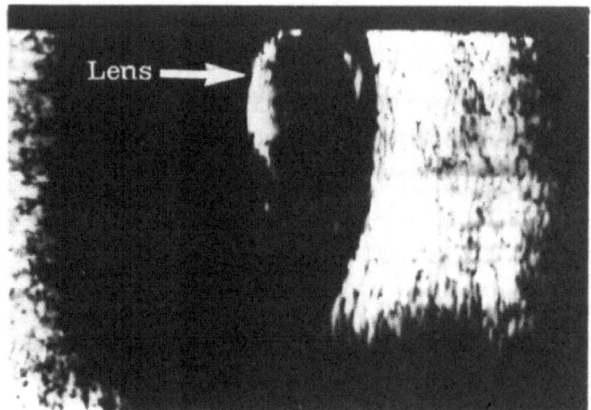

FIGURE 7.17

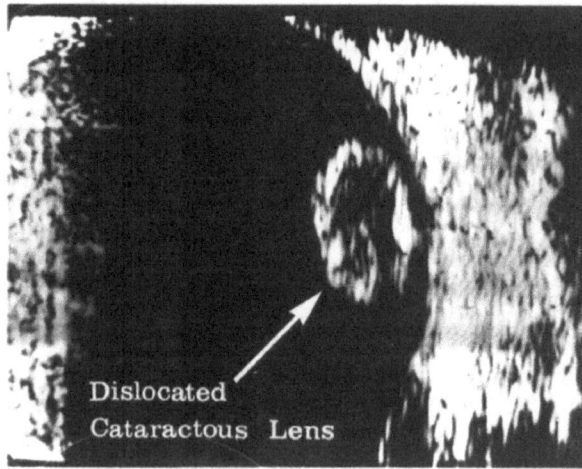

FIGURE 7.18

ture against the retinal boundary. Usually a sonic shadow is produced in the orbital fat due to a dislocated cataractous lens, which may simulate the pattern of the optic nerve (Figure 7.21).

DISLOCATED CATARACTOUS LENS

The lens may dislocate anteriorly or posteriorly. The posterior dislocation often gives a strongly echogenic and irregular echo pattern in the vitreous with a distal lens border that may be both scalloped and of variable echogenicity. Portions of the lens that are perpendicular to the sound beam are strongly echogenic, while areas that are tangential have weak echoes or none at all (Figure 7.22). The sensitivity study of the cata-

FIGURE 7.17
Posterior dislocation of normal lens with no shadowing.

FIGURE 7.18
Posterior cataractous lens dislocation with no sonic shadow sign.

FIGURE 7.19
Anterior border of dislocation lens simulating sheet-like band.

FIGURE 7.20
Posterior lens simulating collar-button type of malignant melanoma.

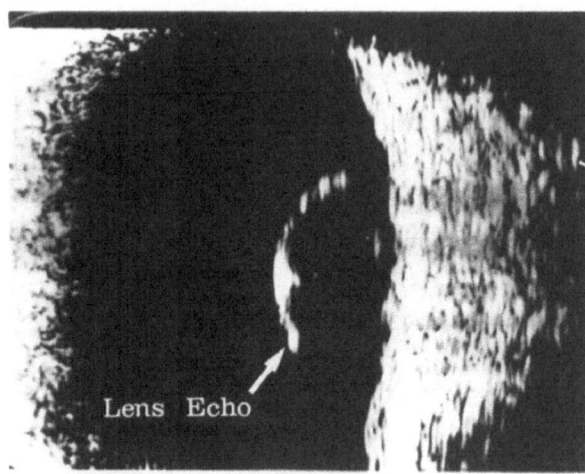

FIGURE 7.19

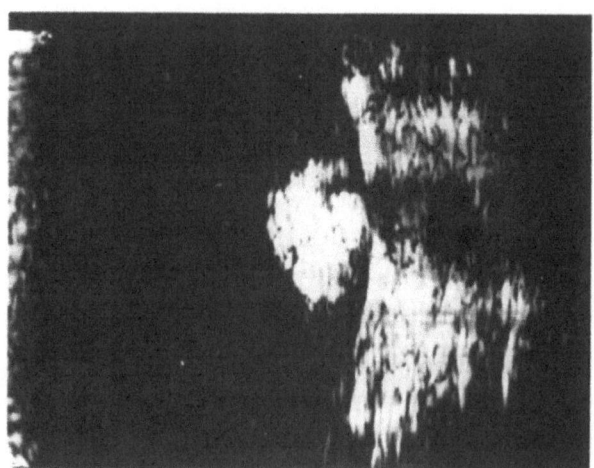

FIGURE 7.20

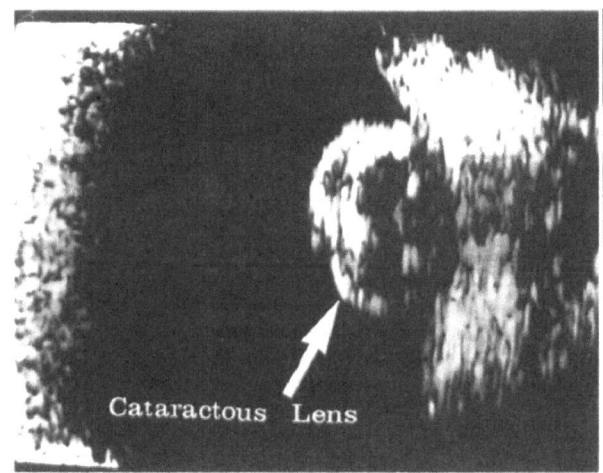

FIGURE 7.21

ractous lens is extremely important to differentiate this condition from other pathological entities such as tumors and focal hemorrhage.

At 80 dB the entire dislocated lens with a cortical cataract is filled with echoes and has a strong sonic shadow (Figure 7.23a). When the gain is decreased to 70 dB the nuclear portion of the lens is echo free (Figure 7.23b), since it is less affected by the peripheral cataractous changes.

FIGURE 7.21
Dislocated cataractous lens. Within the posterior vitreous there is an ovoid shaped echogenic structure against the retinal boundary. A sonic shadow is produced in the orbital fat.

FIGURE 7.22
Cataractous lens. Strongly echogenic and irregular echo pattern is noted in the anterior vitreous. Note that the distal border is both scalloped and has variable echogenicity. Portions of the lens that are perpendicular to the sound beam are strongly echogenic while areas that are tangential have weak echoes or none at all.

FIGURE 7.23a
At 80 dB the entire lens is filled with echoes and has a strong sonic shadow.

FIGURE 7.23b
At 70 dB the nuclear portion of the lens is echo-free since it is unaffected by peripheral cataractous changes. The ovoid partly echogenic has been separated from the posterior ocular wall to differentiate from a malignant melanoma by sitting the patient erect.

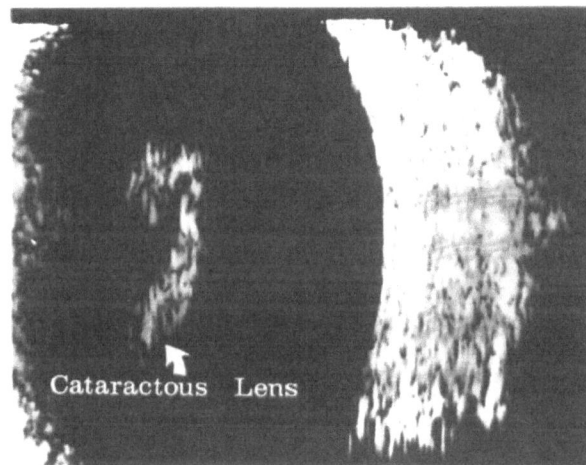

FIGURE 7.22

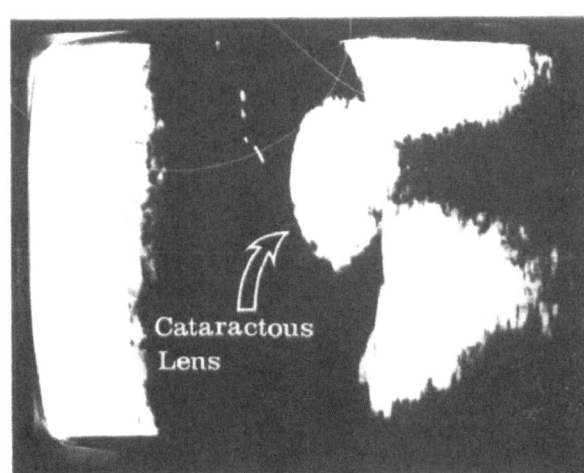

FIGURE 7.23a

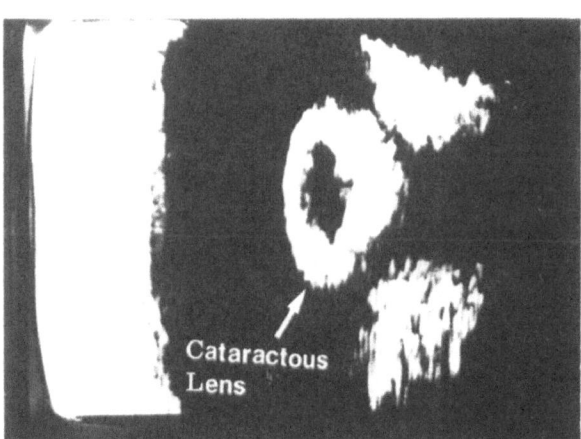

FIGURE 7.23b

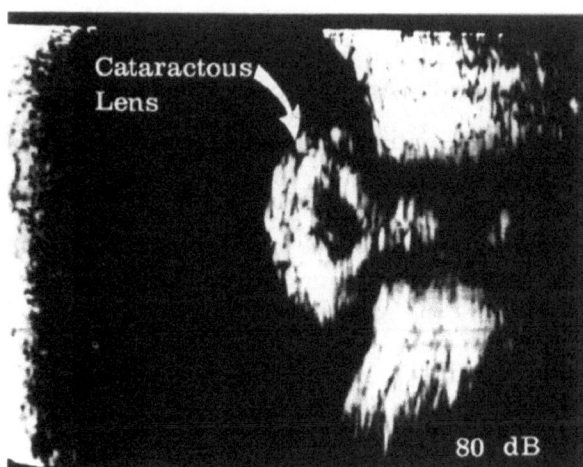

FIGURE 7.24a

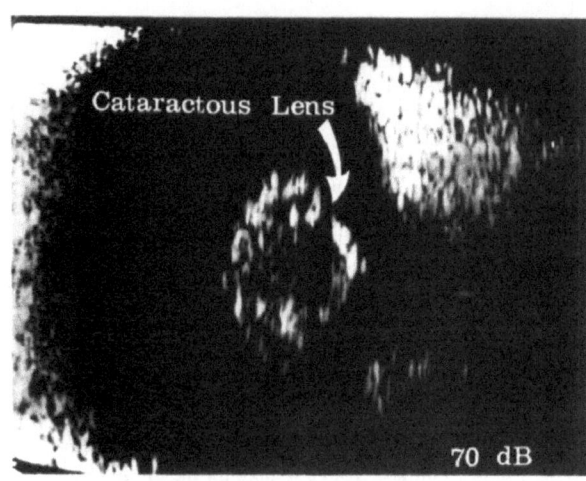

FIGURE 7.24b

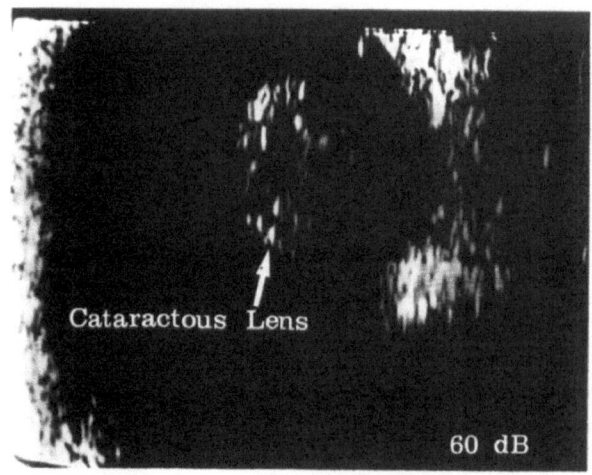

FIGURE 7.24c

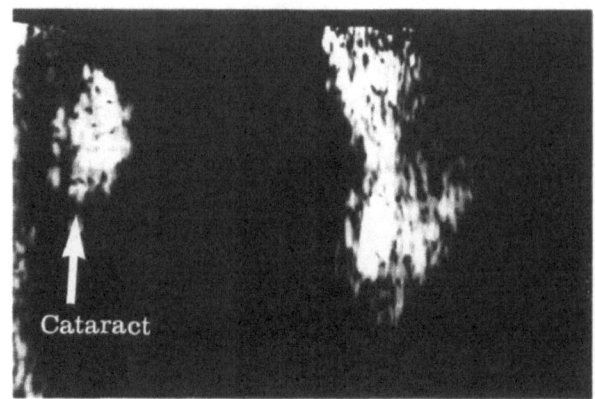

FIGURE 7.25

FIGURE 7.24a
Posterior dislocated cataractous lens at 80 dB.

FIGURE 7.24b
Posterior dislocated cataractous lens at 70 dB.

FIGURE 7.24c
Posterior dislocated cataractous lens at 60 dB.

FIGURE 7.25
There is a posterior depression of the posterior ocular wall which is due to the cataractous lens artifact. Anteriorly is noted a portion of the lens echo. The distal orbital fat echoes are partly visible due to the plane of the scan beam.

As stated previously the dislocated lens should not be confused with malignant melanoma. The lens must be separated by gravitational maneuvers from the posterior ocular wall to differentiate it from a malignant melanoma. Sensitivity study is of great help (Figure 7.24a,b, and c). Sometimes the lens artifact simulates a staphyloma and produces a posterior depression of the posterior ocular wall (Figure 7.25). A portion of the lens echo is often noted in the anterior part of the T.V. monitor. Rescanning with the lens away from the sonic beam removes the defect in the posterior ocular wall.

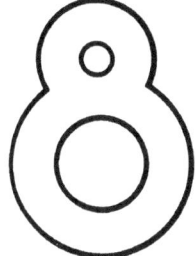

sonography of the vitreous

INTRODUCTION

The vitreous is the road to the retina and the visual pathways. Newer improvements in vitreoretinal surgery now permit vision to be restored in many ocular disorders.

In acute trauma cases, the position of the lens and retina can be easily evaluated, and vitreous hemorrhage or debris may be identified. If there is massive and irreversible disruption of the globe, ultrasound can safely confirm its extent and geographical location. After collecting all the information, the surgeon can undertake the appropriate surgery for immediate enucleation to prevent the risk of sympathetic ophthalmia, or other necessary interventional procedures.

Not only are the changes in the vitreous due to trauma studied, but foreign bodies may be three-dimensionally localized. Additionally, vitreous detachments, opacities, retinal detachments, vitreal membranes and pseudomembranes, traction bands, and fresh and old vitreous hemorrhage may be evaluated.

The location of retinitis proliferans of the diabetic may be noted as well as the presence of a detached retina. The decision to perform a therapeutic vitrectomy may be made with a comprehensive picture of the pathological alterations of the vitreous.

VITREOUS ALTERATIONS WITH AGING

The primary vitreous is associated with a linear funnel shaped canal (Cloquet's canal) which regresses rapidly as the child grows. The secondary vitreous, or definitive adult vitreous body, enlarges in volume as the globe increases in size. With age, the vitreous gel appears rarefied and there is prominence of the fibers in the posterior vitreous.

Liquefaction of the vitreous gel produces cavities called lacunae. These cavities appear dark during ophthalmoscopy due to absence of the Tyndall effect. Senile eyes usually show localized liquefaction involving the posterior vitreous body.

Syneresis, or contraction of particles dispersed within a gel, produces shrinkage of the gel-like vitreous and is part of the aging process. Separation of the liquid from the solid components of the vitreous occurs with this contraction process. Advanced syneresis increases the density of the vitreous gel and decreases its volume resulting in a posterior vitreous detachment from the adjacent retina. The formed vitreous tends to locate anteriorly with the liquid vitreous posteriorly.

VITREOUS DETACHMENT

Separation of the vitreous cortex which is adherent to the wall of the vitreous cavity is called vitreous detachment. The most common form of vitreous detachment occurs in the posterior vitreous and is considered to be part of the aging process, but may occur in patients of any age with prior eye disease or be a manifestation of a generalized disorder in the eye. Floaters and light flashes are common symptoms. Ophthalmologically, one finds vitreous opacities, vitreous hemorrhage, and retinal changes of various types. The location of the vitreous opacities on the surface of the detached cortex helps identify the area of detachment. The degree of collapse of the vitreous body following detachment is variable. Sonographically, the posterior vitreous face presents as a thin, sheet-like echo which is mobile and disappears at 70 dB. Opacities adherent to the vitreous face may persist to 60 dB. When vitreous detachment results from diabetic retinopathy, vitreous hemorrhage and traction retinal detachment are often noted. The mobility of the vitreous face is greatest when liquified gel underlies it and vitreo-retinal adhesions are absent. Mobility is limited in funnel shaped posterior vitreous detachment.

Opacities in the vitreous cavity may be intra-vitreous or retro-vitreous. Vitreous opacities may be due to developmental defects, degenerative disorders (asteroid hyalosis, amyloid, senility, high myopia, and vitreo-retinal degeneration), inflammatory processes of the posterior uveal tract or retina, bleeding from normal or abnormal vessels, and neoplasia involving the vitreous body. Retro-vitreous opacities are in the pre-retinal space, or on the vitreous face or the retinal surface. These are often due to degenerative, hemorrhagic or inflammatory conditions. Exudative vitreous opacities due to inflammation gradually disappear as the process subsides. This clears first from the retro-vitreous space and then from the vitreous gel. Pathologic membranes may occur in any portion of the vitreous or vitreo-retinal junction. These bands result from intraocular disorders associated with inflammation, hemorrhage, degeneration, or trauma. They are generally formed of a hyaline acellular layer coated with cells. They vary in thickness, extent, and location. Intra-vitreal bands are generally innocuous. A membrane becomes a serious finding when it is adherent to the retina and may produce retinal edema, tear, or hemorrhage. Bands in the vitreous gel are associated with severe vitreous inflammation, longstanding vitreous hemorrhage, and retained foreign body. They are often thick and accompany vitreous contraction. Bands in the liquified vitreous are seen with advanced degeneration, chronic inflammation, and high myopia. They may float free or attach to the retina. A membrane is commonly encountered separating the vitreous gel from the liquified vitreous and is often no more than a condensation layer. Pre-retinal membranes line the inner surface of the retina. There is often liquification of the posterior vitreous. This membrane varies in size, shape, and position.

VITREOUS ADHESIONS

Normal adhesions exist between the posterior vitreous and the retina. However, pathologic adhesions may be acquired or congenital. Acquired bands may be due to retinal neovascularization, chorioretinitis, photocoagulation, or freezing. These adhesions firmly bind the retina to the posterior vitreous. Traction at the site of adhesion may result in vitreous hemorrhage and is caused by shrinkage of the vitreous.

Vitreous traction may either stretch the retina or pull it into the vitreous cavity depending on the vector of the exerted forces. Movement of the eye may convert a loose vitreous band into a taut membrane producing traction on the retina. A retina that is degenerated is thin and tears more easily than a healthy retina.

Breaks in the retina may take the form of a retinal hole or a retinal tear with an operculum (flap). A simple retinal hole may remain stationary and lie adjacent to the choroid. It may not progress to retinal detachment in certain instances. Detachment of the retina tends not to occur when the vitreous near the retinal break remains a gel. As the vitreous liquifies, a retinal detachment begins to form. Retinal tears are associated with vitreous traction and follow a progressive course to a retinal detachment.

VITREOUS HEMORRHAGE

The bleeding into the vitreous is broadly divided into sub-vitreal hemorrhage and intra-vitreal hemorrhage. Sub-vitreal hemorrhage is also called sub-hyaloid hemorrhage when blood is present between the internal limiting membrane and the posterior "face" of the vitreous. Blood in this compartment may take from weeks to months to clear. Intra-vitreal hemorrhage occurs with blood in the vitreous body and may take months to years to clear, depending on the condition of the vitreous and the tendency of the lesion to rebleed. Often, bleeding occurs in both compartments.

The blood may clear spontaneously or various complications may ensue. Organization of the blood may produce fibrous membranes lying on the internal surface of the retina. These preretinal membranes may produce a so-called "cellophane" retina. The debris associated with the hemorrhage may obstruct the outflow of aqueous humor precipitating an acute open angle glaucoma called hemolytic glaucoma. Secondary retinal detachment may result from vitreous retraction. Fibrous and fibro-vascular membranes (retinitis proliferans) will contract and tend to pull the retina centrally.

CAUSES OF VITREOUS HEMORRHAGES

Many conditions produce vitreous hemorrhage, including blunt and penetrating trauma, retinal tears, vitreo-retinal separation, hypertensive retinopathy, sickle cell retinopathy, Eale's disease (primary perivasculitis of the retina), retinal neovascularization of any cause, disciform degeneration of the macula, blood dyscrasias, leukemia, uveitis, malignant melanoma, retinoblastoma, metastatic intraocular tumors, retinal angioma, juvenile retinoschisis, subarachnoid hemorrhage, and choroidal hemorrhage with extension.

PATHOPHYSIOLOGY OF VITREOUS HEMORRHAGE

Vitreous hemorrhage is basically due to rupture of a vessel in or near the vitreous cavity. Trauma may be direct as in a penetrating foreign body or

91

indirect as in ocular contusion. Vitreous traction, especially on the fragile retinal vessels accompanying neovascularity, are a frequent cause of bleeding. Increased intravascular pressure may follow retinal vein occlusion resulting in rupture of vessels. Intraocular tumors may compress retinal or choroidal vessels producing pressure necrosis of the vessel wall. Diabetic neovascularization and fibrous proliferation develop along the course of the major retinal vessels and on the surface of the optic disc. Fibrovascular tissue may proliferate on the surface of the detached vitreous cortex and grow into the gel in front of the optic disc. The resulting traction on the new and delicate vessels gives rise to recurrent vitreous hemorrhage. Extensive and recurrent bleeding in the vitreous gel produces dense hemorrhagic vitreous membranes which tend to be multilayered and often permanent.

The diagnosis of recent vitreous hemorrhage is simple when the media is clear. However, long-standing vitreous hemorrhage becomes transformed into a white opaque mass that may simulate inflammatory exudate of uveitis, parasitic endophthalmitis, intraocular foreign body, or retinoblastoma. Blood accumulating in the retrovitreal space is unclotted and shifts with gravity. Red cells in this sub-hyaloid space usually resolve. The mechanism whereby blood in the vitreous resolves is not year clear, but posterior vitreous hemorrhage resorbs faster than central or anterior vitreous hemorrhage due to the nature of the gel. Unclotted blood resolves faster than clotted blood.

Lacunae within the vitreous body form as part of the aging process of the vitreous and contain liquid vitreous. Hemorrhage within the space of a lacuna is partly clotted and partly free. The clotted portion is globular while the unclotted blood is mobile. Blood inside the gel clots readily and forms fingerlike processes extending from the source of bleeding into the gel as it clots along the planes of the vitreous fibers. This is fixed and shifts with eye movements only when the gel begins to liquify.

SONOGRAPHIC PATTERN OF VITREOUS HEMORRHAGE

As mentioned earlier, the vitreous humerous is clear and appears as a sonolucent area between the anterior segment and the retina. When cellular aggregations of a certain size appear in the vitreous, B-scan sonography detects these interruptions in the sonic beam as multiple reflections displayed in the form of dots and small thick lines of varying size. These reflected echoes have a gray-white color when they are visualized on the T.V. monitor. Using gray-scale technique, the sonodense tissue gives the strongest reflection and appears as sonopaque or white, while the weaker echoes have varying shades of gray depending on the strength of the returning signals (Figure 8.1). Vitreous hemorrhage may have many different echo patterns. The most interesting part is that a fresh vitreous hemorrhage may not be imaged during routine sonography.

In our experience for the past five years we have found that vitreous hemorrhage may mimic many conditions of the vitreous. However, the most common types of hemorrhage produce a sonographically identifiable echo pattern:

A thin linear membrane may be noted (Figure 8.2).

A thick linear band may be imaged (Figure 8.3).

The membrane may be interrupted (Figure 8.4).

The band may be sinuous (Figure 8.5a and b).

The membrane may be concave anteriorly (Figure 8.6).

The membrane may be concave posteriorly (Figure 8.7).

The vitreous hemorrhage may appear circular (Figure 8.8).

A triangular mass may occur (Figure 8.9).

A round mass may be noted (Figure 8.10a, b, and c).

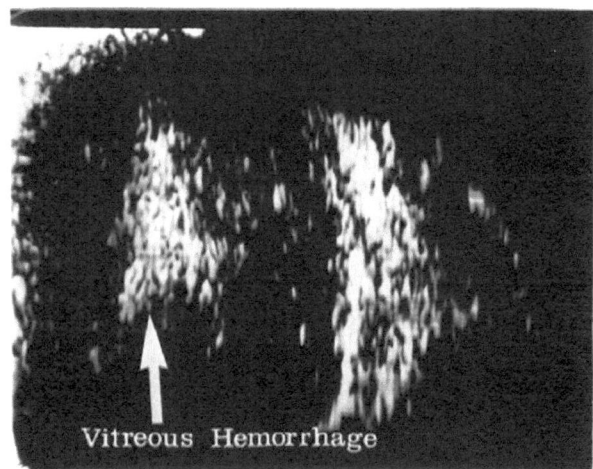

FIGURE 8.1
Vitreous Hemorrhage. The reflectivity of an area of intra-vitreal bleeding depends somewhat upon the angulation of the reflecting surfaces to the interrogating sound beam. Vitreous hemorrhage should be studied in multiple scan planes.

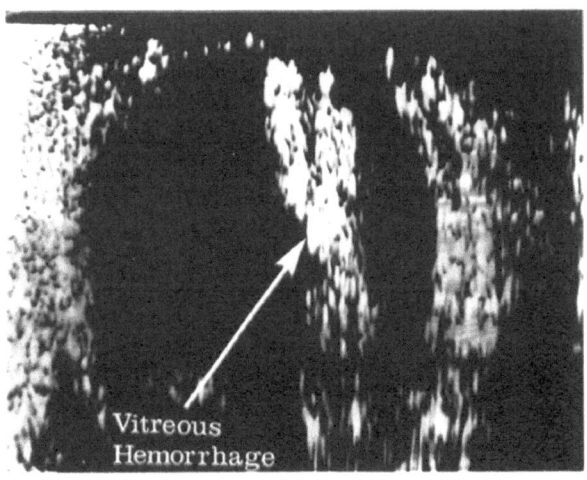

FIGURE 8.3
Vitreous Hemorrhage. A thick linear band may be imaged with varying echo strengths.

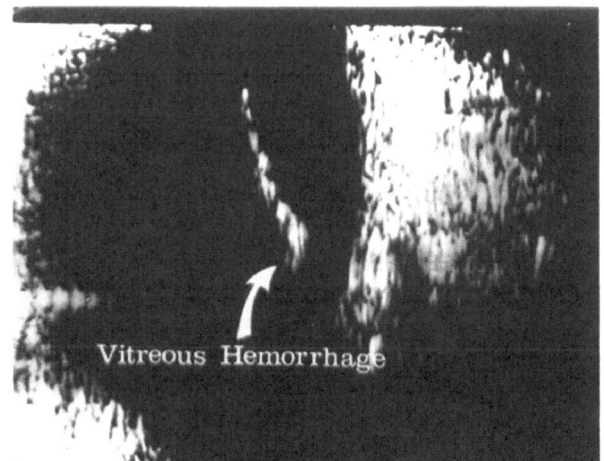

FIGURE 8.2
Vitreous Hemorrhage. The area of bleeding may assume the configuration of thin linear membrane.

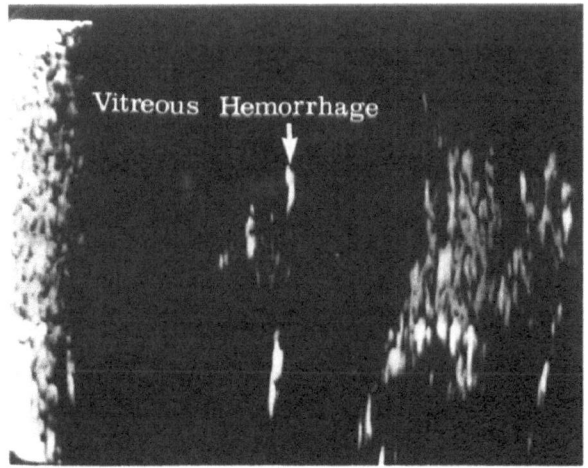

FIGURE 8.4
Vitreous Hemorrhage. The echogenic membrane may appear interrupted at various points and have a varying echo pattern.

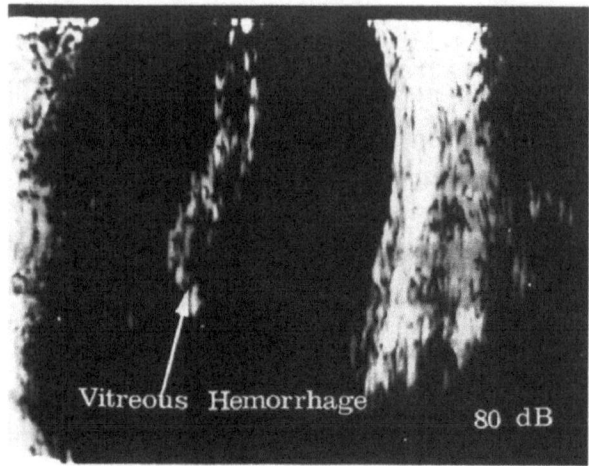

FIGURE 8.5a

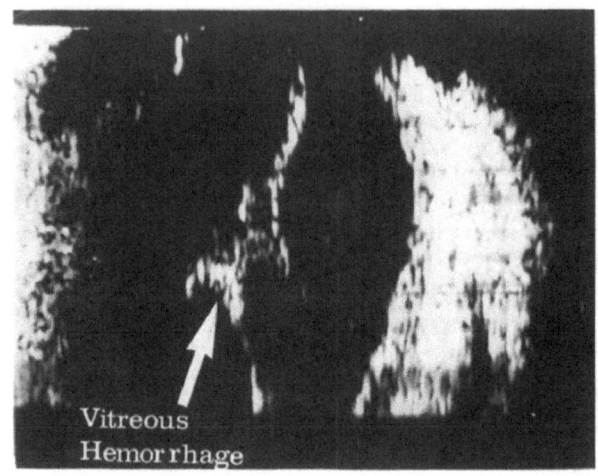

FIGURE 8.7

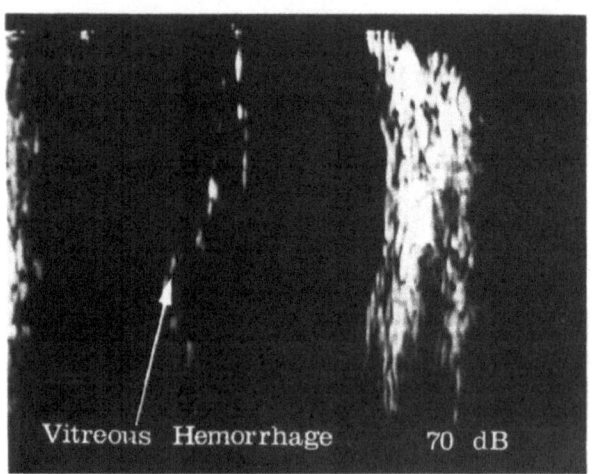

FIGURE 8.5b

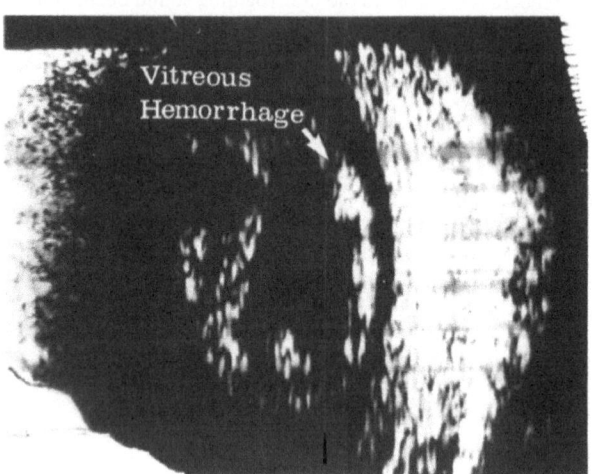

FIGURE 8.8

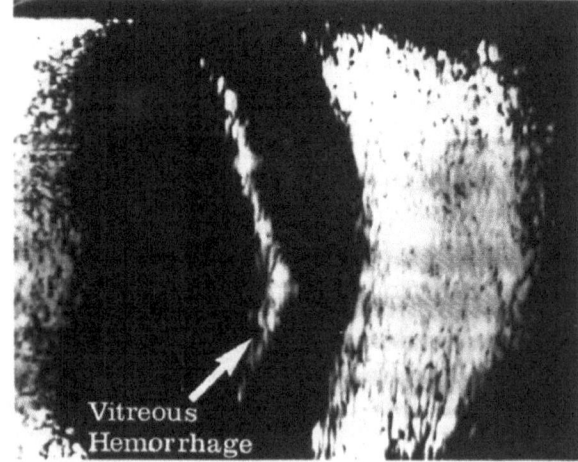

FIGURE 8.6

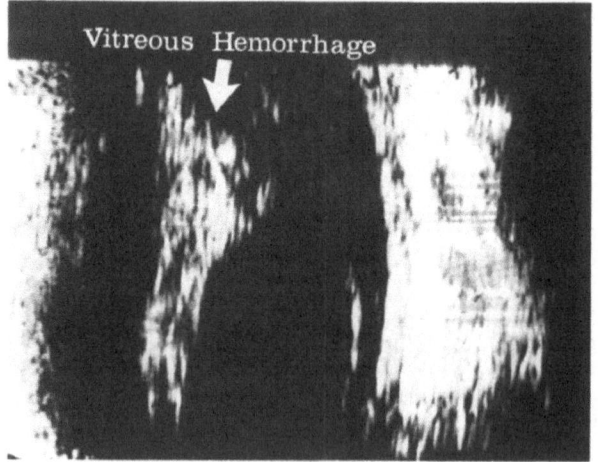

FIGURE 8.9

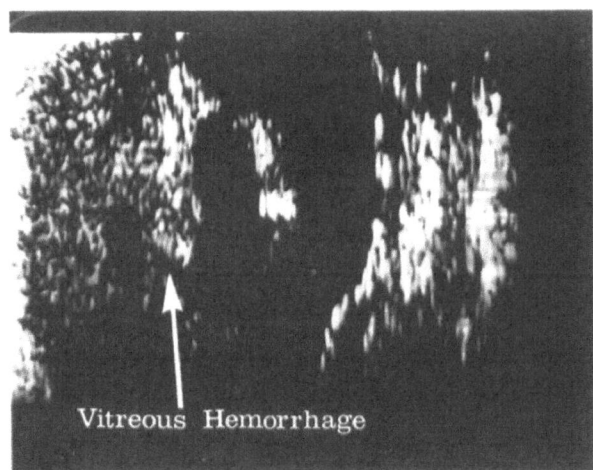

FIGURE 8.10a

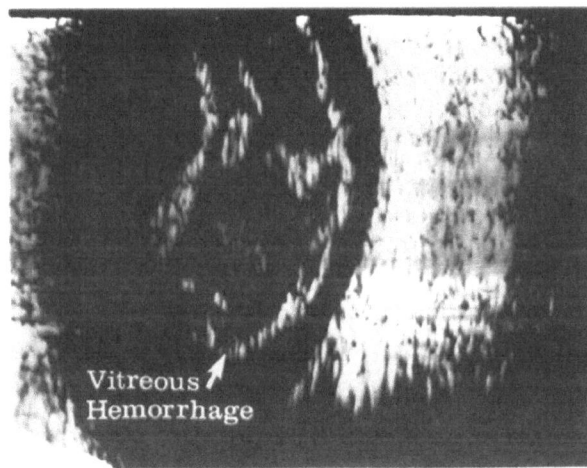

FIGURE 8.10b

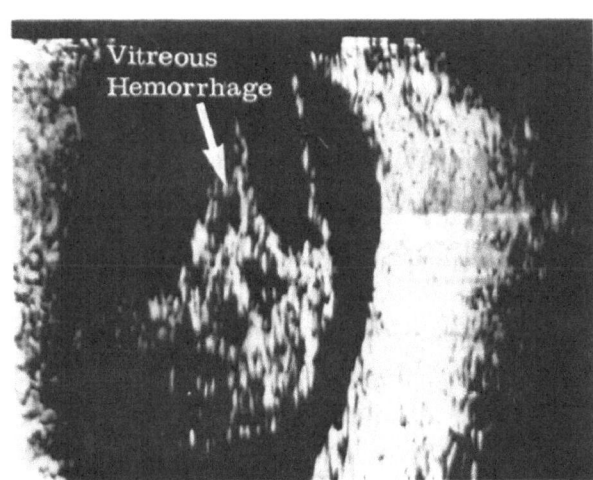

FIGURE 8.10c

FIGURE 8.5a
Vitreous hemorrhage. The echogenic band may be sinuous in configuration. Scan at 80 dB.

FIGURE 8.5b
Scan at 70 dB.

FIGURE 8.6
Vitreous hemorrhage. The membrane formed by intravitreal bleeding may be concave anteriorly.

FIGURE 8.7
Vitreous hemorrhage. The band of echogenic red cells may be concave posteriorly.

FIGURE 8.8
Vitreous hemorrhage. The appearance of the bleeding may produce a circular set of echoes.

FIGURE 8.9
Vitreous hemorrhage. The organizing blood may form an irregular or triangular shaped outline.

FIGURE 8.10a
Vitreous Hemorrhage. The collection of echoes may assume a rounded form which may simulate other types of pathology.

FIGURE 8.10b
Vitreous Hemorrhage. The echo pattern may assume a network appearance.

FIGURE 8.10c
Vitreous Hemorrhage. The echo pattern may assume a conglomerate and complex appearance.

The mass may be echo-dense (Figure 8.11).

The mass may be echo-poor (Figure 8.12).

The border may appear scalloped (Figure 8.13).

The ring may be echo-poor (Figure 8.14).

The ring may be echogenic (Figure 8.15).

The mass may appear layered (Figure 8.16).

The mass may be localized and echogenic (Figure 8.17).

The mass may be moderately well circumscribed and highly echogenic (Figure 8.18).

The mass may be diffuse and echo-poor (Figure 8.19).

The mass may be diffuse and echogenic (Figure 8.20).

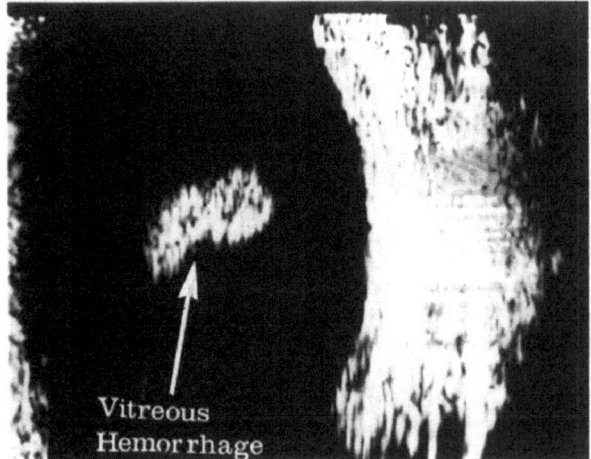

FIGURE 8.11

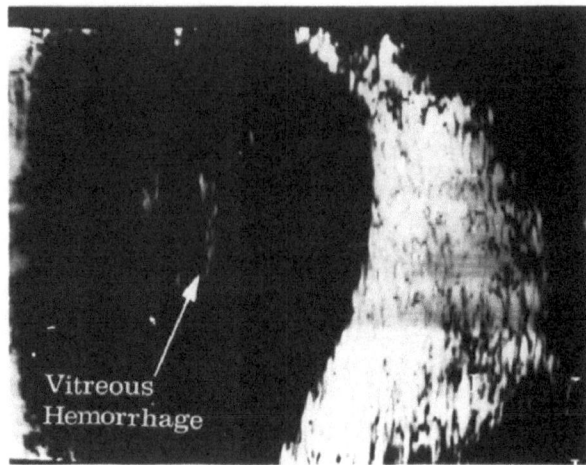

FIGURE 8.14

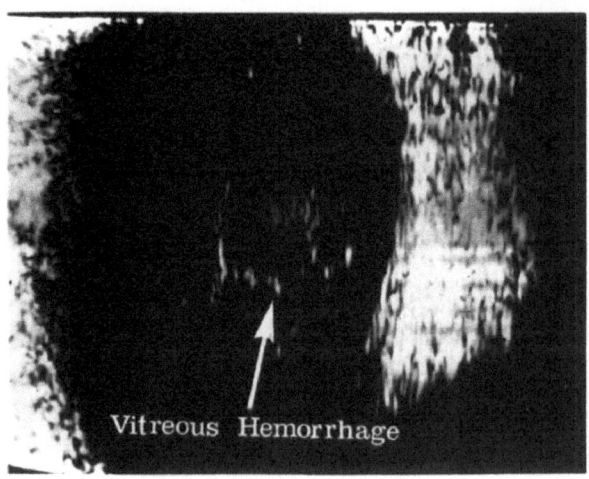

FIGURE 8.12

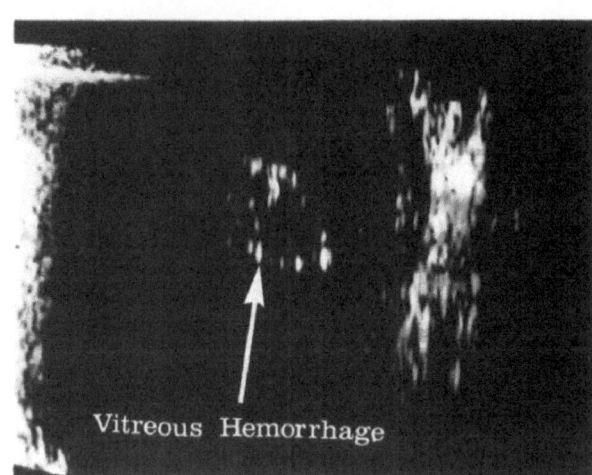

FIGURE 8.15

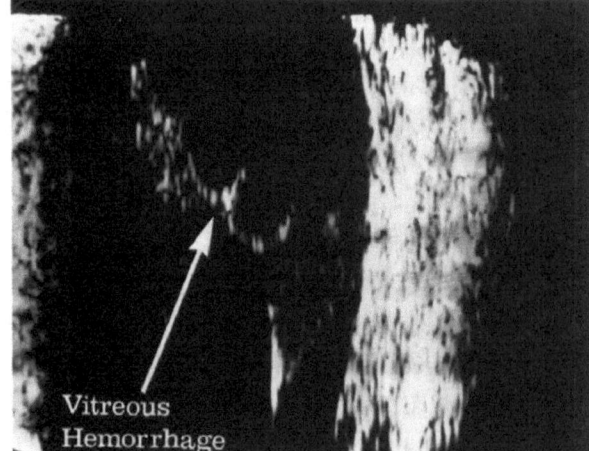

FIGURE 8.13

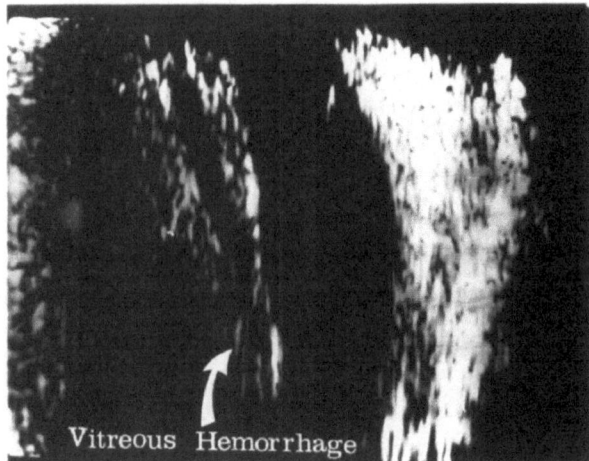

FIGURE 8.16

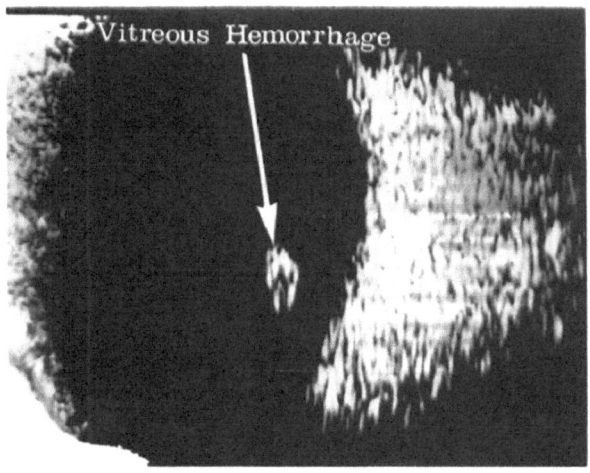

FIGURE 8.17

FIGURE 8.11
Vitreous Hemorrhage. At a fixed sensitivity setting the collection of echoes may be echo-dense.

FIGURE 8.12
Vitreous Hemorrhage. At a given gain setting the echo pattern may be echo-poor.

FIGURE 8.13
Vitreous Hemorrhage. The borders of the collection of echoes may appear scalloped in outline.

FIGURE 8.14
Vitreous Hemorrhage. A ring shaped outline which is echo-poor may be noted.

FIGURE 8.15
Vitreous Hemorrhage. A ring shaped collection of echoes of the blood may be echogenic.

FIGURE 8.16
Vitreous Hemorrhage. The mass of echoes from the intra-vitreal blood may appear layered.

FIGURE 8.17
Vitreous Hemorrhage. Areas of bleeding may be quite localized and echogenic.

FIGURE 8.18
Vitreous Hemorrhage. The mass of organizing blood may be moderately well circumscribed and highly reflective.

FIGURE 8.19
Vitreous Hemorrhage. The collection of echoes may be diffuse and echo-poor consisting of low amplitude reflecting interfaces.

FIGURE 8.20
Vitreous Hemorrhage. The bloody contents may be diffuse and echogenic with a mixed echo pattern.

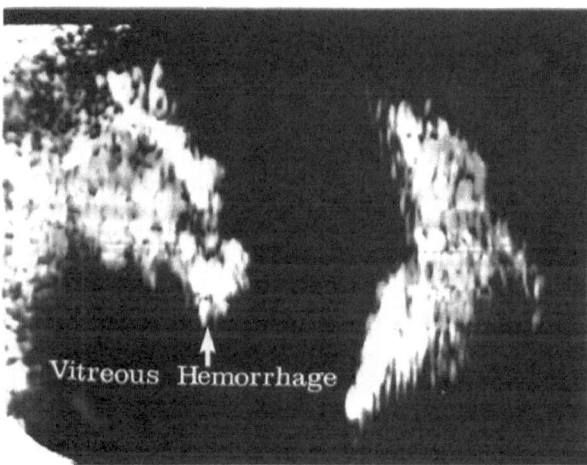

FIGURE 8.18

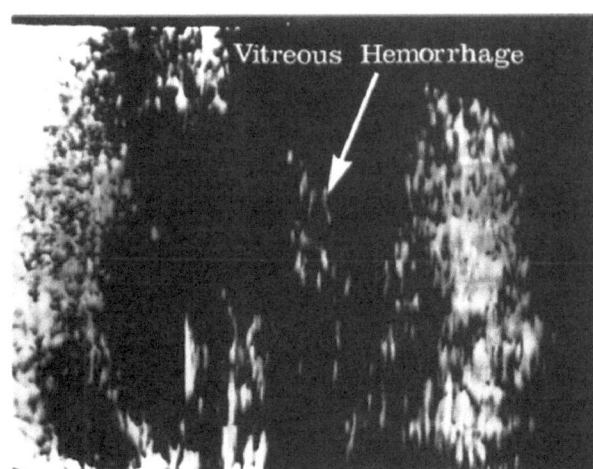

FIGURE 8.19

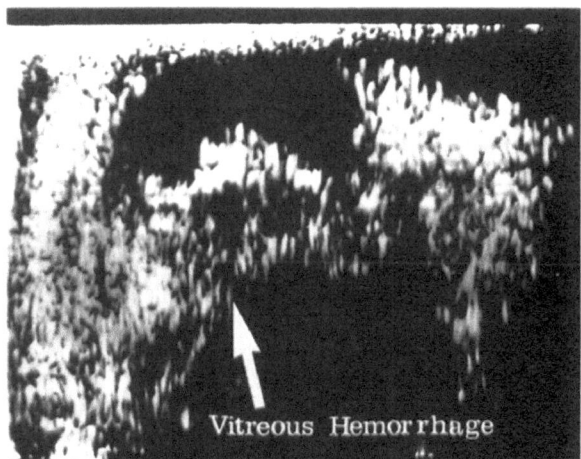

FIGURE 8.20

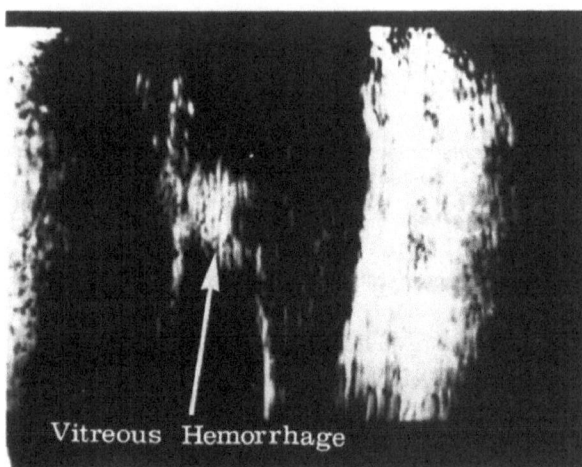

FIGURE 8.21

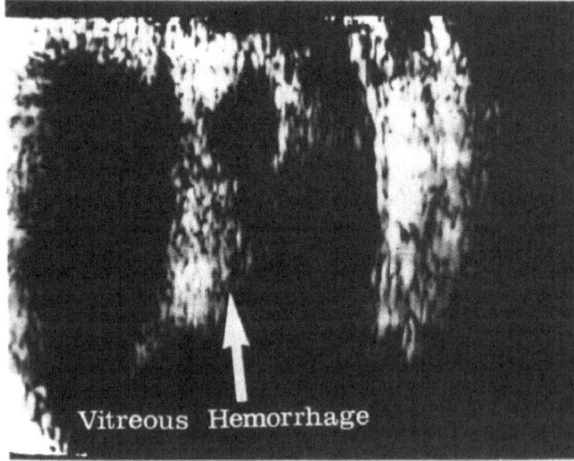

FIGURE 8.22a

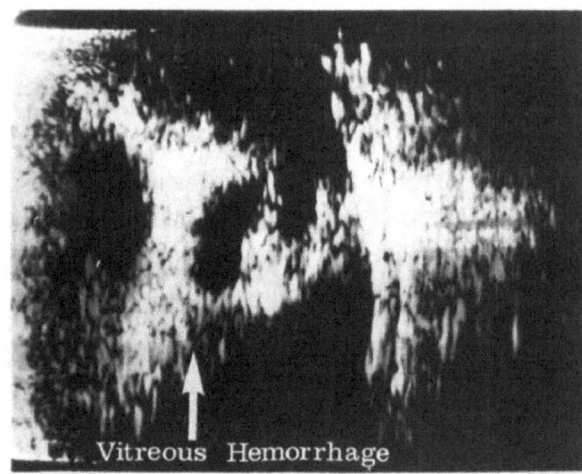

FIGURE 8.22b

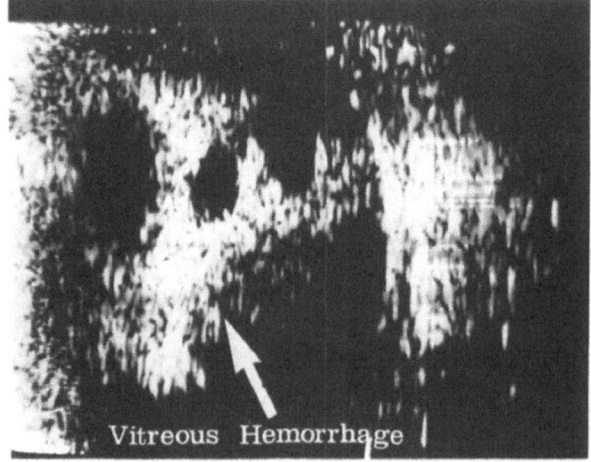

FIGURE 8.22c

Echogenic and echo-poor areas may occur together (Figure 8.21).

Vitreous hemorrhage may have a cystic appearance (Figure 8.22a,b, and c).

Retinal detachment may accompany the bleeding (Figure 8.23).

The hemorrhage may appear attached to the posterior lens capsule or to another anterior structure (Figure 8.24).

One of the most common reasons for our patient referral is for the evaluation of vitreous hemorrhage. Vitreous hemorrhage and certain inflammatory debris cannot be differentiated by sonography at the present time. We examine the patient through a closed lid. To avoid the attenuation of the sonic beam by the lens, the vitreous is studied out of the plane of the lens to allow for

FIGURE 8.21
Vitreous Hemorrhage. Echogenic and echo-poor regions may appear in adjacent areas of the vitreous body.

FIGURE 8.22a
Vitreous Hemorrhage. The clot may have an echo-free center which may appear as an open circle.

FIGURE 8.22b
Vitreous Hemorrhage. The blood may have an ovoid cystic center.

FIGURE 8.22c
Vitreous Hemorrhage. The echo-free center may be smooth and rounded and simulate a true cyst.

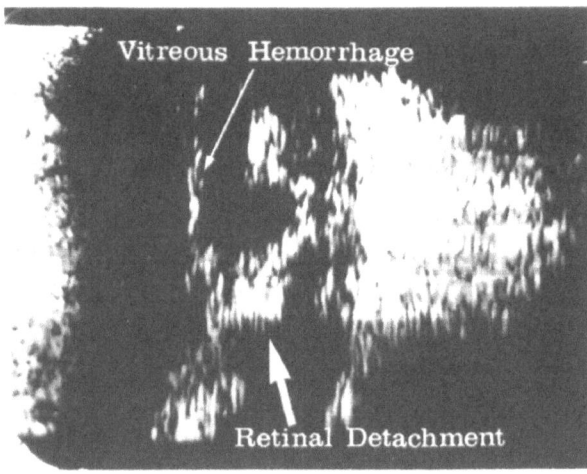

FIGURE 8.23
Retinal Detachment with Vitreous Hemorrhage. A wedge shaped echo pattern extends from the retina with weaker and more mobile echoes surrounding this retinal detachment and representing associated vitreous hemorrhage.

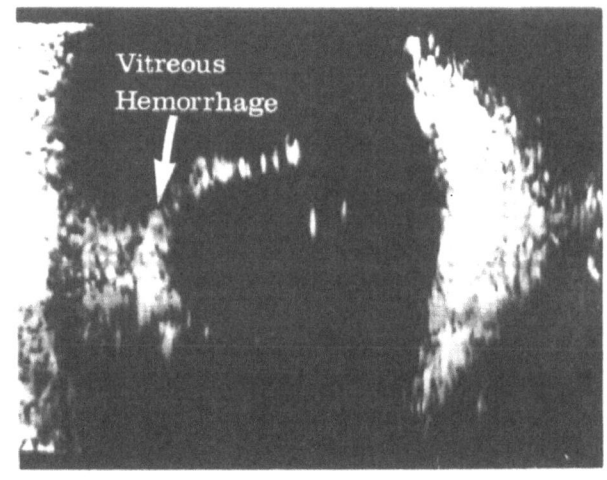

FIGURE 8.24
Vitreous Hemorrhage. Organization within the blood and its vitreous surroundings may form attachments to various structures such as this fibrous band connecting with the posterior lens capsule of a cataract.

optimal passage of the ultrasonic waves. To best accomplish this, the examining ultrasonic probe is placed at proper position or close to the ocular equator. Delayed clearing of vitreal hemorrhage is prognosticated when the hemorrhage is in the formed vitreous. More rapid resorbtion of blood occurs in the more posterior fluid vitreous. (To cover the entire vitreous cavity, the transducer is moved slowly from the equatorial position posteriorly, anteriorly, and in all quadrants.)

To evaluate these patients completely, the main consideration should be as to whether any unsuspected intraocular tumor or foreign body is present, and in the meantime, to evaluate the state of the vitreous, lens, and retina. The diagnosis of intraocular tumor is often straightforward. On the other hand, difficulty may arise in the case of fresh bleeding with rapid organization of the vitreous hemorrhage. Scanning at 80 dB may reveal blurring of the posterior ocular interface by a concave, poorly mobile lesion with a strong echo pattern. Adjacent to this are low amplitude echoes with vigorous aftermovements. This condition in our experience is usually seen in longstanding vitreous hemorrhage.

MINIMAL VITREOUS HEMORRHAGE

Minimal posterior vitreous hemorrhage usually accumulates on the detached posterior vitreous face. As a result, amorphous echoes may appear similar to the retinal detachment (Figure 8.25), but of lower echo amplitude. As previously noted, early vitreous bleeding may not produce any echoes in certain instances.

MILD VITREOUS HEMORRHAGE

In these cases, the maximum information can be gained by positioning the transducer head at the upper lid in appropriate position, because the ultrasonic evidence of hemorrhage will be found in the most gravity dependent portion of the globe, usually between 5 and 7 o'clock. On the other hand, focal vitreous hemorrhage may appear as a localized discrete echogenic area over

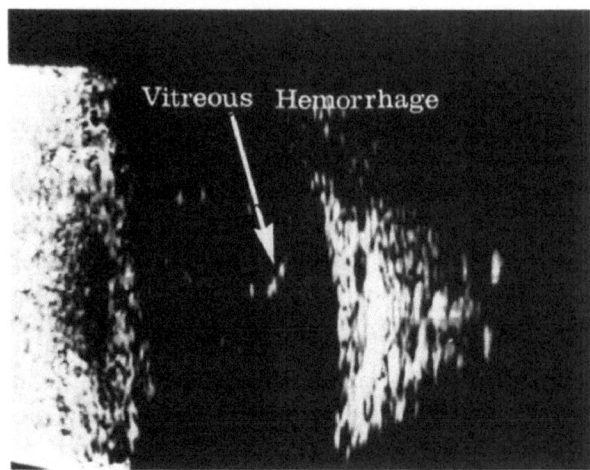

FIGURE 8.25

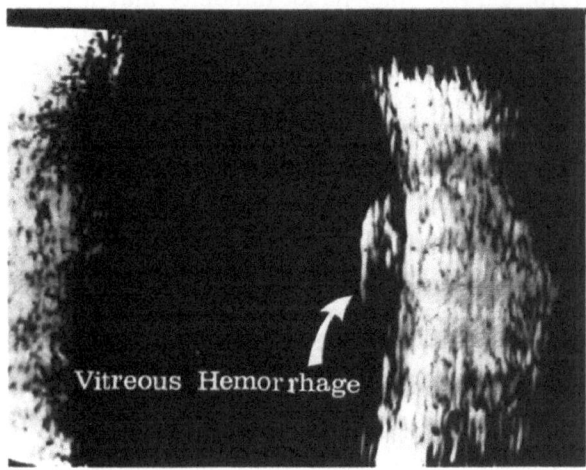

FIGURE 8.26a

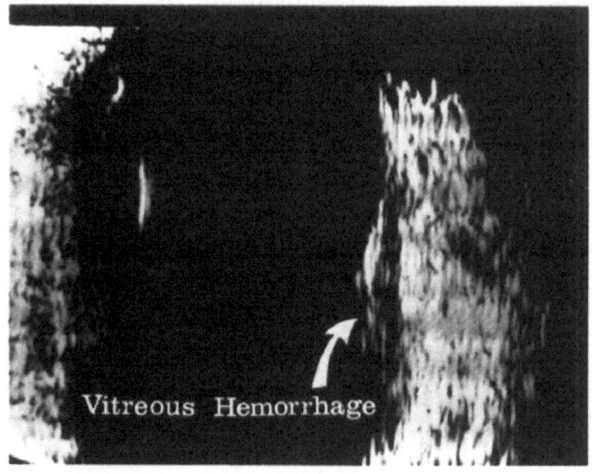

FIGURE 8.26b

FIGURE 8.25
Minimal Vitreous Hemorrhage. Ring shaped echoes in the posterior vitreous may simulate a morning glory retinal detachment but are of lower amplitude.

FIGURE 8.26a
A Vitreous Hemorrhage Simulating Tumor. Echoes protruding from the posterior ocular interface were found to be mobile and disappeared at 60 dB.

FIGURE 8.26b
Vitreous Hemorrhage Simulating Retinopathy. This flat lesion disappeared at 70 dB and moved into the vitreous freely with voluntary eye movements.

the posterior ocular wall simulating a tumor or retinopathy. This lesion is best evaluated by motility studies showing that it moves from the retinal interface and sensitivity changes demonstrating that the echoes disappear at 60 dB (Figure 8.26a and b).

Further bleeding or extensive inflammatory change shows more reflected echoes and the extent of the involvement can be determined. Vitreous flow can be easily evaluated by commanding voluntary movements of the patient's eye. By moving the eye, the gel-like portion of the vitreous appears to undulate and dance in the liquid pools. When the globe is stopped abruptly, the movement will continue. The examination of aftermovements usually adds considerable information as to the pathology of the vitreous. The extent of adhesions formed between the vitreous and the ocular wall as well as membrane formation within the vitreous cavity can be estimated. In scanning the vitreous, the presence of a detachment or other retinal conditions may be made by using the above method.

MASSIVE VITREOUS HEMORRHAGE

In massive vitreous hemorrhage, the shape and echo pattern vary widely. These are related to the location of the hemorrhage and the state of the vitreous (Figure 8.27). If both the liquid vitreous and the formed vitreous are present, both may be involved. Formed vitreous is usually found anteriorly in the vitreal cavity, while the liquid pools are found posteriorly. In the case of advanced and massive vitreous hemorrhage

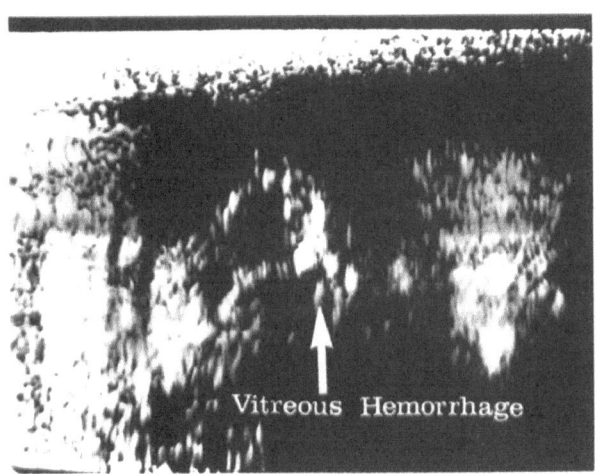

FIGURE 8.27

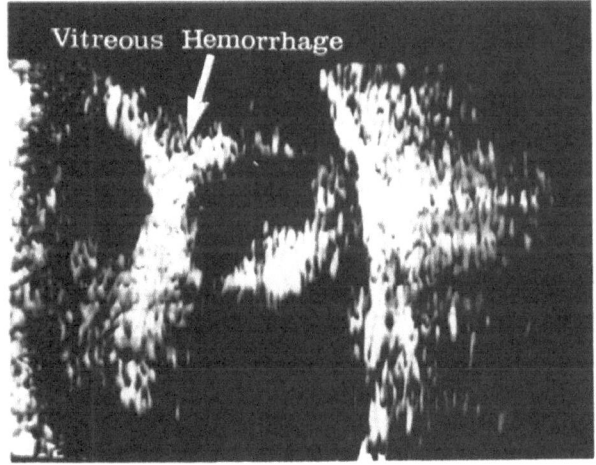

FIGURE 8.28

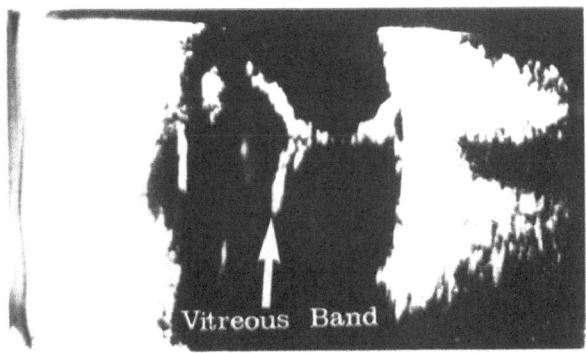

FIGURE 8.29

FIGURE 8.27
Massive Vitreous Hemorrhage. The entire length of the globe is filled with low, medium, and high amplitude echoes in multiple scan planes.

FIGURE 8.28
Fibrosed Vitreous Hemorrhage. Thickened bands inside the vitreous are of high amplitude echoes and move poorly with rapid eye movements. This is common in longstanding disease with advanced fibrotic changes.

FIGURE 8.29
Vitreous Hemorrhage with Vitreous Band. Sheet-like echoes may enter the optic nerve head region simulating a retinal detachment. Motility studies are necessary to resolve this problem.

echoes of medium amplitude are noted, and persist to 60 dB in places. Usually in massive vitreous hemorrhage the vitreous is filled with high and low amplitude echoes. Aftermovements are minimal in the case of longstanding massive vitreous hemorrhage with fibrosis (Figure 8.28). Moderate aftermovements are suggestive of organized vitreous hemorrhage rather than retinal detachment although this may simulate retinal detachment to the novice sonographer. However, echoes may enter the optic nerve head region and simulate a retinal and choroidal detachment (Figure 8.29).

VITREOUS HEMORRHAGE SIMULATING RETINAL DETACHMENT

A circular array of echoes are noted with a retinal detachment scanned perpendicularly. Ring shaped echoes which are highly mobile and disappear at 70 dB are characteristic of vitreous hemorrhage. Three-dimensional scanning will show this appearance to be a localized vitreous hemorrhage (Figure 8.30). The sheet-like echoes are relatively weak in comparison with the echoes of the retinal detachment.

By changing the sensitivity from 80 dB to 70 dB, these low amplitude, reflected echoes will disappear. If there are dense clots, some echoes will still persist to 60 dB. To obtain further information about the accumulation of the red blood cells on the completely separated vitreous face, it should be kept in mind that there is no attach-

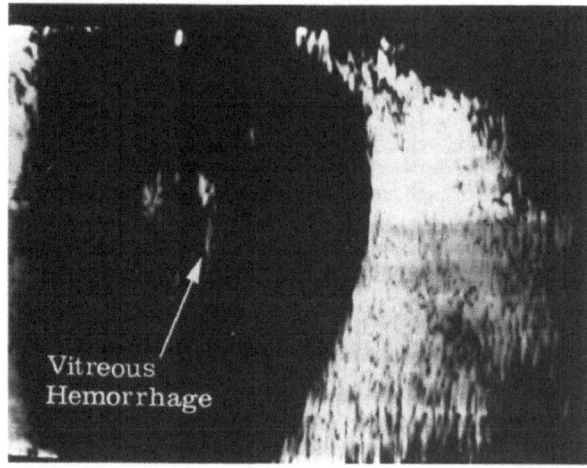

FIGURE 8.30
Ring Shaped Vitreous Hemorrhage. In one plane vitreous hemorrhage may simulate a morning glory retinal detachment. Three-dimensional reconstruction usually clears this question.

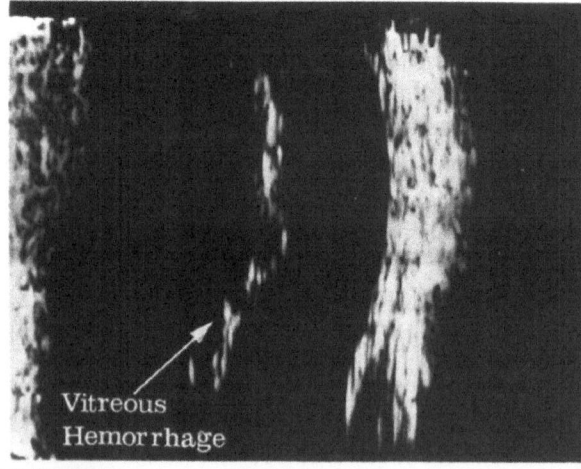

FIGURE 8.31
Vitreous Face Detachment. Low amplitude echoes of vitreous hemorrhage lying against the vitreous face may simulate a retinal detachment but do not insert into the optic nerve head.

ment of the linear echoes of blood to the optic nerve which differentiates hemorrhage from a retinal detachment. When vitreous hemorrhage simulates a retinal detachment, a curved area of echoes is usually seen, but these do not insert into the optic nerve head and disappear totally at 60 dB (Figure 8.31). Aftermovements are marked following rotational maneuvers. If the vitreous face is partially detached, it is possible to ultrasonically demonstrate a sheet-like echo inserted at the optic nerve. In this circumstance there may be confusion with a partial retinal detachment. To overcome this problem, the patient is asked to voluntarily move the globe while the examiner observes the area in question on the T.V. monitor. If the sheet-like echo has a quick motion, it represents cell accumulation on the vitreous face as contrasted to the slower undulating pattern seen in the retinal detachment. The next step is the sensitivity study. If there is a retinal detachment, it will be displayed even at 60 dB because the retina is a strong reflector, while sheet-like echo patterns of vitreous disappear at 70 dB. Vitreous hemorrhage almost always disappears at 60 dB. Estimating the extent of the vitreous hemorrhage is vitally important for the prognosis of spontaneous clearing and for preoperative planning for vitrectomy in cases where the hemorrhage does not clear. In formed vitreous hemorrhage, a long time is required for spontaneous clearing. With sonography, membraneous attachments from the hemorrhage to the ocular wall can be easily localized, and the position of the retina determined for preoperative estimation of long-standing vitreous hemorrhage.

VITREOUS HEMORRHAGE SIMULATING RETINITIS PROLIFERANS

It must be continually borne in mind that frond-like projections emanating from the posterior ocular wall and echogenic at 80 dB may be greatly reduced in both number of echoes and echo amplitude at 70 dB and even move away from the posterior ocular wall. Thus a presumptive diagnosis of retinitis proliferans may be changed to that of a vitreous hemorrhage when

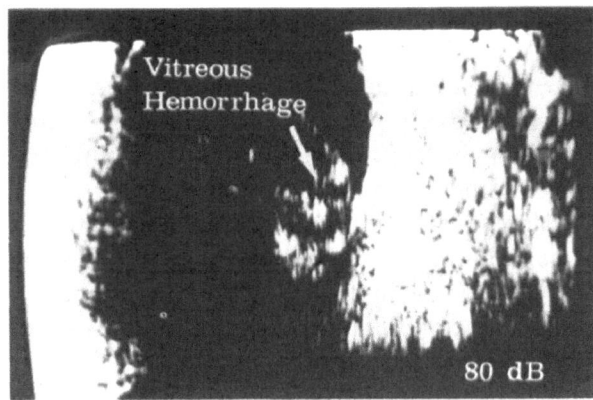

FIGURE 8.32a

FIGURE 8.32a
Vitreous Hemorrhage Simulating Retinitis Proliferans. Frond-like echoes extend from the posterior ocular wall which are poorly mobile but do not insert into the optic disc.

FIGURE 8.32b
Vitreous Hemorrhage Simulating Retinitis Proliferans. Same picture at 70 dB reveals significant decrease in the number of echoes present consistent with organizing vitreous hemorrhage.

FIGURE 8.33a
Vitreous Hemorrhage Simulating Dislocated Lens. Irregular discoid echoes are noted against the posterior ocular wall appearing like an irregular cataractous lens.

FIGURE 8.33b
Vitreous Hemorrhage Simulating Dislocated Lens. Same scan taken at 70 dB shows few echoes remaining.

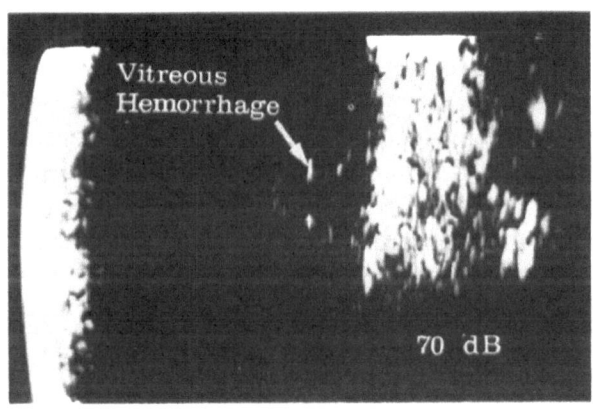

FIGURE 8.32b

the sonographer obtains the maximum information from the examination (Figure 8.32a and b).

Sometimes a focal area of clumped vitreous hemorrhage near the posterior ocular wall may assume the shape of an irregular cataractous lens and have a similar motility to that of a dislocated lens. However, the echoes of advanced cataractous lens tend to remain to 60 dB while most vitreous hemorrhage will disappear by 60 dB (Figure 8.33a and b).

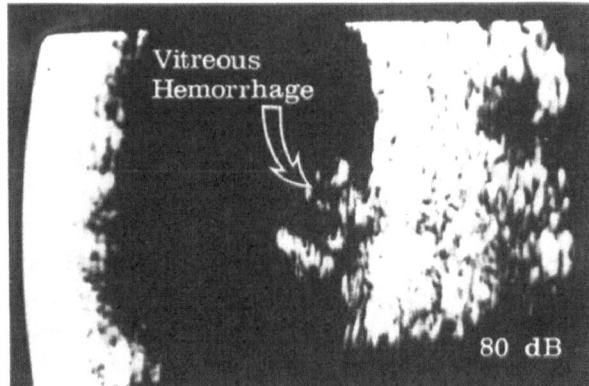

FIGURE 8.33a

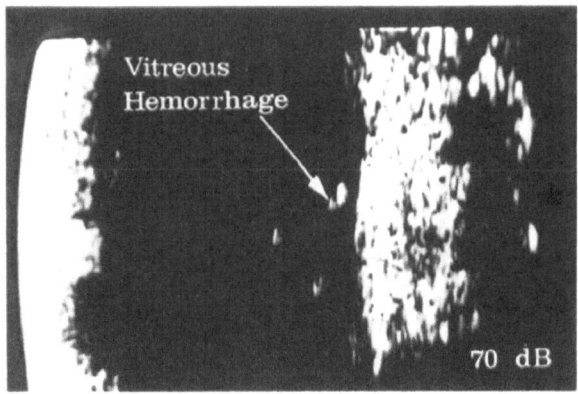

FIGURE 8.33b

SONOGRAPHY IN VITRECTOMY

The introduction of new diagnostic procedures such as the bright flash ERG and the addition of better instrumentation and operative techniques to the surgeon's armamentarium have revolutionized the approach to vitreous disease. The great progress in the field of vitreous surgery has made previously hopeless disorders now amenable to therapy. The operating surgeon needs ultrasonic verification of the status of the vitreous, location and extent of the lesion, echo pattern and type of lesion, status of the retina, and mobility of the lesion. When all the information has been accumulated from physical examinations, physiological tests including the bright flash ERG, and ultrasonography, the surgeon can then select the type of patient who may benefit from vitrectomy, and reject those who cannot be helped by this procedure. The type of instruments for the procedure may be chosen with greater care when the anatomic mapping of the lesion has been outlined by the ultrasonic scanning. Similarly, with the exact location of the lesion and associated retinal changes available, the operative approach and the decision to operate only on the vitreous or to extend the surgery to the retina may be made preoperatively. In the same way the preoperative approach is planned, the postoperative vitrectomy patient may develop a complication producing difficulty in visualizing the globe such as a choroidal effusion. The only simple means of evaluation of the postoperative eye is by ultrasound examination. Diabetic retinopathy with secondary vitreous hemorrhage is the most common condition for operative vitrectomy.

Sometimes, the differentiation between fibroproliferative membrane from retinal detachment with traction is difficult, and on some occasions it is impossible. If the proliferative vessels grow out into the vitreous from the optic nerve head, or perpendicular to the retina, the diagnosis is easy. On the other hand, if multiple areas grow out along the surface of the retina as a sheet, the diagnosis is extremely difficult. At this point, the new tissue formation may simulate a retinal detachment, and, if it has the same accoustically

reflective nature as the retina, the appearance on the T.V. will be similar to the retina. In many circumstances, the proliferating tissue can produce traction type retinal detachments which mix into the fibrous membrane. The ultrasonic pattern study is extremely helpful, but one point of interest is that with all caution taken, proliferative phenomena can still be missed during the examination. This is a common occurrence when the abnormality is small, or in circumstances when the tissue is elevated less than one millimeter from the retina. The accuracy of sonography is more limited when an unexperienced sonographer examines the eye. As a result, some early and progressive capillary disease, specifically in diabetes, may go undetected.

ASTEROID HYALOSIS

Asteroid hyalosis is identified by the presence of spherical white bodies in the vitreal cavity. Basically asteroid hyalosis is a degenerative process and may be seen in diabetes and hypercholesterolemia.

About 75% of asteroid hyalosis is unilateral and the majority occurs in males and older age groups. In our experience in a large number of cases it is unrelated to ocular problems and may be an incidental finding. Patients with asteroid hyalosis are usually asymptomatic and these patients frequently have no decrease in visual acuity.

There are many causes of vitreous opacities; however, asteroid hyalosis produces an ultrasonically characteristic picture. Asteroid hyalosis is a collection of calcium soap scattered throughout the vitreous. Crystals of calcium, sulfur, and phosphorous are embedded in an amorphous matrix and attached to the vitreous framework. This is considered a degenerative phenomenon. White colored particles are seen with the ophthalmoscope in the vitreous body. They are irridescent with edge illumination. These spherules move with the oscillation of the collagenous framework of the vitreous. They are

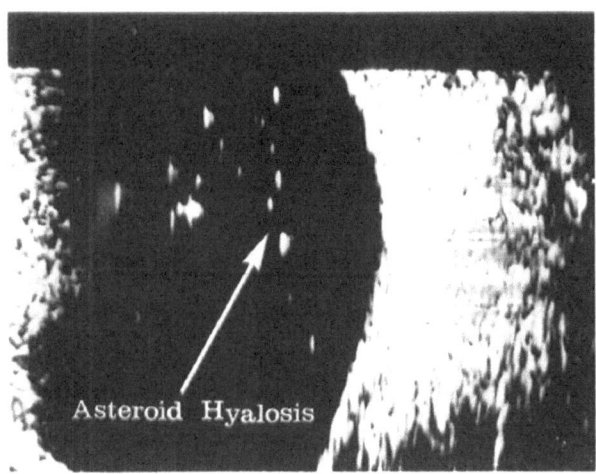

FIGURE 8.34a
Asteroid Hyalosis. Scan at 80 dB shows strongly reflective particulate echoes in the mid-vitreous.

often monocular, do not obstruct vision and are found in the geriatric age group. While considered a benign disease, they are frequently associated with retinal detachment. Ultrasonically, the disease may be minimal and the echo pattern may not be diagnostic. Hyalosis may be marked and then it can be easily detected. The echoes are scattered throughout and actually hang in the substance of vitreous like small stars because the calcium soap particles are excellent reflectors of the ultrasonic beam and produce strong interfaces with multiple areas of discontinuity. As a result, on the T.V. monitor of the unit, it appears as multiple sonopaque foci in the background of the sonolucent vitreous. By changing the sensitivity of the unit from 80 dB to 70 dB, the weaker echoes disappear, while the stronger echoes remain displayed on the monitor. As stated in the usual case the scan at 80 dB shows strongly echogenic particulate matter scattered throughout the mid-vitreous (Figure 8.34a and b). A 70 dB scan shows few remaining focal echoes which totally disappeared at 60 dB. At 60 dB most of the sonopaque echoes disappeared, but still, there were many echoes which were captured by the polaroid film. In vitreous hemorrhage, the echoes completely disappear at 60 dB. The scattered mid-vitreous echoes with characteristic aftermovements and no visual impairment proven to be asteroid hyalosis may be strongly or weakly echogenic at a fixed sensitivity setting (Figure 8.35a and b). The second part of the study includes the dynamic pattern of the eye movement. If the patient is instructed to move the eye voluntarily, all the sonopaque echoes in the background of the sonolucent vitreous move in a smooth, flowing motion.

The sensitivity study is the most important part and should be done in all patients suspected of having asteroid hyalosis in order to avoid confusion with vitreous hemorrhage. Asteroid hyalosis remains as multiple discrete echogenic foci in the mid-vitreous with a flowing motion at 60 dB while vitreous hemorrhage disappears at 60 dB.

At 80 dB the echoes appear suspended in the vitreous. At 60 dB a few particulate areas still

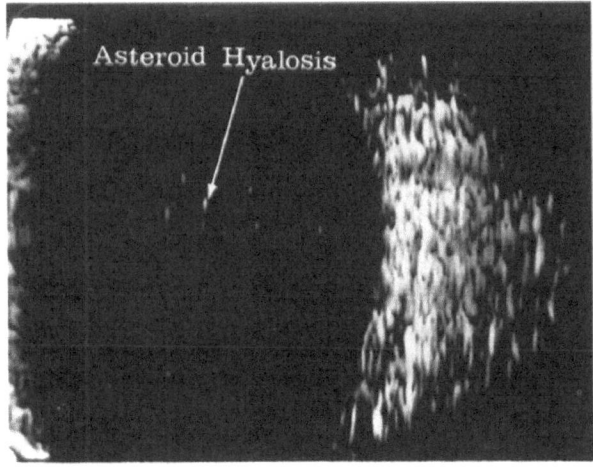

FIGURE 8.34b
Asteroid Hyalosis. Scan at 60 dB demonstrates few particulate echoes remaining. Motility study showed characteristic aftermovements.

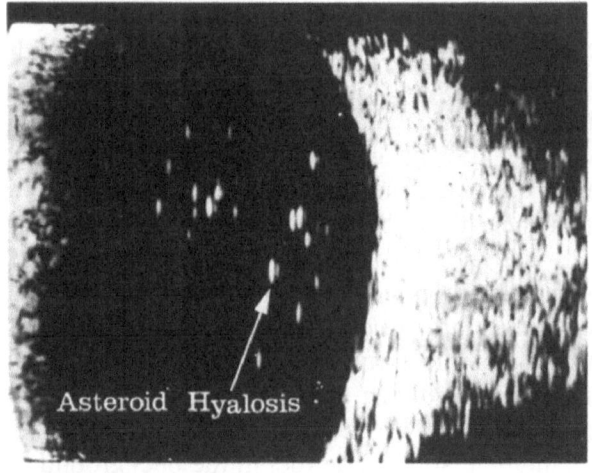

FIGURE 8.35a
Asteroid Hyalosis. Scan at 80 dB show highly echogenic reflecting surface which are similar in size and shape.

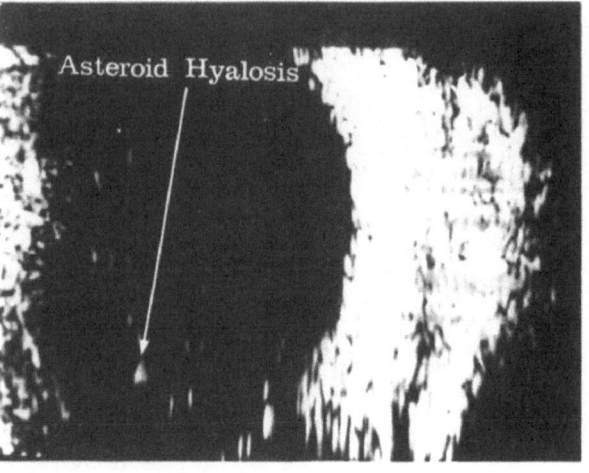

FIGURE 8.36a
Asteroid Hyalosis. Asteroid hyalosis may be located in the anterior portion of the vitreous.

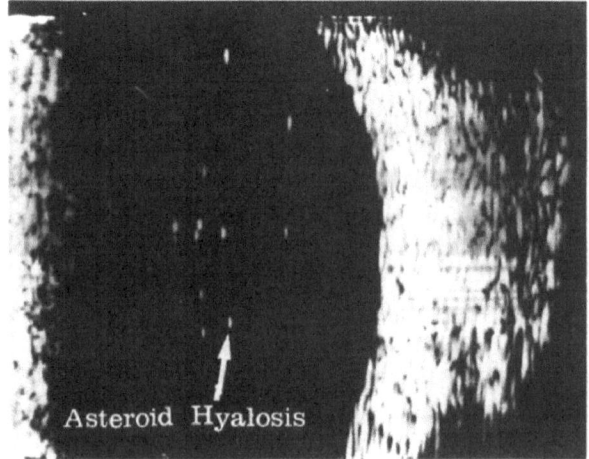

FIGURE 8.35b
Asteroid Hyalosis. Scan at 80 dB in another case demonstrates scattered homogeneous reflectors which are minimally echogenic demonstrating that asteroid hyalosis may have a spectrum of echo patterns.

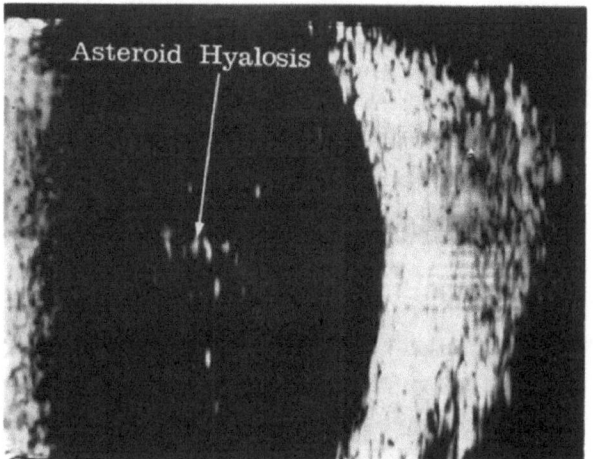

FIGURE 8.36b
Asteroid Hyalosis. The most common form is in the mid-vitreous in location.

106

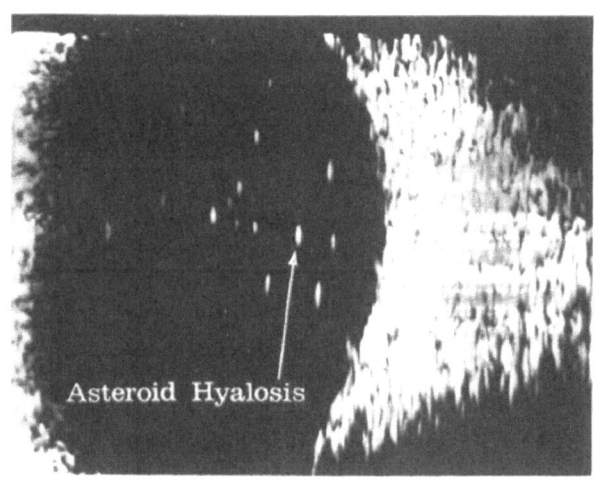

FIGURE 8.36c
Asteroid Hyalosis. Asteroid hyalosis echoes may be predominantly located in the posterior vitreous demonstrating a wide variety of possible positions of this entity.

remain. If vision is obstructed and ophthalmoscopy cannot be performed, both sensitivity study and dynamic study allow a definite diagnosis. However, although asteroid hyalosis is most commonly noted in the mid-vitreous, it may be located predominantly in the anterior or posterior vitreous (Figure 8.36a,b, and c).

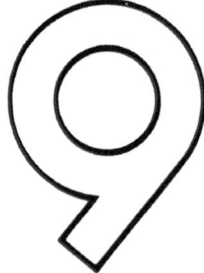

sonography of the retina and choroid

GENERAL INTRODUCTION

The retina is the mirror of the mind. Through this complex layer pass all the visual images we perceive. The retina is divided into various anatomic and functional areas so that a tiny lesion in the macula lutea may visually cripple a patient while a massive, gradual loss of peripheral retinal tissue may go unnoticed. Certain diseases have a predilection for the central retinal area like diabetes, while others tend to the peripheral retina such as sickle cell disease. Both of these entities produce retinopathy and neovascularization. A large number of generalized diseases may be manifested in the retina besides ocular pathology.

The choroid layer of the eye nourishes the sensory retina. This highly vascular layer is the site of most of the primary and metastatic tumors of the eye. This delicate zone may swell markedly in size due to decreased intraocular pressure and is frequently the site of unrecognized effusions following eye trauma and surgery. Ultrasonography is of great value in localizing the pathology to a given area of the choroid or retina and focusing on a particular disease entity which may have structural and geographic hall marks.

RETINAL DETACHMENT

Complete or partial separation of the retina from the choroid is called retinal detachment. Usually, at first the detachment is partial, but if left untreated becomes complete. Particular emphasis is placed on the diagnosis of retinal detachment since this is a potentially preventable cause of blindness. Early detection and prompt surgery can preserve the vision in an eye that would otherwise become irreversibly blind. Clinical detection of retinal detachment is often possibly by the patient's complaints. The sudden breakthrough of blood cells and retinal pigment into the vitreous produce a burst of vitreous floaters. The tear in the retina that allowed the floaters to occur may not produce an immediate retinal detachment and many of these tears occur at the equator in the far periphery of the eye so that they are generally out of the field of vision. The blood and pigment cells in the vitreous will quickly settle in response to gravity although they may not clear for years entirely. More rapid clearing occurs in the vitreous that is more fluid.

Vision usually improves as the cells in the vitreous settle and clear. Then the patient notes a gradually enlarging peripheral field defect which responds to the advancing retinal detachment caused by the intraocular fluid extending subretinally. The retina that is removed from the choroid layer that provides its nutrition ceases to function. The condition is painless. Ophthalmoscopy shows the elevated retina and the presence of subretinal fluid which obscures the background details of the choroid vessels and pigment markings that are normally visible. Early peripheral detachments and small retinal holes are difficult to evaluate clinically. Retinal detachment occurs after ocular injury and in patients with high myopia. Many retinal detachments occur in aphakic patients who have had cataract extractions. Retinal detachment is due to vitreous disease. Vitreous traction causes both the

hole in the retina to form and pulls the membrane off the choroid layer. Diabetic changes produce scarring in the vitreous body which may pull off the retina. The type of retinal detachment produced by a hole in the retina from vitreous traction is called rhegmatogenous retinal detachment. Rhegma is derived from the Greek word meaning "tear". Nonrhegmatogenous retinal detachments have no tears or holes in the retina. They are caused by the leakage of fluid from the choroidal or retinal vessels. This occurs in primary and metastatic tumors, sympathetic ophthalmia, and severe inflammatory and traumatic conditions.

CAUSES OF RETINAL DETACHMENT

Retinal detachment occurs most commonly in myopes (especially those about -5 to -8 diopters). It is a frequent complication after trauma.

Accumulation of fluid beneath the intact sensory retina due to Harada's disease, Coat's disease, malignant hypertension, eclampsia, choroidal malignant melanomas, and subretinal hemorrhages will detach the retina. As previously noted, traction bands produce the majority of retinal detachment and are found in posttraumatic vitreous condensation and fibrosis, complications of cataract surgery and vitreous bands in diabetes mellitus. Accumulation of fluid beneath a broken retina is associated with vitreous traction.

SONOPATHOLOGY OF RETINAL DETACHMENT

Detection of retinal detachment may be extremely simple or the most difficult diagnosis in ophthalmic sonography. In a nonopaque lens, the diagnosis of retinal detachment can be made through ophthalmoscopy. When the lens is opaque, the clinician is unable to detect any pathology behind the lens including retinal detachment. In this situation, sonography gives fascinating results. The diagnosis of a retinal

109

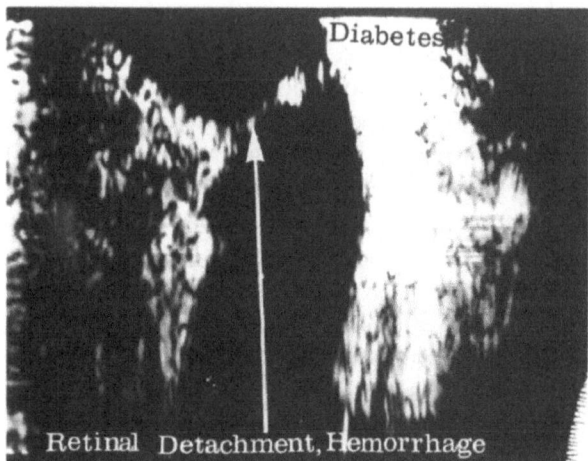

FIGURE 9.1a

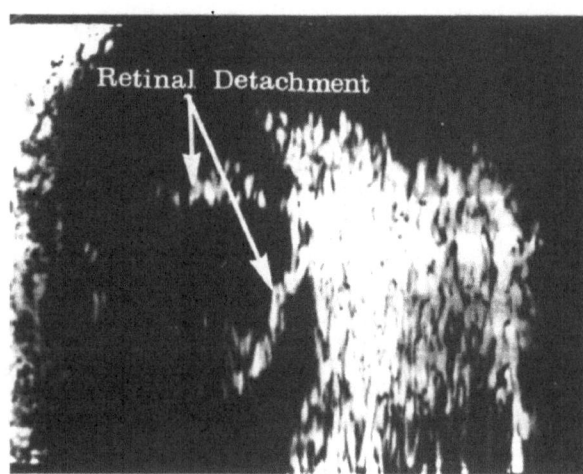

FIGURE 9.1b

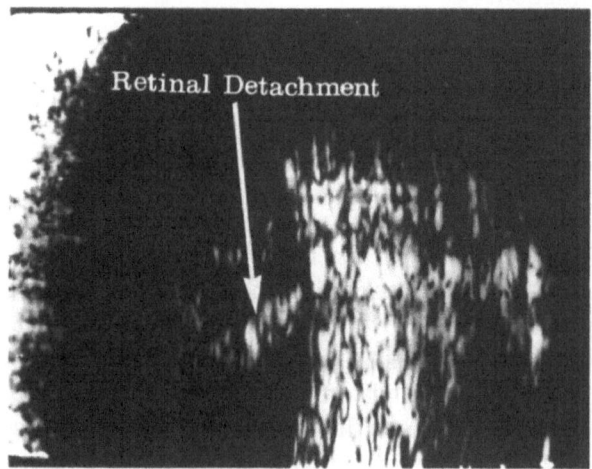

FIGURE 9.1c

FIGURE 9.1a
Retinal detachment with vitreous hemorrhage. Trauma frequently produces low amplitude anterior vitreal echoes adjacent to high amplitude retinal echoes.

FIGURE 9.1b
Simple retinal detachment scanned perpendicularly is thin, echogenic, and sharp.

FIGURE 9.1c
Simple retinal detachment scanned at oblique angle often has thick and fuzzy outline with low amplitude echoes which may simulate traumatic vitreous hemorrhage.

detachment is easy in the presence of a mature cataract.

In cases of recent ocular trauma, the contact B-scanner is the simplest method for evaluating a detached retina.

The scan of a retinal detachment with vitreous hemorrhage due to trauma shows an anterior section of the vitreous with scattered low amplitude echoes which is surrounded by a region of high amplitude echoes (Figure 9.1a). The vitreous is filled with highly echogenic retinal tissue. In the case of a simple retinal detachment scanned perpendicularly (Figure 9.1b) the vitreous shows a hazy low amplitude retinal outline due to deviation from right angle scanning (Figure 9.1c).

Retinal detachment may occur after very powerful miotics, thinning choroidal scars, or contracting vitreous bands. Also, retinal detachment is one of the complications of phthisis bulbi, foreign bodies, and inflammatory disease.

Retinal detachment may have a wide variety of patterns:

A. Partial detachment close to the posterior ocular wall (Figure 9.2).

B. More extensive partial detachment separated from the wall with irregular pattern (Figure 9.3).

C. Total detachment diverges widely from the optic nerve (Figure 9.4).

D. Total detachment may diverge with narrow angle from the nerve (Figure 9.5).

110

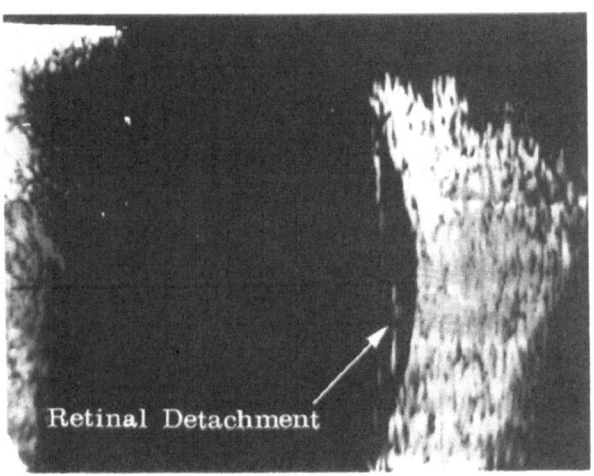

FIGURE 9.2

FIGURE 9.2
Partial retinal detachment. The echogenic membrane lies near the posterior ocular wall and does not insert into the optic nerve head.

FIGURE 9.3
Retinal detachment. A more extensive retinal detachment demonstrating the echogenic band separated from the posterior ocular wall with irregular pattern.

FIGURE 9.4
Retinal detachment. Total retinal detachment diverges from the optic nerve head with a wide angle.

FIGURE 9.5
Total detachment. Leaves of the echogenic retinal detachment emanate from the optic disc with a narrow angle and appear less echogenic than expected.

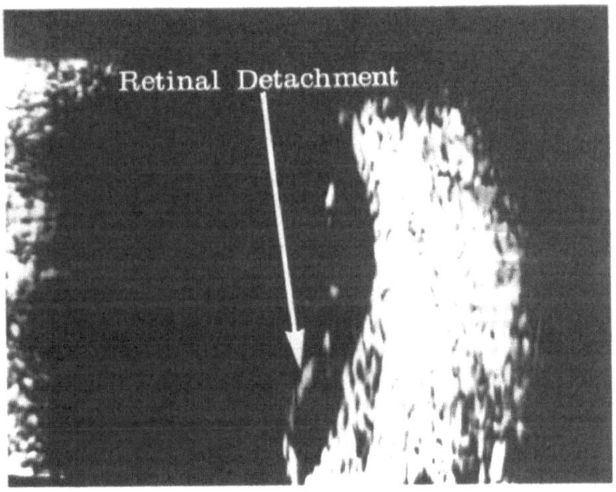

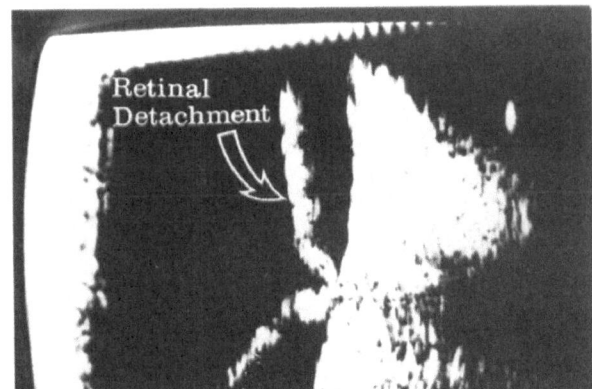

FIGURE 9.3

E. Leaves of detachment may be concave towards the lens (Figure 9.6).

F. Leaves of detachment may be convex towards the lens (Figure 9.7).

G. Leaves of detachment may be parallel to equator of eye (Figure 9.8).

H. Leaves may be S-shaped or sinuous (Figure 9.9).

I. Leaves may be thin (Figure 9.10).

J. Leaves may be thick (Figure 9.11).

K. Leaves may be frond-like (Figure 9.12).

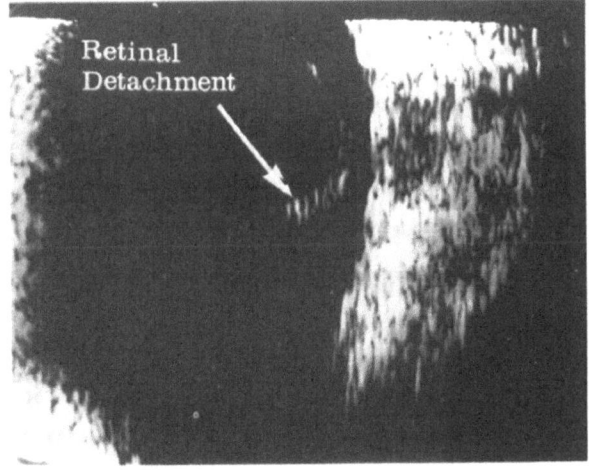

FIGURE 9.4

FIGURE 9.5

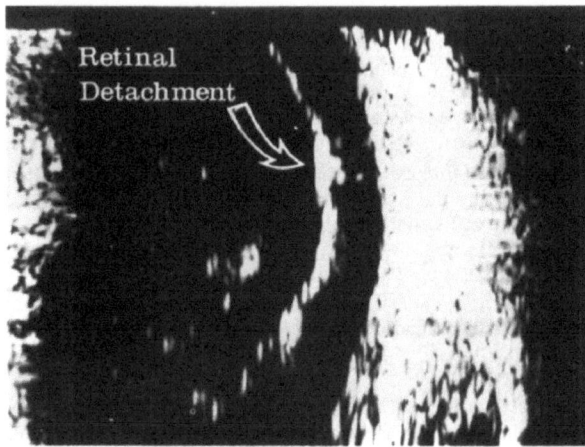

FIGURE 9.6

FIGURE 9.6
Retinal detachment. Leaves of the detached retina may be concave towards the lens.

FIGURE 9.7
Retinal detachment. Leaves of the retina may be convex towards the lens.

FIGURE 9.8
Retinal detachment. Leaves of the retina may be parallel to the equator of the eye.

FIGURE 9.9
Retinal detachment. Leaves of the detachment of the retinal membrane may be S-shaped or sinuous.

FIGURE 9.10
Retinal detachment. The leaves of the retinal detachment may be very thin. Note well outlined choroid layer.

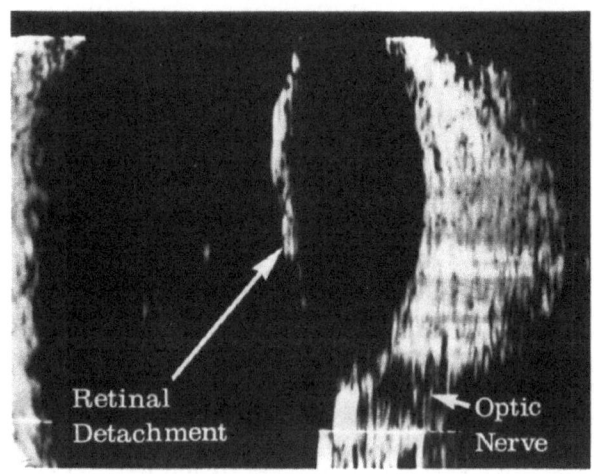

FIGURE 9.7

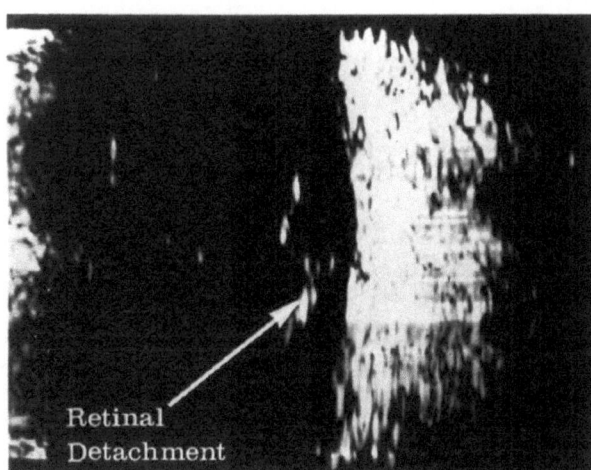

FIGURE 9.9

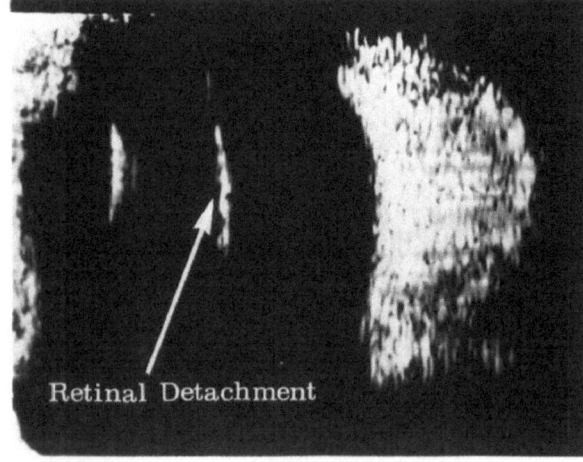

FIGURE 9.8

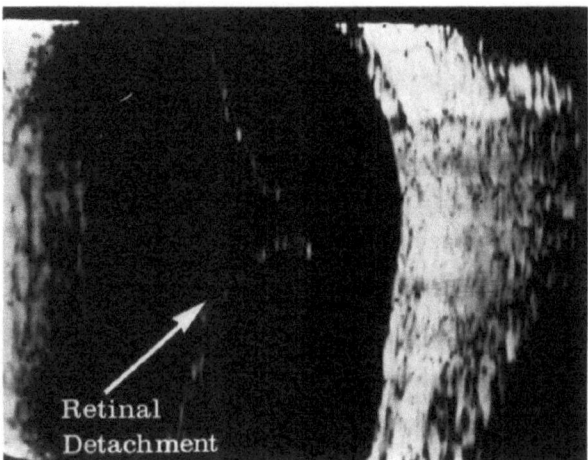

FIGURE 9.10

FIGURE 9.11
Retinal detachment. The leaves of the detached retina may be thick and highly echogenic.

FIGURE 9.12
Retinal detachment. The leaves of the retinal detachment may be irregular and frond-like.

FIGURE 9.13a
Retinal detachment. The leaves of the retinal detachment may be thin and poorly echogenic simulating a vitreous detachment.

FIGURE 9.13b
The retinal detachment may be mobile simulating vitreous hemorrhage. Same case as 9.13a following eye movement.

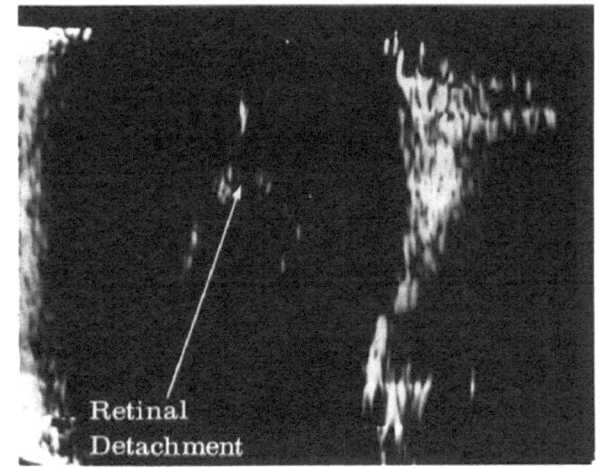

FIGURE 9.13a

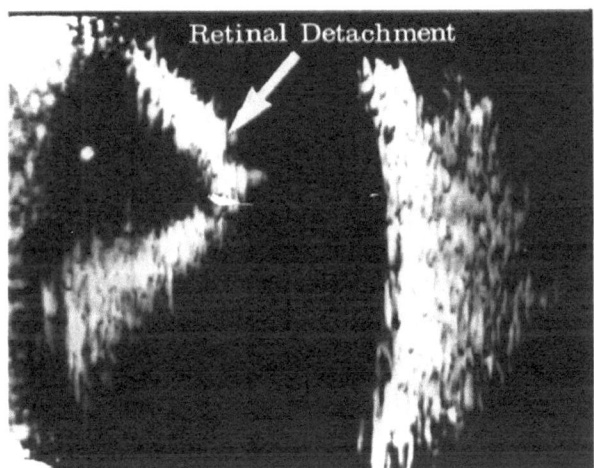

FIGURE 9.11

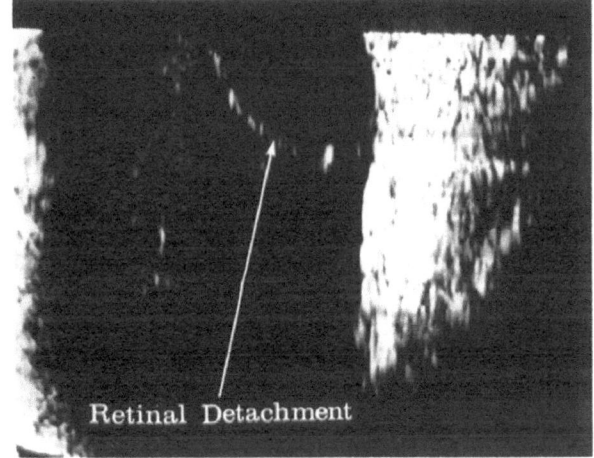

FIGURE 9.13b

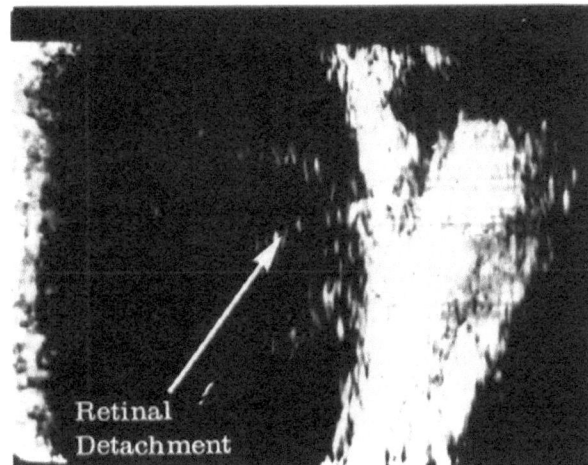

FIGURE 9.12

L. Leaves may be highly mobile simulating vitreous detachment (Figure 9.13a and b).

M. A thin cyclitic membrane may be present (Figure 9.14).

N. A thick cyclitic membrane may be present (Figure 9.15).

O. Leaves may not be traceable back to optic nerve head if not sectioned properly by scanning beam (Figure 9.16).

P. Amorphous detachment may simulate vitreous hemorrhage (Figure 9.17).

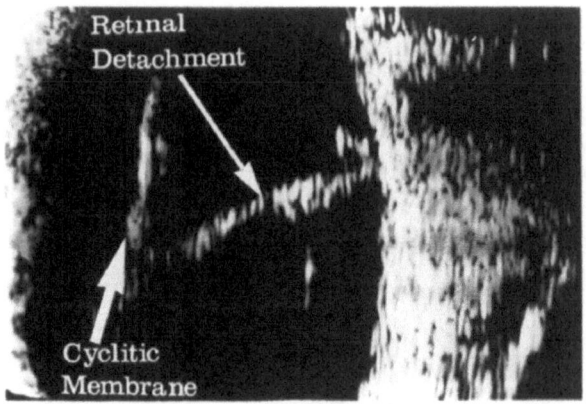

FIGURE 9.14

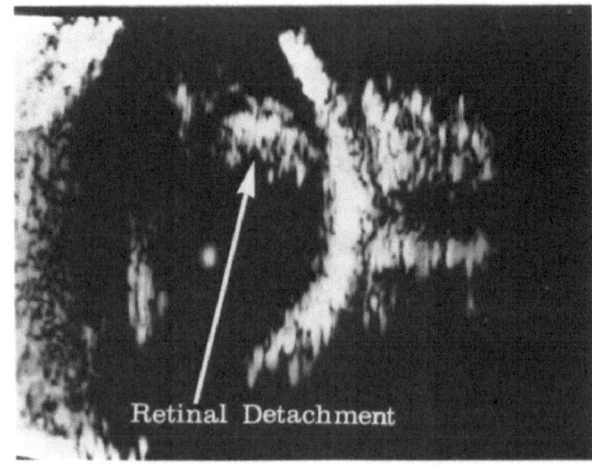

FIGURE 9.17

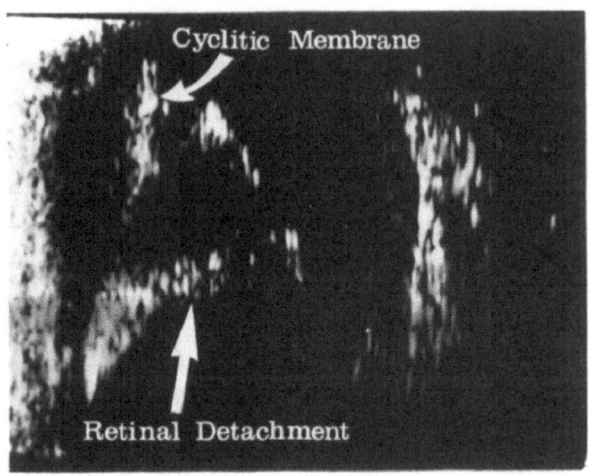

FIGURE 9.15

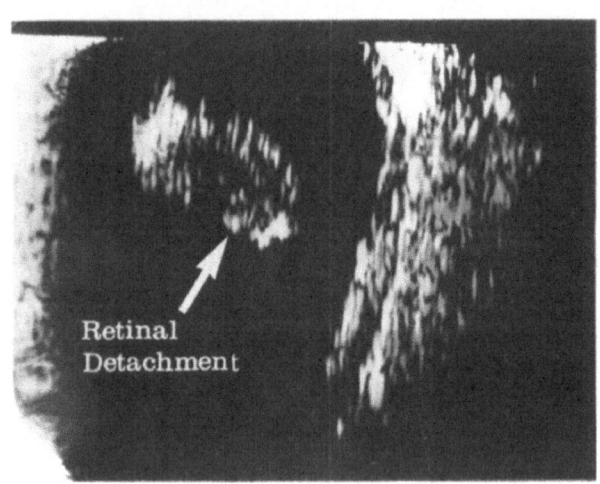

FIGURE 9.18a

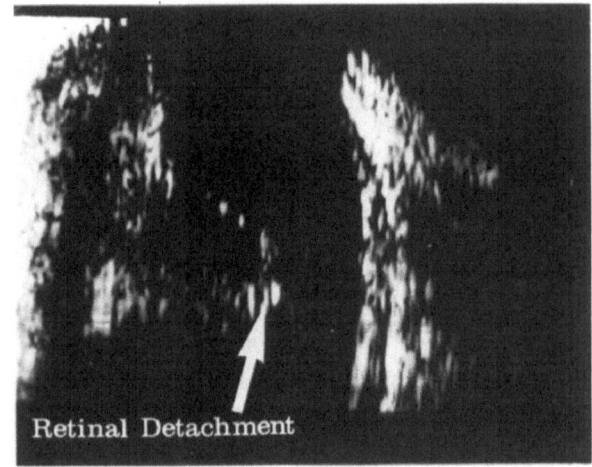

FIGURE 9.16

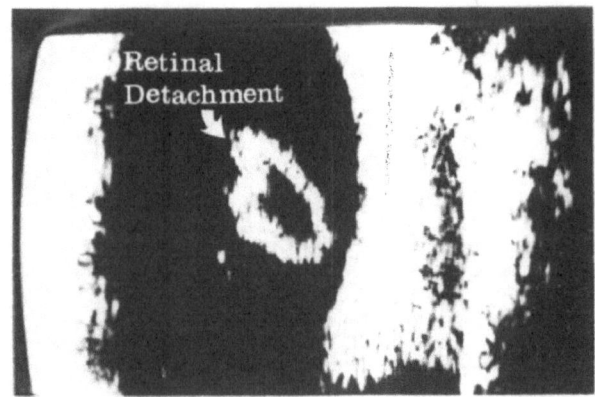

FIGURE 9.18b

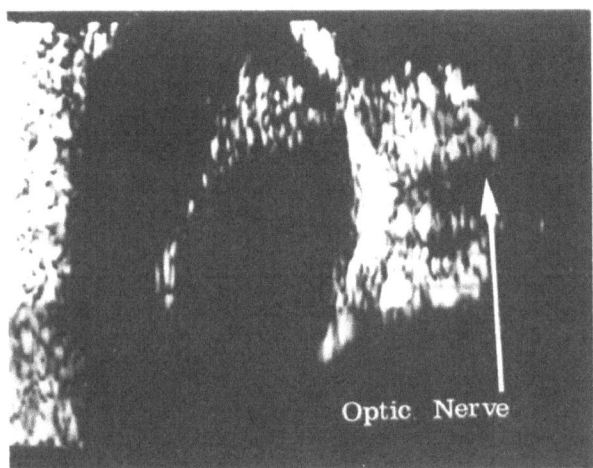

FIGURE 9.19

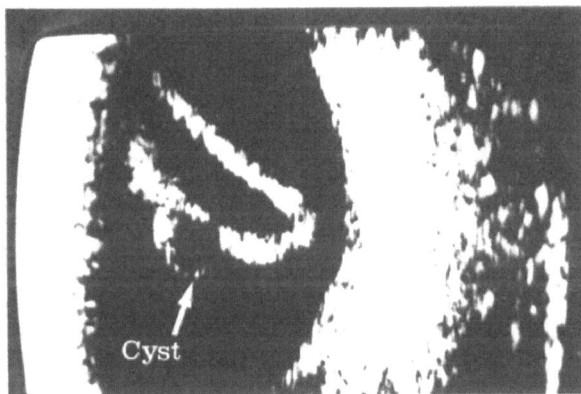

FIGURE 9.20a

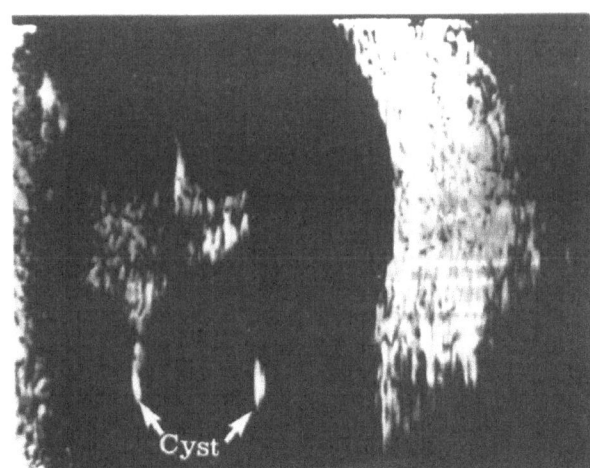

FIGURE 9.20b

FIGURE 9.14
Cyclitic membrane. The membrane lying at the anterior face of the retinal detachment is thin and well delineated.

FIGURE 9.15
Cyclitic membrane. The band adjacent to the open end of the leaves of the retinal detachment is thick and poorly outlined.

FIGURE 9.16
Retinal detachment. The leaves of the retinal detachment may converge in the posterior vitreous rather than the optic disc if scanned in an oblique manner.

FIGURE 9.17
Amorphous retinal detachment. The leaves of a disorganized retinal detachment may simulate a vitreous hemorrhage.

FIGURE 9.18a
Retinal detachment. Oblique scanning may show the diverging leaves as an ovoid echogenic lesion.

FIGURE 9.18b
Cross section of a retinal detachment may appear circular in outline.

FIGURE 9.19
Retinal detachment with vitreous band. The anteriorly located echogenic vitreous membrane exerts traction on the retina producing a detachment.

FIGURE 9.20a
Cyst formation. Longstanding retinal detachment with echo-free cystic lesion along inferior margin.

FIGURE 9.20b
Cyst formation. A disorganized echo array from a longstanding retinal detachment is noted. At the inferior portion of the film are the anterior and posterior highly echogenic borders of a retinal cyst.

Q. Oblique scanning may depict a circular image (Figure 9.18a and b).

R. Traction bands may be identified anteriorly (Figure 9.19).

S. Cystic transformation may occur (Figure 9.20a and b).

T. Vitreous bands may be indistinguishable from the leaves of a retinal detachment (Figure 9.21).

Patients with vitritis usually have traction bands from vitreous inflammatory tissue pulling off the retina in the region of the optic head nerve. This band should not be confused with a retinal detachment (Figure 9.22). In the traumatic form of retinal detachment we may note a retinal detach-

115

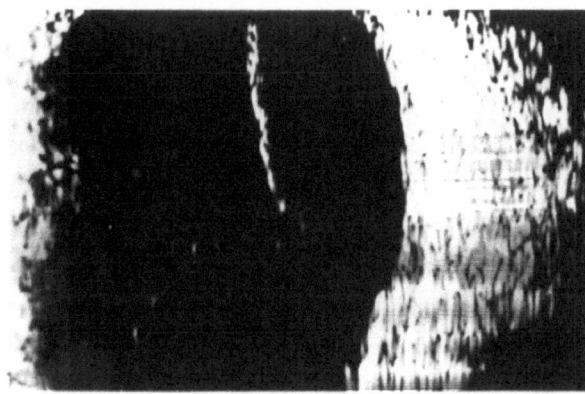

FIGURE 9.21

FIGURE 9.21
Vitreous band. Linear vitreous band did not enter the optic nerve head but remained echogenic until 60 dB.

FIGURE 9.22
Vitreous band. A localized retinal detachment occurs from the posterior ocular wall by an echogenic vitreous traction membrane.

FIGURE 9.23a
Traumatic retinal detachment. Scan shows a V-shaped retinal detachment with echogenic subretinal blood and scattered low amplitude intravitreal echoes.

FIGURE 9.23b
Perpendicular scan demonstrates the low amplitude intravitreal echoes and the more highly echogenic subretinal hemorrhage with a ring-shaped echogenic outline of the retina.

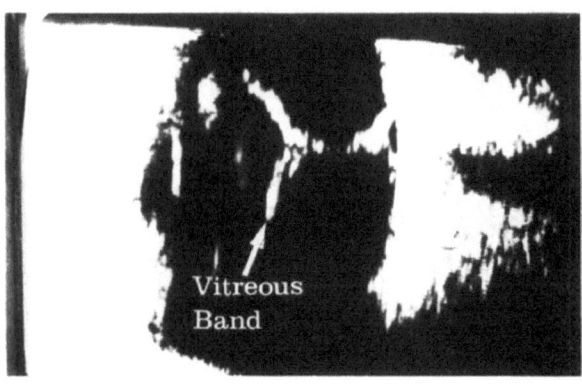

Vitreous
Band

FIGURE 9.22

ment with vitreous hemorrhage and subretinal bleeding existing together. Scanning parallel to the optic nerve plane shows an echogenic V-shape of retinal detachment with low amplitude echoes within the vitreous, and medium amplitude echoes within the subretinal space (Figure 9.23a). Intra-vitreal and subretinal echoes show appropriate motion for hemorrhagic material in this disorder. A cross-section scan shows an oblong shape to the retinal detachment totally surrounded by the subretinal and vitreal echo pattern (Figure 9.23b). By gravity and motion subretinal fluid can be shifted and in some cases easily be detected. This technique involves scanning the patient in the supine position which shows the echogenic sheet-like membrane that usually lies close to the posterior ocular wall with the transducer head in the longitudinal posi-

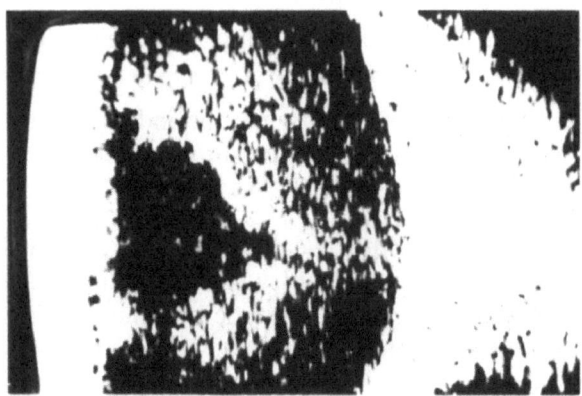

FIGURE 9.23a

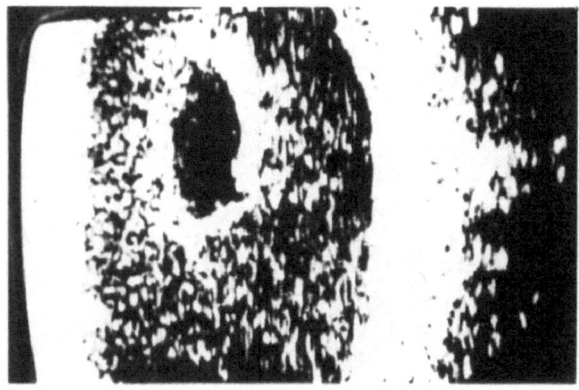

FIGURE 9.23b

FIGURE 9.24a
Shifting method. Supine scan. The retinal detachment leaves lie close to the posterior ocular wall in the dependent position.

FIGURE 9.24b
Erect scan. The mobile subretinal fluid pushes the inferior retina further into the vitreous as it accumulates in the graviationally dependent position.

FIGURE 9.25
Nonrhegmatogenous retinal detachment. The snake-like retina flows in the vitreous. A large choroidal tumor is noted inferiorly to be the etiology of this detachment.

FIGURE 9.26
Old retinal detachment. Fibrotic and degenerative changes produce a disorganized echo pattern to this retinal detachment. Incidentally noted is thickened choroid.

tion. In the erect position, the inferior segment of the retina shifts anteriorly as the subretinal fluid moves to a more dependent position (Figure 9.24a and b). By sonography, not only may a retinal detachment be detected, but we may at times differentiate between rhegmatogenous retinal detachment and detachment secondary to tumor (Figure 9.25). When a retinal detachment is present with other pathological conditions its source should be carefully investigated. In a retinal detachment that is longstanding, the usual clean edges are no longer present due to concomitant degenerative changes (Figure 9.26). Retinal detachment may be associated with choroidal detachment. For example, in some cases

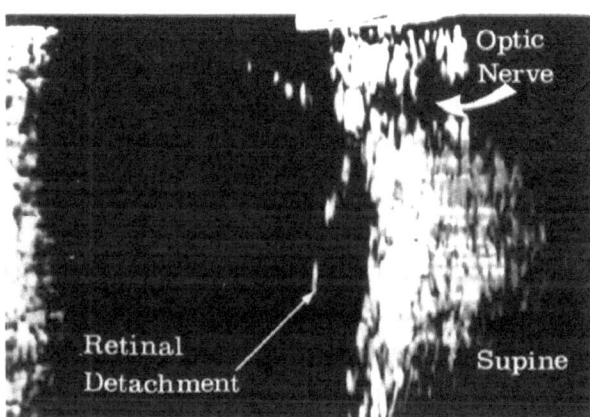

FIGURE 9.24a

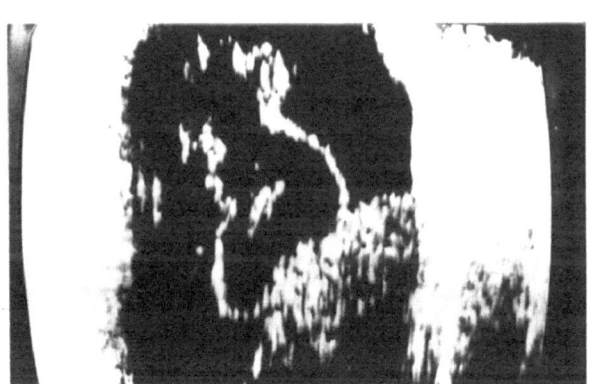

FIGURE 9.25

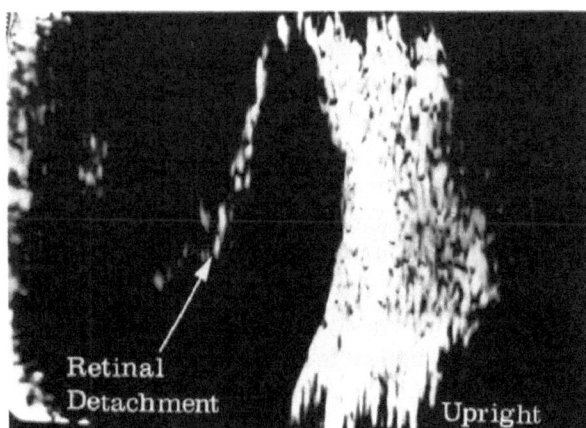

FIGURE 9.24b

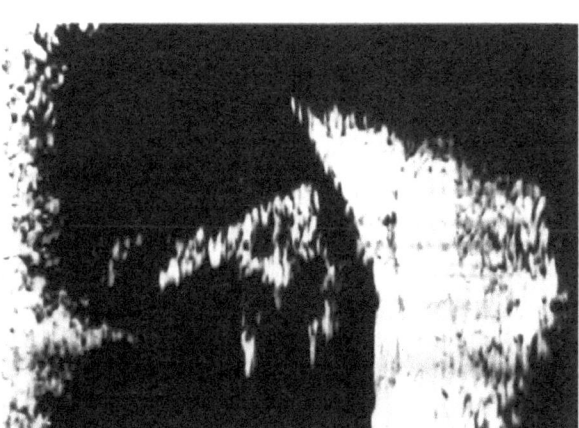

FIGURE 9.26

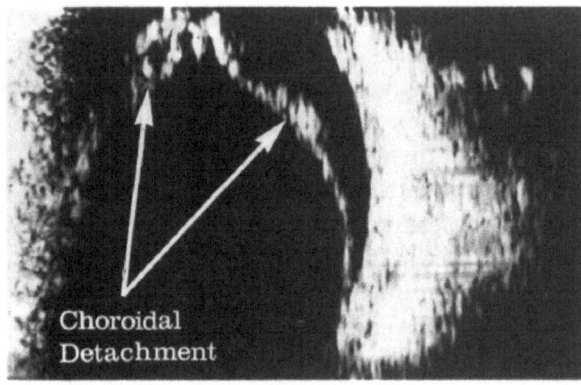

Choroidal
Detachment

FIGURE 9.27

FIGURE 9.27
Choroidal detachment. Choroidal effusion extends from the posterior ocular wall to its attachment near the equator by the vortex vein in an arc shape.

FIGURE 9.28
Retinal and choroidal detachment. Both the curvilinear outline of the retinal detachment and the abrupt step-sign of the superior choroidal detachment are noted.

FIGURE 9.29
Focal retinal detachment. A linear membrane inserts into the posterior ocular wall and lies at a distance from the optic nerve head.

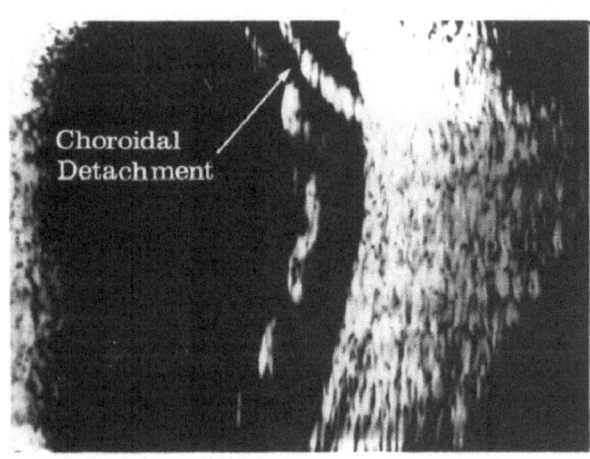

Choroidal
Detachment

FIGURE 9.28

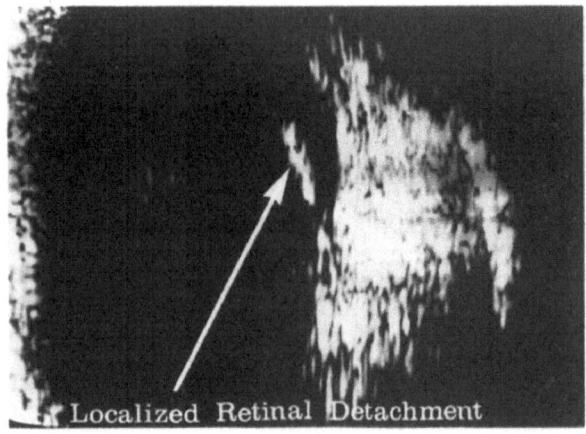

Localized Retinal Detachment

FIGURE 9.29

the choroid layer is pushed centrally in a 360 degree manner and appears as an arc-shaped structure at the periphery of the picture (Figure 9.27). Within the vitreous the irregular echoes of a total retinal and choroidal detachment may be detected (Figure 9.28), and be readily evaluated. For example, if multiple echoes arise from the subretinal fluid space, hemorrhage or tumor must be suspected.

Focal retinal detachment seen often in diabetes may have a normal optic nerve head pattern. The localized area of retinal detachment appears as a linear membrane contacting the retinal layer at various points on the posterior ocular wall (Figure 9.29). Sometimes, the source of retinal detachment in the region of the macula can be evaluated. The macula may show elevation of the retina with an echogenic structure adjacent to a sheet-like echogenic area with an echo free interior which is due to macular degeneration with partial retinal detachment. With sonography, vitreous hemorrhage can be differentiated from the detached retinal architecture. As a result, retinal detachment can be differentiated from vitreous hemorrhage or it can be detected in the presence of vitreous hemorrhage. Irregular thick echogenic membranes noted with vitreous hemorrhage may extend from the optic nerve head anteriorly, persist to 60 dB, have poor motility and a transverse anterior moderately echogenic membrane representing a cyclitic membrane (Figure 9.30a,b, and c). The presence of a cyclitic membrane supports the

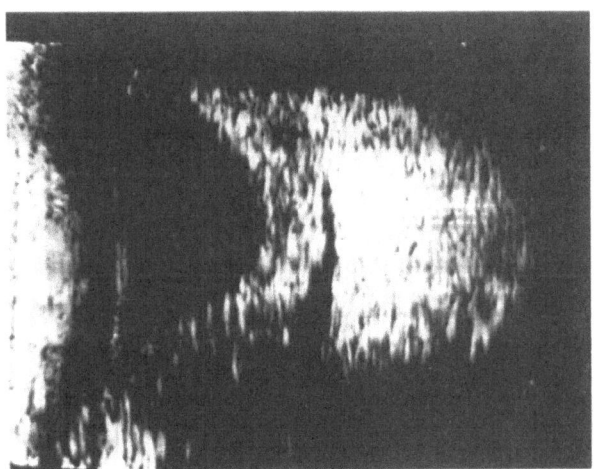

FIGURE 9.30a

FIGURE 9.30a
Vitreous hemorrhage simulating retinal detachment. Long-standing vitreous hemorrhage may have a cyclitic membrane.

FIGURE 9.30b
The echoes of vitreous hemorrhage may be poorly mobile.

FIGURE 9.30c
Echoes of a vitreous hemorrhage may emanate from the region of the optic nerve head.

FIGURE 9.31
Artifactual subretinal echoes. Cross-section scan through retinal detachment shows ovoid outline. Adjacent to choroid are amorphous light area which may be mistaken for choroidal mass. Light artifacts.

possibility of a longstanding retinal detachment, but may be seen with old vitreous hemorrhage. When evaluating retinal detachment the presence of artifacts must be taken into consideration, since a retinal detachment with focal amorphous subretinal echoes may be noted (Figure 9.31). The presence of vitreous echoes with a retinal detachment is common due to the associated vitreous hemorrhage. Subretinal echoes suggest the presence of tumor. In this case the irregular subretinal echoes are artifactual due to room lighting. An echogenic but amorphous retinal echo pattern may be mistaken for vitreous blood. However, the retina is poorly mobile and may be associated with choroidal detachment. Also, choroidal thickening due to early phthisis bulbi (Figure 9.32) may be noted in longstanding retinal detachment.

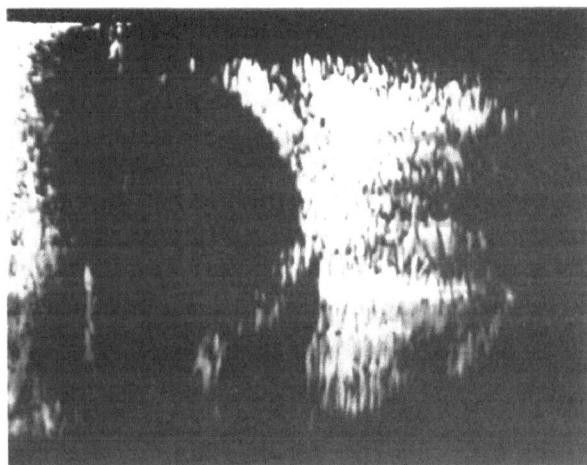

FIGURE 9.30b

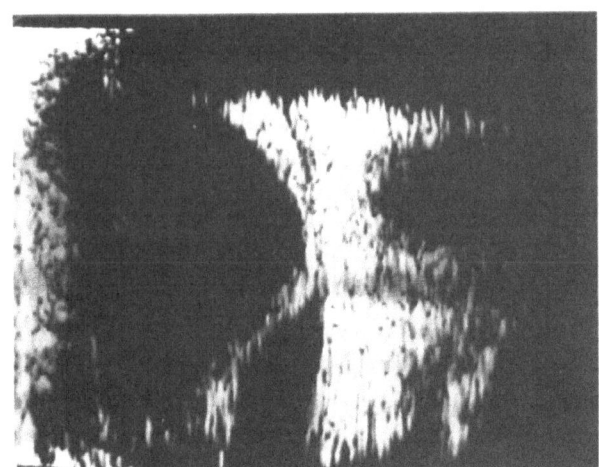

FIGURE 9.30c

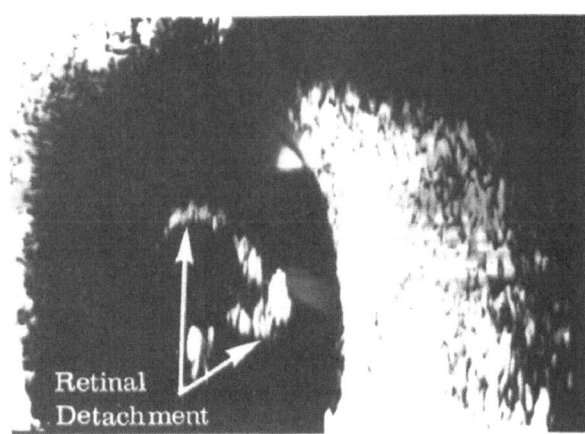

Retinal
Detachment

FIGURE 9.31

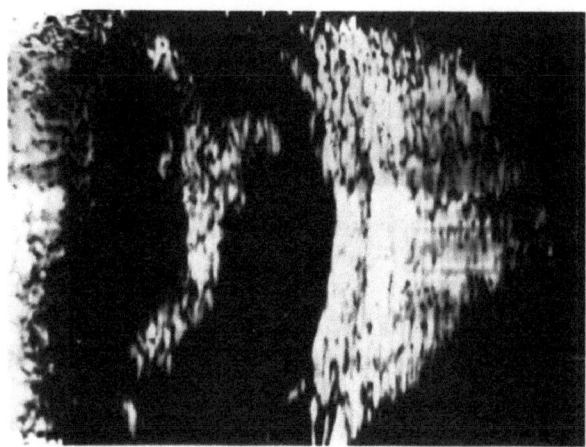

FIGURE 9.32
Retinal detachment with choroidal thickening. Thick irregular retinal detachment simulating vitreous hemorrhage is associated with choroidal thickening in this pre-phthisical eye.

When surgery is contemplated, preoperative evaluation of the retina by sonography is important, because the decision for surgery may be completely altered by this study. Before surgery it is important to perform sonography to evaluate the retina in the following conditions: Opaque cornea, occlusio or seclusio papillae, cataract, secondary membranes, vitreous hemorrhage, vitreous implantation, and choroidal detachment.

In detecting the retinal detachment the sensitivity of the unit should be 80 dB. By moving the probe over the globe or changing the patient's angle of gaze, the extent of the detachment can be determined.

Points of detachment should be seen clearly. The mental integration of a three-dimensional image in the mind of the examiner is extremely helpful. This may be simple or difficult depending on the pathologic morphology of the eye. Anterior and posterior portions of the detached retina should be carefully evaluated. After confirmation of retinal detachment the sensitivity setting should be changed. If the sheet-like abnormal echoes disappear or if there is no attachment to the optic nerve, this would indicate a vitreous hemorrhage rather than a retinal detachment. The retinal detachment persists at 70 dB and is even seen to 60 dB. If the probe is perpendicular to the detachment, this gives maximum reflection and the echoes are always stronger than in vitreous hemorrhage.

The duration and nature of the retinal detachment can be judged because the movement can be recorded by the real-time scanner when the patient shifts his gaze medially, laterally, up, or down. The resultant movement or lack of movement yields information about the nature of the detachment. The aftermovements of a vitreous hemorrhage are rapid and jerky, while movements of a detachment are of a slow and sinuous fashion. Another detection technique is to shift the subretinal fluid. To accomplish this, the patient's position should be moved from supine to upright, and in this manner, move the position of the membrane by shifting the subretinal fluid.

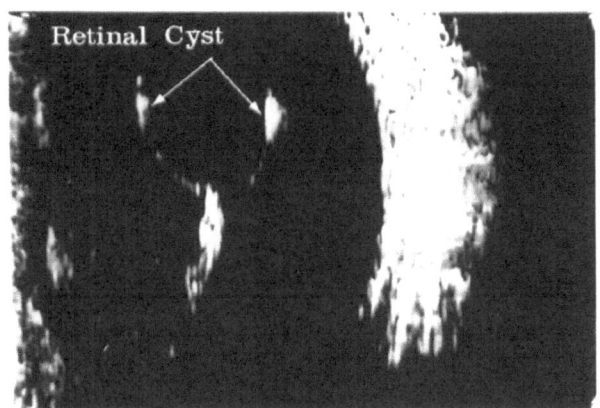

FIGURE 9.33a
Retinal cysts. A large retinal cyst is noted adjacent to a midvitreal portion of the detached retina.

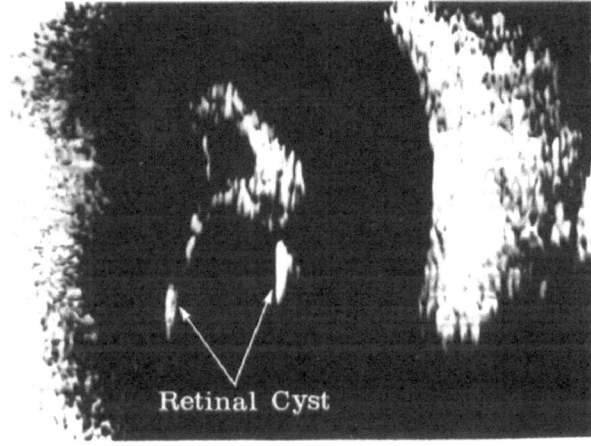

FIGURE 9.33b
Greater angulation demonstrates a second cyst closely related to the large cyst of the retina.

Subtotal or localized detachments appear as a solitary sheet which may not be traced to the optic nerve, and again, this membrane should be differentiated from the vitreous hemorrhage.

The retinal detachment is a strong reflector and will persist to 60 or 50 dB while a vitreous hemorrhage always disappears. In total detachment, insertion of the detached retina into the optic disc can always be traced. The most difficult problem is the detached retina with an accompanying vitreous hemorrhage. The detachment gives strong echoes and the hemorrhage gives weaker echoes with more gray shades. If the bleeding is dense, the echoes may still persist at 70 dB and the lack of attachment to the optic nerve is extremely helpful. The retinal detachment with cystic transformation should also kept in mind, since this may produce a confusing picture (Figure 9.33a and b).

Multiple imaging planes are necessary to fully outline the full extent of the pathological change. Longstanding total retinal detachment with a membrane crossing the ciliary body over the most anterior portion of the retinal detachment is called a cyclitic membrane (Figure 9.34a and b).

B-contact sonography can be used daily after treatment of retinal detachment to evaluate the status of the attached retina and choroid whether or not the fundus is visible. Finally it should be kept in mind that the iris may simulate retinal

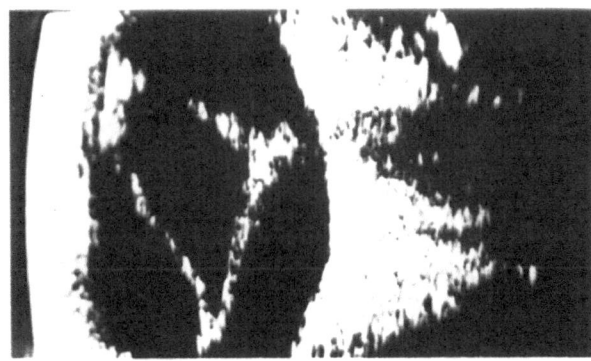

FIGURE 9.34a
Cyclitic membrane. Cyclitic membranes form anteriorly across the ciliary body and appear as a linear echogenic band that is usually thin.

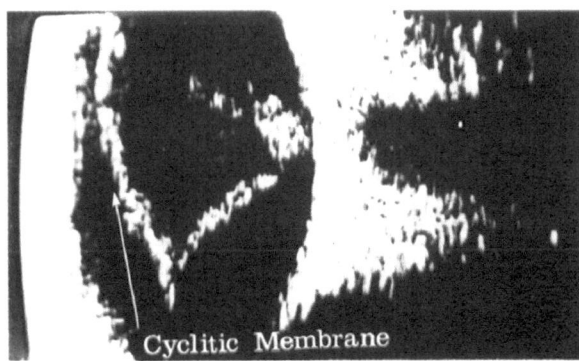

FIGURE 9.34b
The anterior echogenic membrane may thicken in longstanding pathological processes.

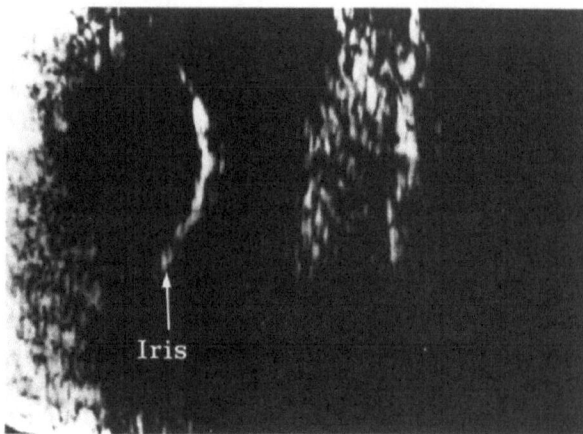

FIGURE 9.35a

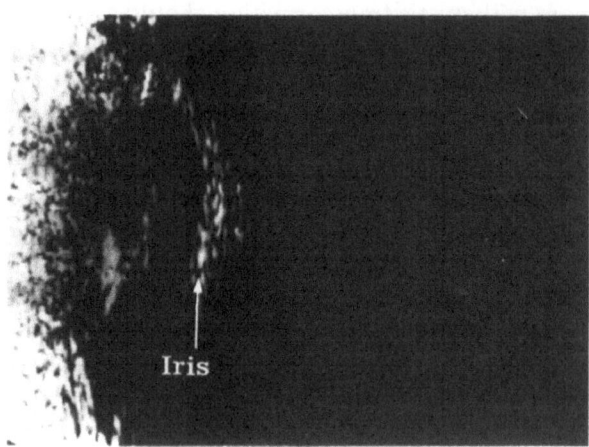

FIGURE 9.35b

FIGURE 9.35a
Iris simulating retinal detachment. The dilated pupil scanned tangentially shows a curvilinear echo pattern. Note that the orbital fat echoes are markedly attenuated.

FIGURE 9.35b
Scanning more tangential to the pupil will demonstrate the inner and outer walls of the iris musculature. The orbital fat echoes are no longer imaged.

FIGURE 9.36a
Subretinal hemorrhage. There is elevation of the posterior ocular wall near the disc with low amplitude echoes at 80 dB.

FIGURE 9.36b
At 70 dB the echoes of the blood are almost not imaged. This entity may produce retinal detachment.

detachment. The iris appears as a semicircular strongly echogenic structure noted anteriorly. The echo-poor nature of the orbital fat indicates that the scan plane is tangential to the orbital fat causing marked attenuation (Figure 9.35a).

Rescanning this area by angling the transducer head more anteriorly usually demonstrates a double set of concentric echoes corresponding to the outer and inner margins of the iris (Figure 9.35b). In detecting early retinal detachment the sonographic finding of subretinal bleeding should be followed serially. In subretinal hemorrhage a localized elevation is noted in the retina which at 80 dB is an echogenic homogenous area that is

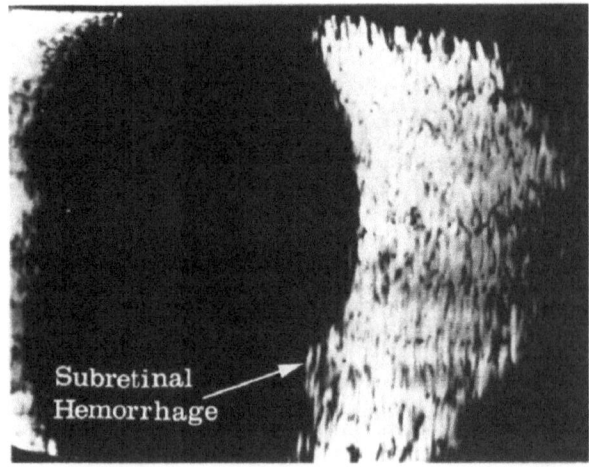

FIGURE 9.36a

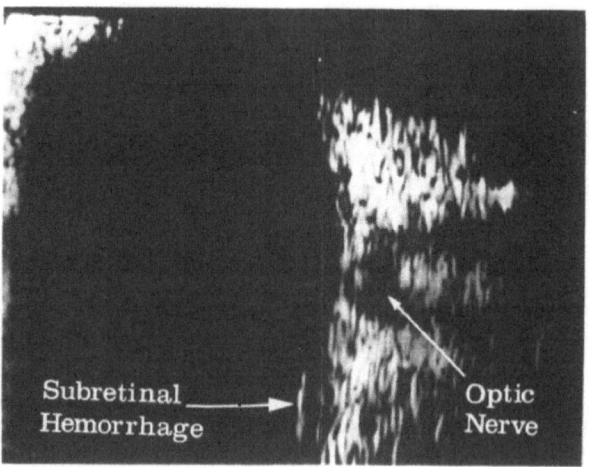

FIGURE 9.36b

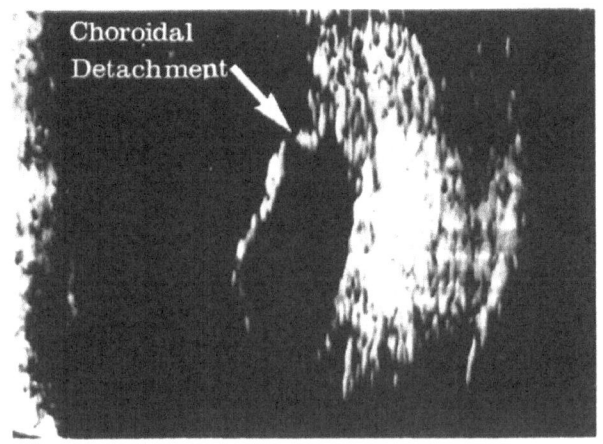

FIGURE 9.37
Choroidal detachment. The thickened choroid layer is noted against the posterior ocular wall and a thin echogenic membrane has good mobility in the vitreous area.

sharply delimited with no shadowing and at 70 dB the outer limiting membrane is echogenic but the hemorrhagic contents are not present at this sensitivity setting (Figure 9.36a and b).

CHOROIDAL DETACHMENTS

Detachment of the choroid is a common transient complication following intraocular surgery. It results most often from hypotony of the globe. It is sometimes called hydrops of the choroid and is an edematous state of the loose outer layers of the choroid and ciliary body. It is more like an intrachoroidal effusion than a true detachment. The outer layers of the uveal tissue are spread out and the space adjacent to this is filled with an eosinophilic coagulum. The separation of the choroidal layers is due to the operated eye having lower intraocular pressure. When the choroidal detachment occurs, the flat or hypotonic eye is further aggravated by a slowing or cessation of aqueous production by the edematous ciliary body.

CHOROIDAL THICKENING

There are multiple causes of thickening of the choroid. Irregular thickening of the choroid layer may be seen with Harada's disease. A very common condition with an enlarged choroidal layer is in phthisis bulbi with lowered intraocular tension. Sympathetic ophthalmia may develop and engorge the choroid in response to the injury from the exciting eye. Finally, leukemia may give choroidal infiltrates.

SONOPATHOLOGY OF CHOROIDAL DETACHMENT

To the beginner in ultrasonography the choroidal detachment is very similar to the subtotal retinal detachment—there is a thickened, moderately echogenic area corresponding to thickened choroidal tissue. Usually there is a membrane taking off from the choroidal layer with good mobility typical of a choroidal detachment (Figure 9.37).

123

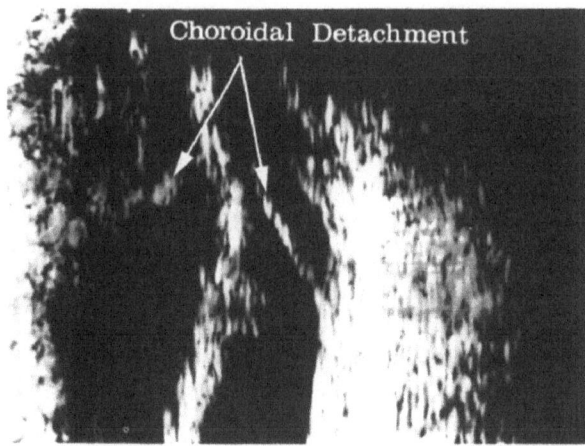

FIGURE 9.38

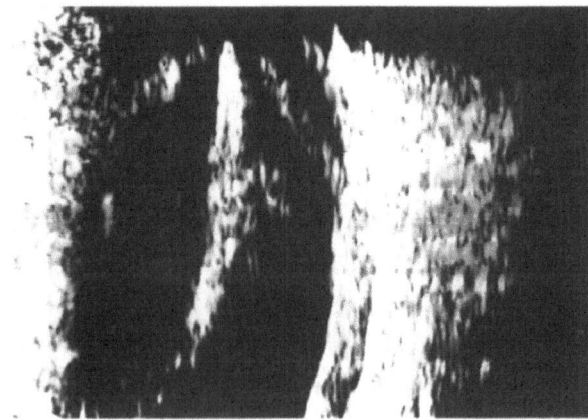

FIGURE 9.39

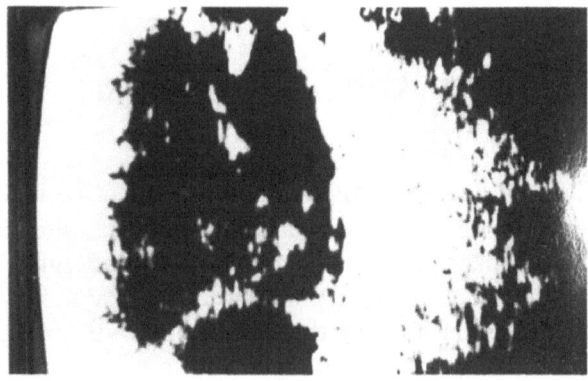

FIGURE 9.40

FIGURE 9.38
Choroidal detachment. Associated vitreous hemorrhage with low amplitude echoes is noted along with a distinct take-off of the choroid from the choroid layer.

FIGURE 9.39
Choroidal detachment. The detached choroid layer is thickened as well as the choroid adjacent to the sclera which is of lower amplitude than the scleral echoes.

FIGURE 9.40
Choroidal detachment with retinal detachment. The choroidal effusion appears at both peripheral areas of the film. Echogenic material within the vitreous represents retinal detachment.

There is no practical difference in the reflecting echo pattern, except in cases of choroidal thickening where the membrane is more echogenic and the choroid usually thickened to twice its normal size.

The choroidal effusion may show scattered vitreal echoes present from mild concomitant vitreous hemorrhage (Figure 9.38), or there may be associated widening of the choroid layer which fills in the low pressure area produced by the shortened globe. Usually the choroidal echo pattern is separate from the posterior scleral echoes (Figure 9.39). Choroidal detachments usually have smooth shapes and extend anteriorly to the ora. In the typical case the choroid layer is pushed centrally in a 360 degree manner and appears as an arc-shaped structure at the periphery of the picture. Within the vitreous irregular echoes of a total choroidal detachment may be noted (Figure 9.40). The described echo pattern and patient history may be of great help for differential diagnosis. It should be pointed out that in the majority of choroidal detachments the echo pattern demonstrates an echogenic sheet-like echo that inserts into the posterior ocular wall near the disc margin and merges with the echo-producing choroid layer (Figure 9.41). When the choroidal detachment is extensive this pattern is usually seen throughout the screen. The completely detached choroid is pushed medially to circumferentially surround the periphery of the eye. This appears as an echogenic membrane running perpendicular to the equator of the globe (Figure 9.42). The nature of a choroidal detachment is usually demonstrated in the

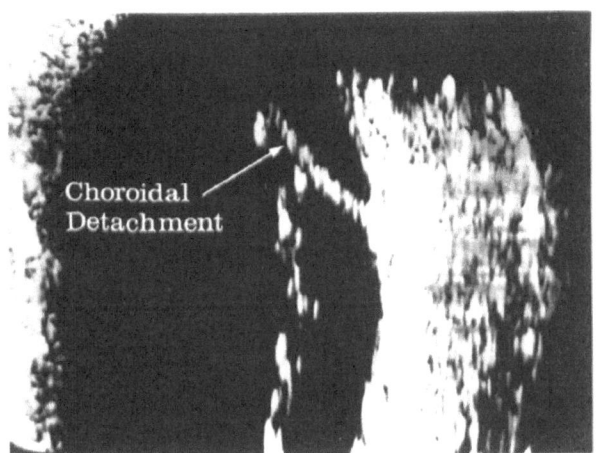

FIGURE 9.41

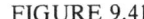

FIGURE 9.41
Choroidal detachment. The choroidal detachment appears as a linear echogenic band inserting into the posterior ocular wall at a distance from the optic nerve head.

FIGURE 9.42
Choroidal effusion. The usual effusion appears as a smoothly arcing membrane at the upper and lower borders of the film. Incidentally noted is a retinal detachment.

FIGURE 9.43
Choroidal detachment. The arc of the effusion is interrupted as the choroid is fixed to the sclera by the insertion of the vortex veins near the equator of the globe.

FIGURE 9.44
Step sign. The take-off of the choroidal detachment produces an echogenic elevated area at the choroid layer.

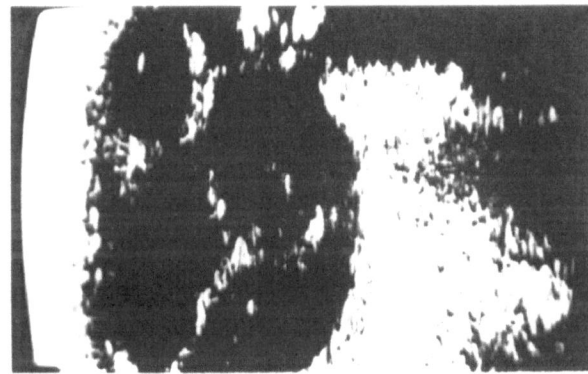

FIGURE 9.42

oblique scan to show that the choroidal effusion is limited by the insertion of the four vortex veins near the equator of the eye (Figure 9.43). One of the most important signs in choroidal detachment is the "step" sign which appears as a highly echogenic elevation of the choroid due to the origin of the detachment. The typical step sign of the detachment can be seen anywhere except in the optic nerve head. Retinal detachments often extend to the center of disc, but choroidal effusions stop at the optic disc margin (Figure 9.44).

An extensive circumferential choroidal effusion may show the arc-shaped membranes to meet at a common point. This pattern is called "kissing" choroidal detachment (Figure 9.45).

Echoes appearing beneath the choroidal detachment may signify hemorrhage or necrotic debris.

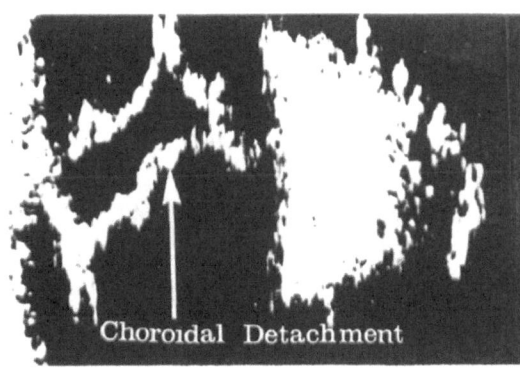

FIGURE 9.43

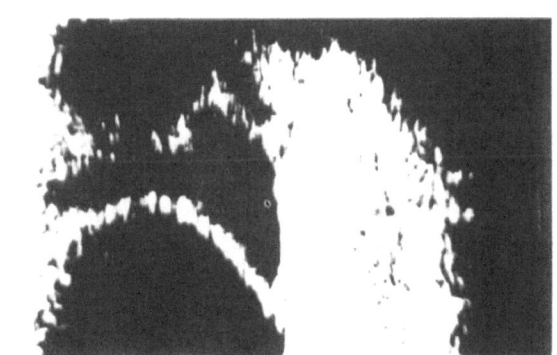

FIGURE 9.44

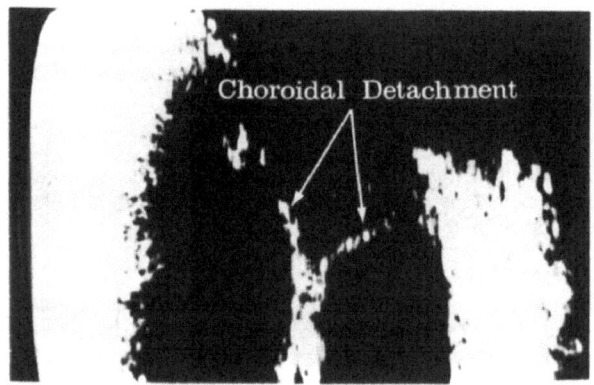

FIGURE 9.45
Kissing choroidal detachment. Oblique scan demonstrates the walls of large circumferential choroidal effusions to approximate in the center of the picture.

However, extreme care should be taken to exclude tumor. In the follow up study of a choroidal detachment this echo pattern may be seen to have subsided. Serial examination may be useful in the evaluation of choroidal detachments.

STAPHYLOMA

Among the many locations of staphylomas, those involving the sclera and the cornea are of greatest clinical significance. Staphylomas must be differentiated from ectasias. Staphyloma and ectasias of the sclera are bulgings of the sclera occurring due to increased intraocular pressure or local decrease in the resistance of the sclera to stress.

Ectasias involve the sclera only, while staphylomas are lined with uveal tissue. An ectasia may be total or partial. Total ectasia is seen in congenital glaucoma when the entire globe is enlarged. Partial ectasia occurs at the posterior pole in severe myopia and at the lamina cribrosa in glaucomatous excavation of the optic cup.

Staphylomas involve localized regions of the globe where the sclera is penetrated by blood vessels or nerves (Figure 9.46). Staphyloma may present itself as a mild depression (Figure 9.47) or in a bizzare pattern (Figure 9.48). They divide

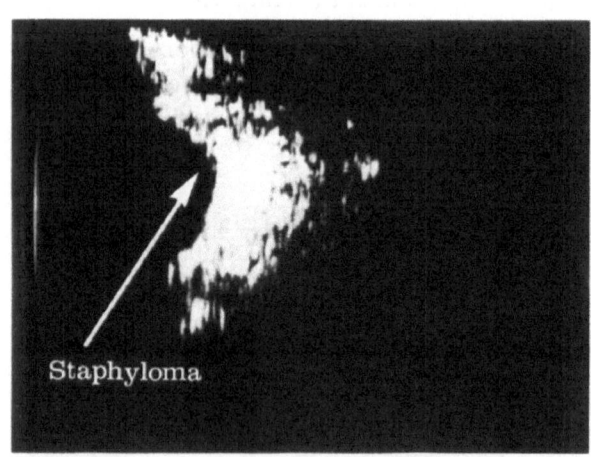

FIGURE 9.46
Staphyloma. Bulge of the sclera posteriorly occurs near the optic nerve head and appears well localized.

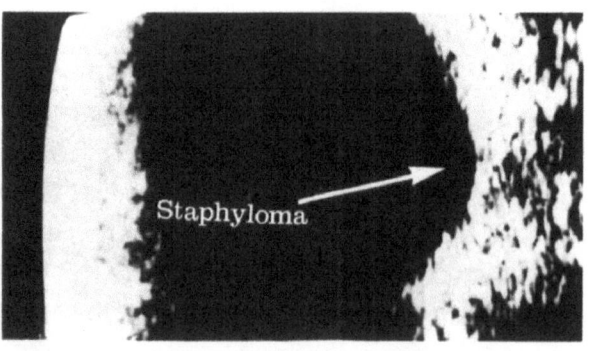

FIGURE 9.47
Staphyloma. Posterior bulge of the ocular wall is noted which may simulate a lens artifact. Scanning out of the plane of the lens verifies this condition.

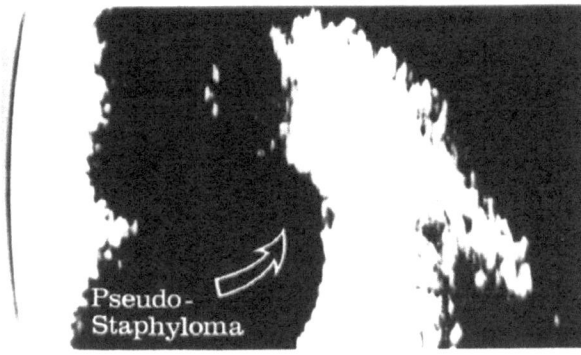

FIGURE 9.48
Pseudostaphyloma. Elevation of the adjacent ocular wall produces a simulated depression to the normal area of the vitreoretinal interface.

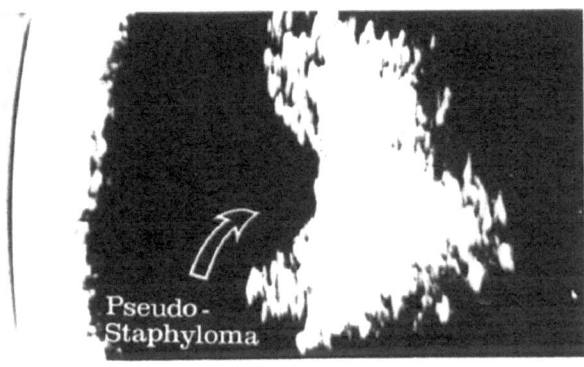

FIGURE 9.49a
Pseudostaphyloma. Vitreous hemorrhage lying in a donut shape on the posterior ocular wall produces a simulated depression.

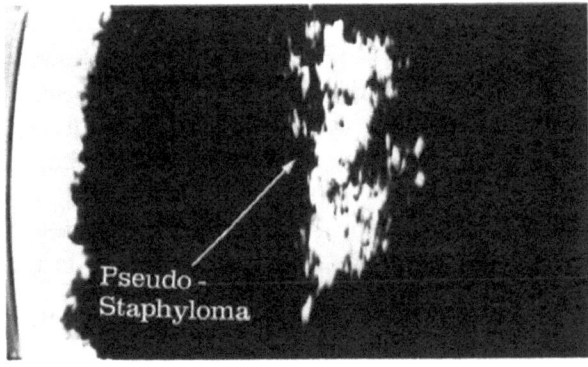

FIGURE 9.49b
Motion of the eye with decrease of the sensitivity effectively removes any resemblance of vitreous hemorrhage to pseudostaphyloma.

into anterior and equatorial staphylomas. Anterior staphylomas occur between the ciliary body and the corneoscleral limbus and are secondary to advanced glaucoma or eye injuries. Equatorial staphylomas occur at the equator of the eye.

Diabetic retinopathy with traction bands often causes pseudostaphyloma. Sometimes a localized area of posterior vitreous hemorrhage appears to have a circular distribution and the irregular echoes of the hemorrhage of the same amplitude of the posterior ocular wall also give the pattern of pseudostaphyloma (Figure 9.49a and b). However, the hemorrhagic echoes tend to scatter following eye movement. Staphylomas should always be verified following motion techniques and sensitivity changes.

COLOBOMA

A coloboma is an embryologic failure of the optic cup to close in the region of the fetal fissure resulting in absence of uveal tissue in the region. They involve the inferior nasal sector and may extend from the optic nerve to the pupil. The retinal pigment epithelium is missing although the sensory retina is present but transparent. The white sclera is seen at the base of choroidal colobomas. Scleral ectasia may be present. A coloboma of the ciliary body may be associated with a notching defect of the lens and ectasias involve the areas near the points of exit of the four vortex veins from the eye. A localized bulging of the sclera may be a factor in retinal separation but this is not detected unless surgical or ultrasonic exploration is performed. Corneal staphyloma is lined with uveal tissue and is an ectasia or bulging of the cornea. It occurs with prolapse of the iris and is found in degenerated eyes following perforation of a corneal ulcer. The anterior chamber is obliterated and secondary glaucoma is present. In the following case of staphyloma there is a localized bulge posteriorly in the posterior ocular wall. This region is removed from the artifact producing area of the lens and represents a defect from previous inflammatory disease (Figure 9.47).

127

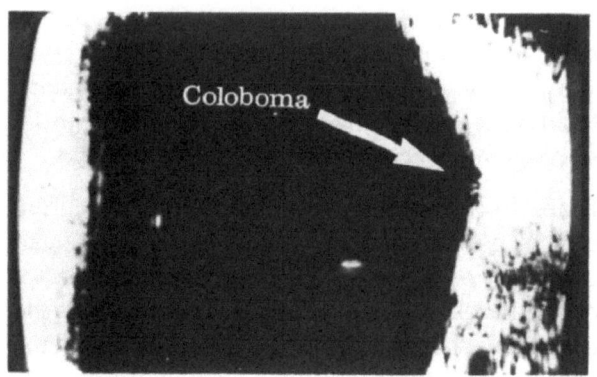

FIGURE 9.50
Coloboma. There is a depression adjacent to the optic nerve head which makes the region of the disc prominent.

PSEUDOSTAPHYLOMA

Pseudostaphyloma is usually due to an elevation of the posterior ocular wall which is pulled in by tractions bands (Figures 9.48 to 9.49a, b). This causes the remaining normal retinal contour to appear outwardly bulging corresponding to the deficient area. The appearance of a coloboma may be due to the prenatal infection, particularly toxoplasmosis. Congenital colobomas of the iris involve the inferior nasal portion and give rise to a defect in the shape of the pupil, which usually simulates a pear.

As mentioned, in coloboma there is a defective area in the retina and choroid surrounding the optic nerve head producing a posterior bulging of the tissues around the disc. Since the optic nerve remains in position, it appears to produce a pseudo-elevation of the disc which may be mistaken for papilledema. The increased axial length of the globe can be seen in cases of coloboma with the disc displayed prominently (Figure 9.50). In some cases near the disc there is a marked posterior depression that increases the axial length of the eye (Figure 9.51).

MACULA

The macula is well imaged by the ophthalmoscope and the ultrasonographer since it is centrally located and approximately 2 DD temporal to the characteristic ultrasonic landmark of the optic nerve head. The macula is an area of great functional importance to the eye, since a small disease process in this area may markedly reduce vision, whereas a large pathologic change in the peripheral retina may be completely asymptomatic. Also, a large variety of systemic diseases manifest themselves by changes in the macula.

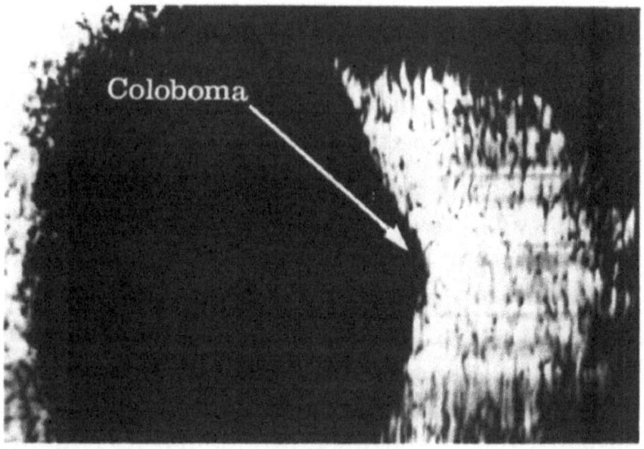

The inner surface of the retina in the region of the macula may produce a membrane in many diseases, but most often in the presence of intraocular inflammation, vaso-occlusive retinal dis-

FIGURE 9.51
Coloboma. The defect has increased the axial length of the eye which is best imaged at 1.5–4.5 cm scan setting.

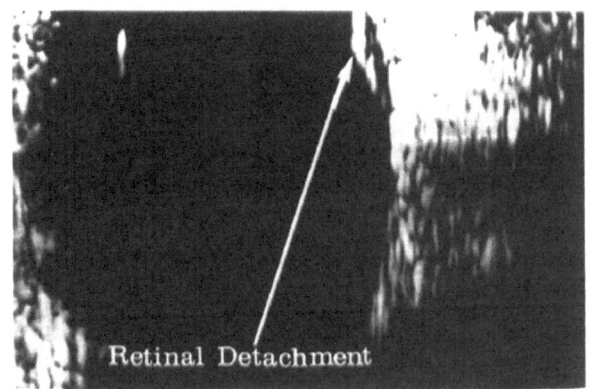

FIGURE 9.52
Macular retinal detachment. Central retinal artery occlusion has produced a subretinal hemorrhage partially detaching the macular retina.

ease, and in degenerative changes of the vitreous interface. The membrane contracts and produces a wrinkled area over the macula. The retinal distortion produced by this membrane is usually permanent. Edema of the entire thickness of the retina is usually post contusion in nature. This edema may affect any portion of the eye, but the patient seeks medical attention when the macula edema affects his central visual acuity. This appears as a dense gray discoloration that completely obscures the vessel pattern of the choroid. The more superficial retinal vessels are not concealed. Contusion edema produces a visual loss that may last for several days. The eye must be carefully examined to rule out a tear in the retina which may evolve to a full retinal detachment later on. Edema of the inner half of the retina is due to occlusion of retinal arterioles with infarction of the inner retina. Characteristically, the distribution of the infarcted area is related to the branching of the affected arteriole. The gray appearance of the retina is most marked in the macula, where it is the thickest. Retinal infarction causes immediate and total, irreversible blindness, due to the death of the retina. Retinal spasm is usually associated with a momentary loss of vision. The usual cause of retinal occlusion or spasm is due to occlusive disease of the internal carotid artery. The sonographer should think of scanning the carotid artery and possibly the cardiac chambers to fully evaluate the sources of retinal emboli. In the case of central retinal artery occlusion, there may be an associated localized retinal detachment (Figure 9.52).

Cystic degeneration of the macula is most commonly due to aging changes. The cysts are sharply defined and may range in size from very small up to ½ DD. Macular lipoid exudates assume a fan shape due to the retinal fibers affected. These are usually seen in hypertensive disorders of many etiologies. The star shaped exudates and the associated marked visual loss from the macular opacities are often reversible if the hypertension is medically controlled. Small microaneurysms are characteristic of diabetic retinopathy and often concentrate in the posterior portion of the fundus in the macula. These may be accompanied by small hemorrhages and neovascularization of the retinal surface. This has become the leading cause of blindness in this country. The presence of severe diabetic changes in the retina signify that life expectancy is not long.

Selective degeneration of the macular cones occurs in older patients and produces a central scotoma of gradual onset. Pigmentary changes are noted and hemorrhages or exudates are scattered.

Peripheral retinal detachments may also involve the macula. Holes in the peripheral retina allow the retinal detachment to progress from the equator towards the macula. Spontaneous degeneration of the peripheral retina usually produces holes in the membrane although this is also noted in myopic eyes after trauma. The enlarging detachment is noted as a progressive visual field loss by the patient, until the macula is involved, producing severe visual impairment.

Ideally, the retinal detachment should be surgically corrected before the macula is affected. A special macular retinal detachment occurs due to central serous choroidopathy. This is most likely inflammatory in nature and resolves in several months. This is produced by a leak of fluid through the lamina vitrea layer, and appears as a sharply circumscribed lesion.

Subretinal exudates are irregularly distributed and may be seen in von Hippel-Lindau disease (inherited systemic angiomatosis) and Coat's Disease (producing pediatric monocular visual loss). Disciform macular degeneration occurs when the lamina vitrea layer is ruptured producing a dark elevation of the macula. This is often accompanied by drusen, and the condition is often bilateral, so both eyes should be examined and scanned by the sonographer since the presence of drusen in the contralateral eye is of diagnostic importance in separating this degenerative phenomenon from clinically similar malignant melanoma.

SONOPATHOLOGY OF MACULAR DEGENERATION

In some macular degeneration there is a localized elevation of the posterior ocular wall just temporal to the optic nerve head. A strong anterior interface is followed by an echo-poor center. This should not be confused with a tumor of the globe (Figure 9.53). Macular elevation may be noted. In macular degeneration the plaque-like irregular elevation is temporal to the optic nerve head (Figure 9.54). No sonic shadow is noted. This entity may simulate a malignant melanoma, but it is distinguished by its typical location and appearance (Figure 9.55). The localized macular changes due to inflammation may separate the rods and cones from the underlying pigment epithelium by accumulating fluid. This is not an ultrasonic entity at the present time. There are conditions where the localized elevation of the posterior ocular wall over the macula could be mistaken for a tumor, but the location and clinical appearance are characteristic for this degenerative phenomenon.

Cyclitic membrane is a post-inflammatory sheet-like echo complex stretching in a linear manner across the ciliary body in the anterior vitreous. This moderately echogenic structure usually disappears at 60 dB. It may be associated with retinal detachment, choroidal detachment, vitreous hemorrhage, or may be seen by itself (Figure 9.56a and b).

SCLERAL BUCKLE

The treatment for a retinal detachment called the scleral buckle procedure may produce a confusing ultrasonic appearance. Since a traction type of retinal detachment may lead to a retinal tear, the scleral buckle is designed to relieve the traction and prevent a rhegmatogenous retinal detachment with its poor prognosis. A retinal tear with or without detachment of the retina may be treated by a scleral buckle. The extrinsic material that pushes the sclera medially is held in position by a small encircling band. This sub-

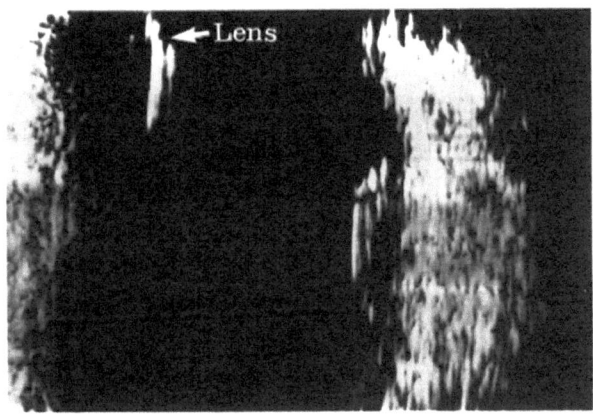

FIGURE 9.53

FIGURE 9.53
Macular elevation. Degenerative changes in the macula may simulate a tumor.

FIGURE 9.54
Macular elevation. The macular area is noted to be raised in its usual location temporal to the optic disc.

FIGURE 9.55
Macular degeneration. Smooth elevation over the macula is noted which may simulate a tumor ultrasonically.

FIGURE 9.56a
Cyclitic membrane. This post-inflammatory sheet-like echo complex stretches in a linear manner across the ciliary body in the anterior vitreous. This moderately echogenic structure disappeared at 60 dB and was poorly mobile.

FIGURE 9.56b
The echogenic cyclitic membrane which across the ciliary body may appear thick.

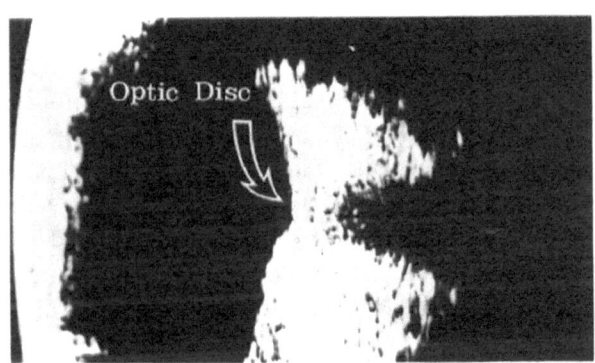

FIGURE 9.54

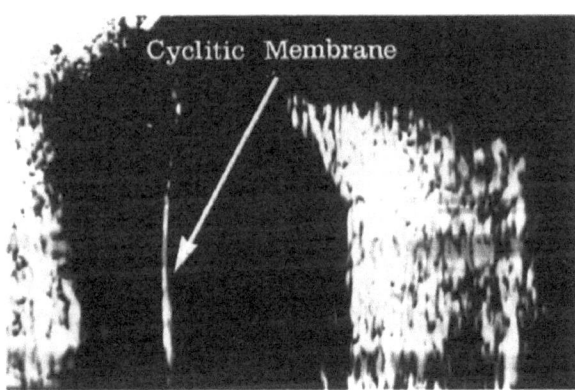

FIGURE 9.56a

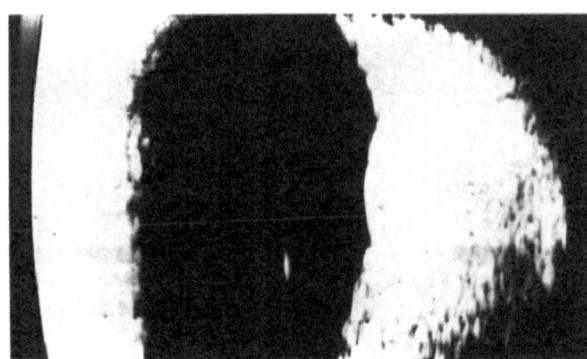

FIGURE 9.55

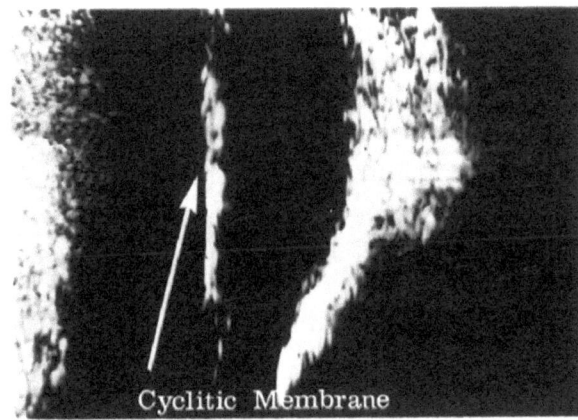

FIGURE 9.56b

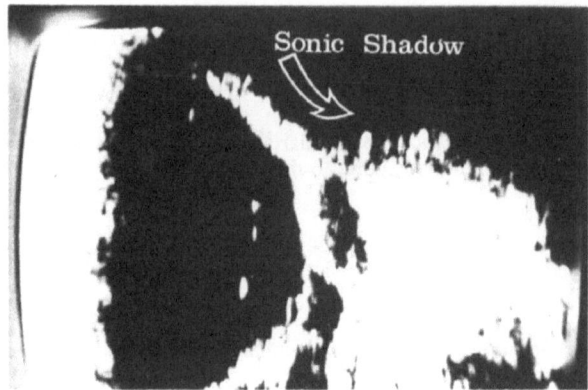

FIGURE 9.57a

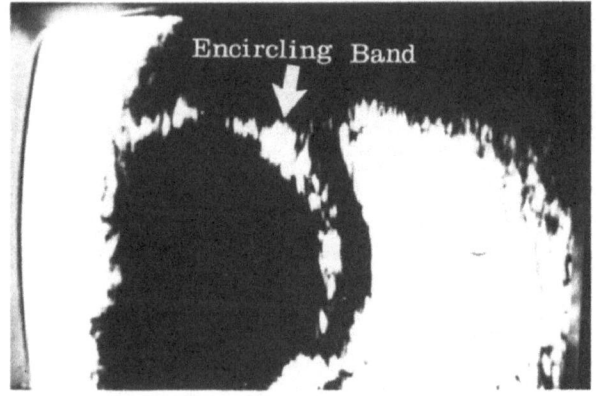

FIGURE 9.57b

FIGURE 9.57a

Scleral buckle. There is a superiorly located echogenic membrane located near the equator. Behind this is a strong sonic shadow indicative of a scleral buckle absorbing the sound beam. The band holding the buckle in place is also noted.

FIGURE 9.57b

Band holding scleral buckle. There is an echo-free zone paralleling the sclera immediately inside the orbital fat echoes which is a device used to held the scleral buckle in position. This band usually encircles the equator of the eye.

FIGURE 9.57c

Scleral buckle. The thick band of echogenic with some distance from orbital fat is secondary to the usage of the device.

FIGURE 9.57d

Scleral buckle simulating choroidal detachment. Posterior echogenic irregular membrane is due to retinal detachment. Towards the inferior portion of the picture, there is a membrane extending anteriorly which terminates in the midvitreous with many strong echoes. There is a sonic shadow produced by the scleral buckle which is not present with a choroidal detachment.

stance is frequently placed near the equator of the eye since this is a common site of early retinal detachment. The material produces a highly reflecting interface in the vitreous and casts a sonic shadow (Figure 9.57a,b, and c). When the buckle procedure is performed near the equator of the globe, it may simulate a choroidal detachment (Figure 9.57d). However, the initial anterior echo from the scleral buckle is much stronger than that of a choroidal detachment and no sonic shadow is produced in the case of an effusion of the choroid layer.

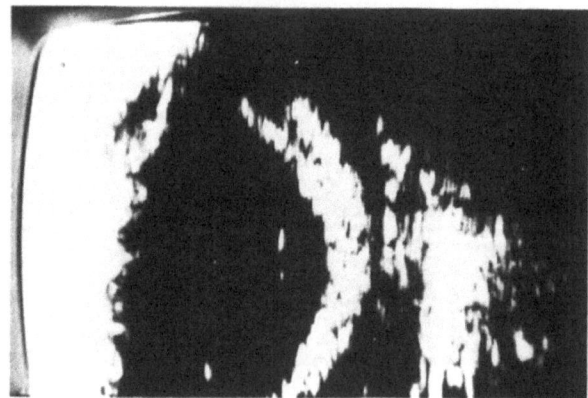

FIGURE 9.57c

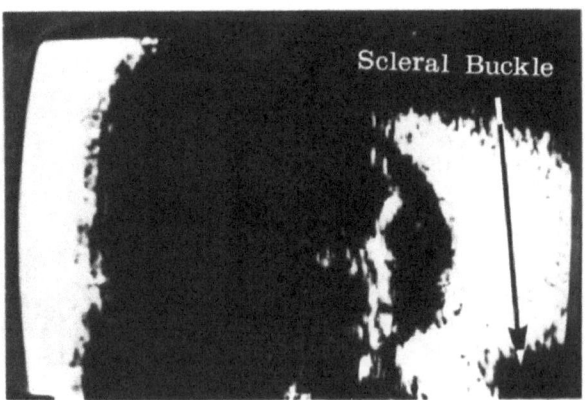

FIGURE 9.57d

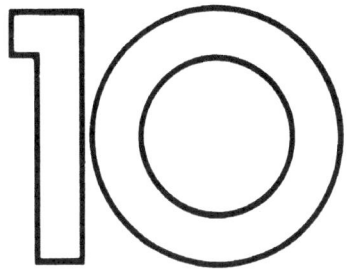

sonography of the optic nerve

GENERAL INTRODUCTION

The optic nerve is a prolongation of the central nervous system from the brain and is the entrance of images into the visual pathways. It is thus subjected to diseases that affect the brain, the orbit, and the globe. Intracranially it is in close relationship to the carotid arteries and regional brain structures. In the orbit it is subject to diseases of orbital infiltration, trauma, and tumors of the nerve coursing through the orbit. The optic nerve head is encompassed by the posterior pole of the globe, and a variety of clinical disorders are noted such as papilledema due to many causes and optic atrophy with its various etiologies.

The optic nerve that is imaged sonographically may have a variety of sizes, shapes, and echo patterns both in health and disease. The nerve may be considered as a flexible attachment to the posterior globe that changes its form and position as the globe moves within the orbit. As the eye moves laterally, the optic nerve will rotate in an opposite manner and lie in a more parallel plane to the medial rectus muscle.

Due to the clinical significance of diseases of the optic nerve, the sonographer should have a comprehensive clinicopathological understanding of this vital area.

PAPILLEDEMA

Papilledema is a swelling of the optic nerve head, usually resulting from increased intracranial pressure, or interference of the venous return from the eye.

Elevation of the optic disc is readily observable both ophthalmologically and sonographically. It is important to differentiate papilledema from other disc abnormalities. As stated, papilledema is the actual edema of the optic nerve resulting from anterior transmission of increased intracranial pressure through the meningeal spaces surrounding the optic nerve. An increase in this pressure partially blocks the draining veins of the optic nerve producing dilatation of the venous system. This venous engorgement is one of the postulated mechanisms of papilledema.

CAUSES OF PAPILLEDEMA

Papilledema is noted in any condition causing increased intracranial pressure, such as brain tumors, hydrocephalus, grade IV hypertension, subdural hematoma, brain metastases, and toxic encephalopathy, to mention the more common conditions. It can also be the result of meningitis, cavernous sinus thrombosis, and severe renal disease. Dilatation and tortuosity of the fine capillaries of the disc and central retinal veins are noted. Hemorrhage, hard exudates, and characteristic field defects also occur.

CLINICAL ASPECTS OF PAPILLEDEMA

In the early stages of papilledema, the vision is not affected. As time passes, the blind spot is enlarged. After a certain duration of untreated papilledema, the blindness ensues due to secondary optic atrophy. The disc is elevated at this point and is detectable by sonography.

SONOPATHOLOGY OF PAPILLEDEMA

The best maneuver for evaluation of papilledema is a lateral approach. However, optimal imaging depends on the examiner's experience and the patient's condition. In certain subjects, an alternate approach may be considered. Papilledema can be evaluated easily ultrasonically when it exceeds the resolution of the equipment of approximately 1 mm (Figure 10.1a,b, and c). The swelling appears as a dome-shaped echogenic protrusion inside the echo-free vitreous in the head of the optic nerve (Figure 10.2). The echogenicity of the edema varies. The boundaries are usually sharp and rounded (Figure 10.3), but may have an irregular border or even a flat appearance. The optic nerve is usually enlarged in these cases and, as a result, in a number of instances it produces a faint sonic shadow sign in the normal orbital fat. As the sensitivity of the unit is decreased, the pattern of echogenicity changes and starts to fade. If papilledema is accompanied by drusen, sonographic evaluation is simple.

DIFFERENTIAL DIAGNOSIS OF PAPILLEDEMA

Other entities simulate papilledema. Optic neuritis produces an inflammatory blockage of the venous outflow and may give an identical picture to that of papilledema (Figure 10.4). The onset of visual loss occurs more rapidly than in papilledema. Pain is common in the affected eye and the lesion is often monocular. Multiple sclerosis and other demyelinating disorders are etiologic in producing optic neuritis. Vascular disorders like ischemic optic neuropathy, occlusion of the central retinal vein, and retinitis proliferans may be confusing (Figure 10.5a and b). Degenerative conditions, namely circumpapillary chorioretinal

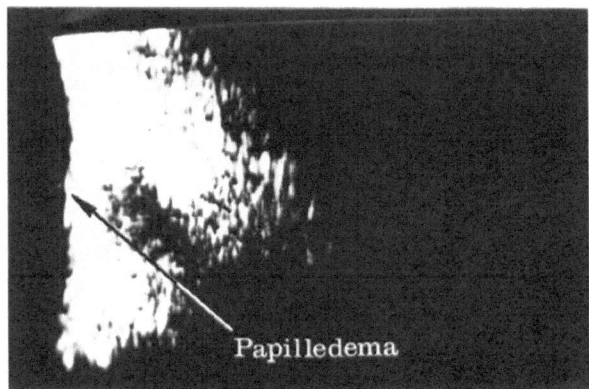

FIGURE 10.1a

FIGURE 10.1a
Papilledema. Early elevation of the optic nerve head must exceed the scanner's resolution and be at least 1 mm high. Scan at 1.5–4.5 cm.

FIGURE 10.1b
Optimal imaging of the edematous nerve head depends on accurate localization of the plane of the optic nerve. Note echogenic slight elevation of the nerve head.

FIGURE 10.1c
Poor imaging of the papilledema occurs as the scan plane passes away from the center of the plane of the underlying optic nerve. The echo of the elevated tissue is of decreased amplitude compared to the more perpendicular scan.

FIGURE 10.2
Papilledema. The protrusion of the optic nerve head into the vitreous often appears dome-shaped and moderately echogenic.

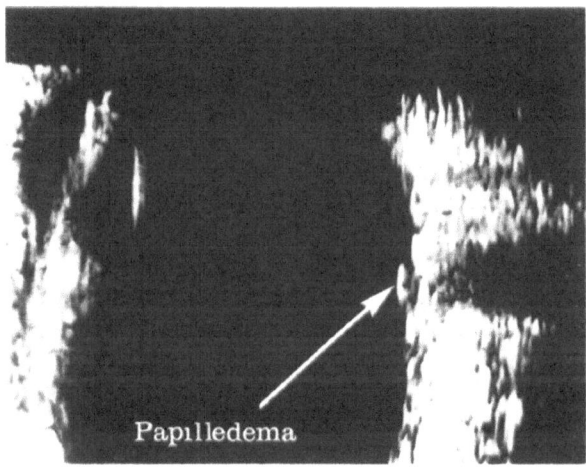

FIGURE 10.1b

atrophy and hyaline deposits (optic nerve head drusen) may produce diagnostic difficulty. Many of the above disorders do not produce the degree of elevation of the optic disc seen in severe papilledema and many have other ophthalmo-scopically distinguishing features. In the sonographic study, elevations above 1 mm may be easily seen. However, in pseudopapilledema, changing the sensitivity does not change the echo pattern of the optic nerve head. Finally, the information gained through sonography in pseudopapilledema should be coupled with clinical data.

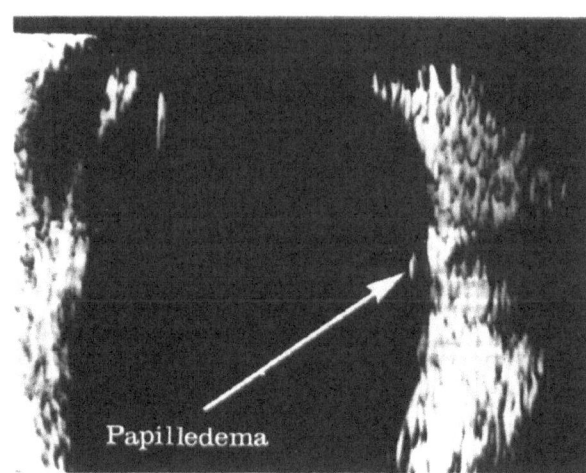

FIGURE 10.1c

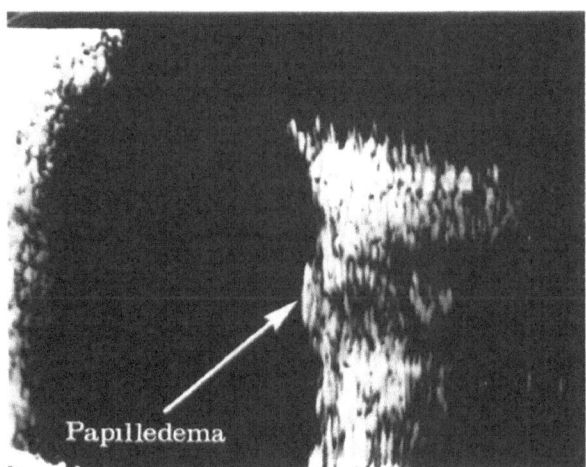

FIGURE 10.2

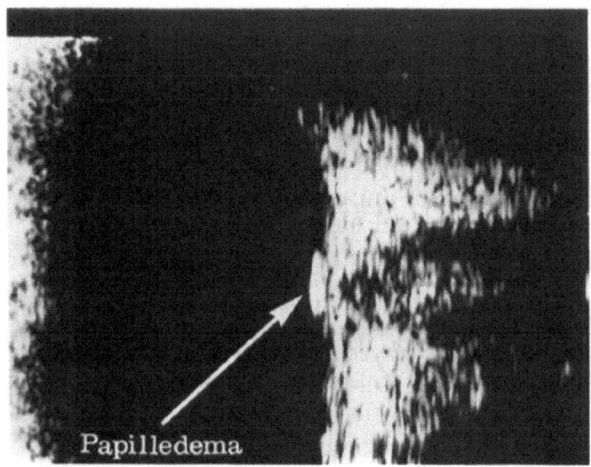

FIGURE 10.3
Papilledema. The anterior outline of the elevated optic nerve head is usually sharply imaged and rounded due to the sudden change in acoustical impedance from the vitreous.

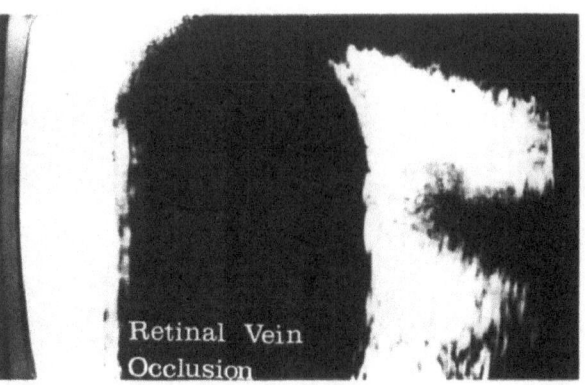

FIGURE 10.5a
Retinal vein occlusion. Projection of the optic nerve head occurs in venous occlusion with engorgement of the optic nerve.

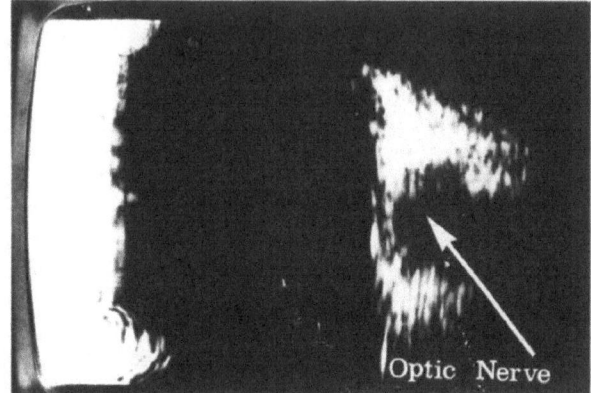

FIGURE 10.4
Optic neruitis simulating papilledema. The outline of the optic nerve is irregular and a portion of the optic nerve head projects into the vitreous cavity.

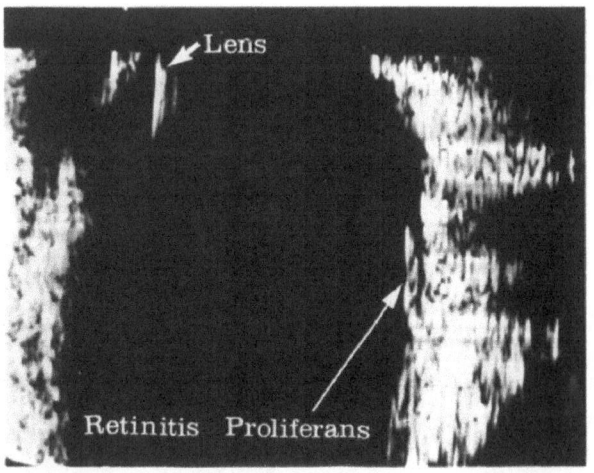

FIGURE 10.5b
Retinitis proliferans. Proliferative, degenerative, and vascular disease may produce an ultrasonic appearance simulating papilledema when the lesions are flat or improperly imaged.

DRUSEN

Drusen are a common degenerative change occurring with aging and are hyaline nodules on the lamina vitrea. They are invisible when tiny, but as they enlarge the overlying retinal pigment epithelium is displaced and they become visible as rounded spots. Drusen are diffusely scattered throughout the retina, but are frequently concentrated near the macula and are often bilateral. Although drusen do not ordinarily affect vision, they are important in that they may be mistaken for other lesions or they may be associated with degenerative local tissue changes which may simulate more serious eye pathology. Their characteristic ultrasonic appearance easily removes this as a source of confusion to the ophthalmologist.

SONOGRAPHY OF DRUSEN OF THE OPTIC NERVE HEAD

In certain disorders such as pseudopapilledema, the drusen of the optic nerve head easily can be seen through ophthalmoscopy. They appear as yellow-white spots in the retina. In this condition, the ultrasound is not necessary. If the drusen are buried deep in the nerve head, they may be in such quantity to produce signs of disc elevation, but not be individually visible to white light. Sonography is of extreme help for the diagnosis. For proper examination, the unit is set at 80 dB; by changing the sensitivity to 50 or 40 dB all echoes disappear except the echoes which originated from the drusen. This is true because drusen of the nerve head often contain calcium and produce strong echoes. (Figure 10.6a,b,c,d, and e). The method of examination is simple. By positioning the transducer vertically at the lateral aspect of the closed lid, the sonic beam is directed from the lateral aspect in the oblique direction through the optic nerve head. Meantime, the assistant changes the sensitivity from 80 dB to 40 dB. The reason for the oblique direction of the sonic beam through the optic nerve is to avoid the sonic shadow sign of the drusen due to the calcium content. In cases of foreign body or dislocated lens, it may be extremely difficult to evaluate drusen. The sonic shadow of drusen is not as extensive as the sonic shadow of calcified dislocated lens, calcified tumors, or foreign bodies.

GLAUCOMA

Glaucoma refers to eye disease associated with increased intraocular pressure which usually produces impairment of vision ranging from slight abnormalities to permanent visual loss. The incidence of this disorder is high, and blindness is preventable if treatment is started early. The population over age 40 is especially susceptible to this affliction and approximately 2% of people in this age grouping have glaucoma. Several types of glaucoma exist, but the most common is chronic simple glaucoma. Glaucoma is resultant to obstruction of the trabecular meshwork and canal of Schlemm mechanism of outflow of the aqueous humor produced by the ciliary body in the angle of the anterior chamber. Loss of trabecular permeability is the pathologic alteration causing chronic simple glaucoma. The elevated intraocular pressure from blockage of the outflow of aqueous produces slow nutritional damage and gradually increasing visual loss in the periphery until the characteristic arcuate scotoma produced in glaucoma encroach on the central visual areas. The disease is usually painless and bilateral. Advanced glaucoma produces ophthalmoscopically visible atrophy and cupping of the optic disc.

Acute glaucoma is explosive and rapidly destroys the eye. Pain and corneal edema occur when the narrowed angle of the peripheral part of the anterior chamber is obstructed by the iris. Aqueous secretion continues and the rapid rise in intraocular pressure stops the circulation of the central retinal artery.

Glaucoma may be congenital due to an abnormally developed filtration angle. This too, is correctible if treated early.

137

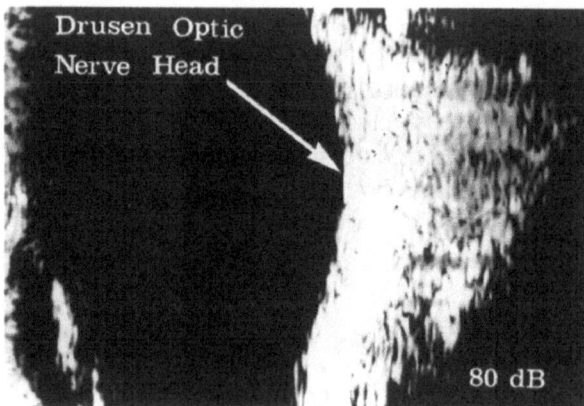

FIGURE 10.6a

FIGURE 10.6a
Optic nerve head drusen. At 80 dB the strongly reflecting drusen is often obscured in the echoes of the adjacent echogenic tissues.

FIGURE 10.6b
Drusen at 70 dB. The echogenic calcium containg drusen begins to stand out as the sensitivity is decreased.

FIGURE 10.6c
Drusen at 60 dB. The drusen nodules in the lamina vitrea appear elevated as the echoes of the retina and choroid layers are no longer imaged.

FIGURE 10.6d
Drusen at 50 dB. Optic nerve head drusen may simulate papilledema but are readily distinguished by scanning with different sensitivities.

FIGURE 10.6e
Drusen at 40 dB. This appearance is pathognomic for optic nerve head drusen if there is no clinical suspicion of a metallic foreign body.

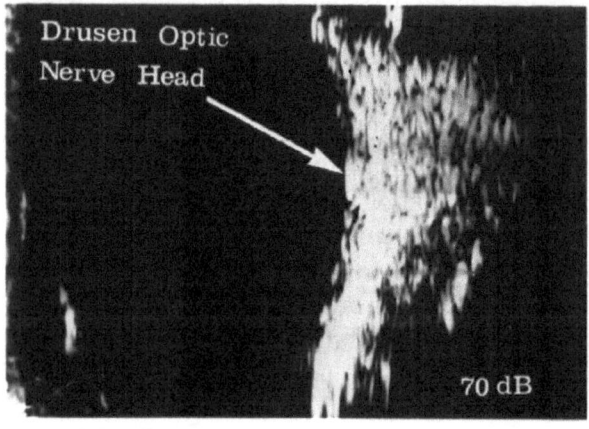

FIGURE 10.6b

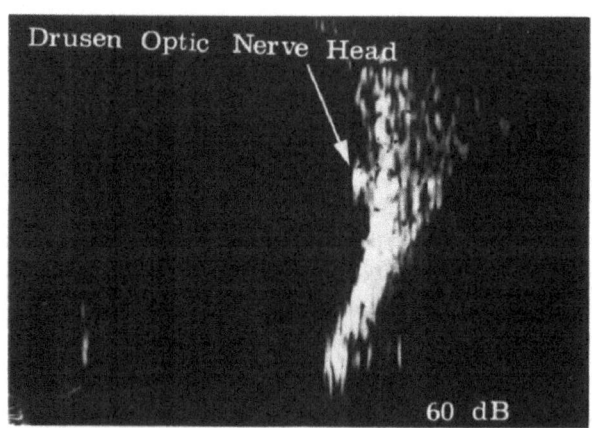

FIGURE 10.6d

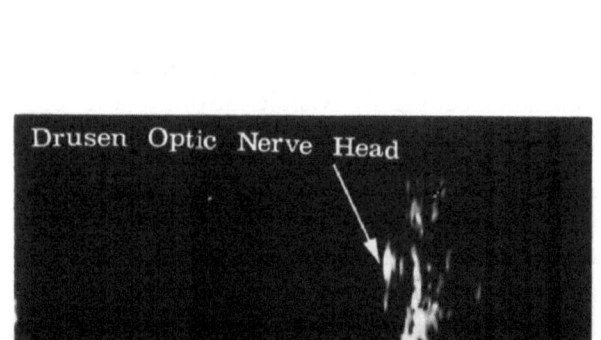

FIGURE 10.6c

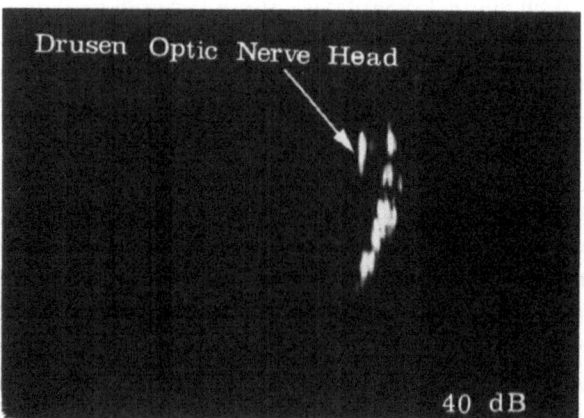

FIGURE 10.6e

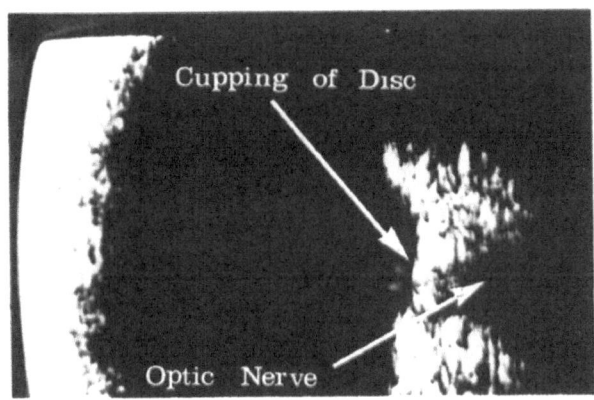

FIGURE 10.7a

Glaucoma. Severe glaucoma with pronounced depression of the optic nerve head will appear as cupping of the optic disc since this must be greater than 1.5 mm to be definitively imaged with the real-time scanner. Note remainder of the optic nerve behind the depressed disc.

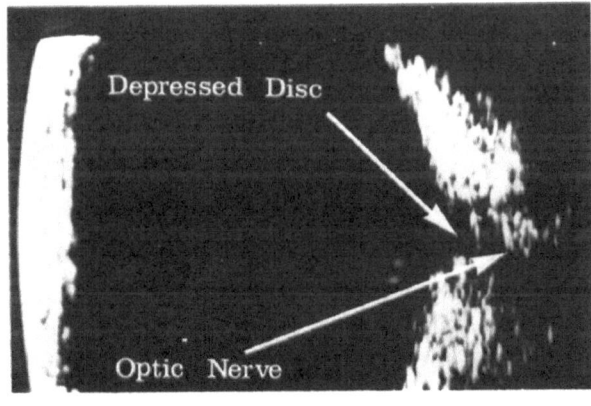

FIGURE 10.7b

Cupping of the disc. The apparent discontinuity in the normally echogenic vitreoretinal interface occurs due to scanning in the plane of the side walls of the depressed optic nerve head which result in a loss of echo return due to lack of perpendicularity of the beam.

ETIOLOGY OF GLAUCOMA

Glaucoma is divided into primary glaucoma and secondary glaucoma. Primary glaucoma may be an acute or chronic congestive (narrow angle) type or chronic simple (wide angle) and congenital glaucoma is also a primary type.

The causes of primary glaucoma are not known. Vasomotor and emotional disturbances, hyperopia, and hereditary factors are among the predisposing elements. Secondary glaucoma refers to elevated intraocular pressure due to other causes of ocular pathology. Aqueous outflow blockage may also occur in iridocyclitis, trauma, severe diabetic retinopathy, total occlusion of the central retinal vein, dislocation of the lens, intraocular tumors, postoperative complications, and facial angioma.

SONOGRAPHY OF GLAUCOMA

In advanced glaucoma there is cupping of the optic disc as the following case demonstrates. There is a significant depression in the optic nerve head due to longstanding increased intraocular pressure in this patient with glaucoma. The depression in the posterior ocular wall appears well circumscribed to the disc (Figure 10.7a and b). If associated with other ocular pathology, the findings depend on the severity of the disease. For example, glaucoma associated with trauma, diabetic retinopathy, or intraocular tumor has a different pattern. The dislocated cataractous lens may produce a sonic shadow and obscure the sonographic findings of glaucoma.

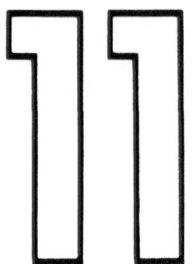

sonography of the orbit

GENERAL INTRODUCTION

The bony orbit houses the extraocular muscles, orbital fat, optic nerve, sympathetic and parasympathetic nerves, and ophthalmic arteries and veins. These structures are far distant from the scanning sound beam and are often difficult to adequately image. In order for the sonographer to take maximum advantage of an orbital examination, the examiner must have a keen understanding of the normal anatomy and the pathophysiologic changes associated with diseases of the orbit, due to local or systemic disorders. Many technical maneuvers must be performed to get the scanning beam to optimally image the various portions of the orbit. The orbit is a treacherous area for the novice ultrasonographer and careful comparison between both retrobulbar areas is imperative. Extensive clinical experience is necessary to fully understand the three-dimensional relationships of the oblique muscles and the muscle cone structures. Subtle alterations of the echo pattern of the posterior orbital fat echoes will determine whether an orbit will be surgically explored or conservatively treated.

ORBITAL LANDMARKS

Proper evaluation of the orbit requires identification of the landmarks within this bony structure. The optic nerve is easily observed in its distal aspect within the orbital fat echoes. At the junction of the optic nerve with the apex of the muscle cone the attenuated sonic beam portrays this conglomerate of structures as a vaguely defined echo-poor region.

Of greatest value to the sonographer in the optimal study of orbital disease are the muscles forming the muscle cone. These may be serially and simply identified with the following localization system. As previously mentioned, the scan head is always positioned with the cap facing either superiorly or nasally with respect to each eye. In scanning the orbit we usually hold the transducer head either in the transverse or longitudinal position. When needed, oblique sections are obtained.

For localization of each muscle we use our identification system which is based on the past five years of practical experience. The right eye is abbreviated OD. When the sector scan is performed transversely it is called TOD. The sector scan in the longitudinal plane is called LOD. (TOD = transverse scan of right eye) (LOD = longitudinal scan of right eye).

Similar terminology is used for the left eye. (TOS = transverse scan of left eye) (LOS = longitudinal scan of left eye).

To identify each muscle we designate the letter M for the medial rectus, L for the lateral rectus, S for the superior rectus, and I for the inferior rectus muscle. As a result, when each specific letter is used in coordination with the above identification system and appears on the films, it is concluded that the specific muscle of interest has been studied. Optimal imaging of the medial rectus muscle occurs when the study is performed in the temporal gaze and the transducer is held transversely at the temporal side. Since the metallic cap of the transducer housing corresponds to the superior portion of the T.V. monitor, the medial rectus muscle appears as linear band at 70 dB passing along the upper aspect of

the T.V. screen and finally will be registered on the upper portion of the polaroid film.

Scanning of the lateral rectus muscle is best accomplished with the eye in the extreme nasal gaze while the transducer is held medially with the cap toward the nasal area and the lateral rectus muscle will appear as a linear band of echoes at 70 dB passing along the lower aspect of the T.V. screen. Similarly, the superior rectus muscle of the eye is best imaged in the maximum inferior gaze while the transducer is held longitudinally and the cap points upward at the most inferior brim of the orbit. The muscle appears as a linear band of echoes at 70 dB passing along the superior aspect of T.V. screen. The inferior rectus muscle is better imaged in the superior gaze. The superior and inferior rectus muscles are usually scanned longitudinally, but can be studied in the transverse plane. For better understanding of the orbital sonographic pattern, it should be kept in mind that in the transverse sector scanning plane with the sound beam traversing a nasotemporal path, the structure appearing as an echo-poor (echo-free at 70 dB) linear band extending supero-posteriorly on the upper portion of the screen will be the medial rectus muscle. The polaroid picture is taken when the muscle is maximally imaged and the assistant is instructed to label the film TOS–M or TOD–M. The letter M designates the medial rectus muscle. Similarly, as the probe scans in the transverse plane from temporal to nasal, an echo-poor image will appear extending from the bottom of the screen infero-posteriorly. This is the lateral rectus muscle and the picture is labelled TOS–L or TOD–L. In the longitudinal scan plane, again with the cap pointing superiorly, the muscle identified along the infero-anterior orbit is the inferior rectus muscle. Since the superior and inferior rectus muscles run at a lateral angle to the sagittal plane of the orbit, special care must be taken to optimally image these muscles. The inexperienced sonographer will easily confuse the more proximally situated and better outlined inferior rectus muscle with the more distal and poorly defined inferior oblique muscle. Similarly, appearing as a mirror image to the inferior rectus will be the superior

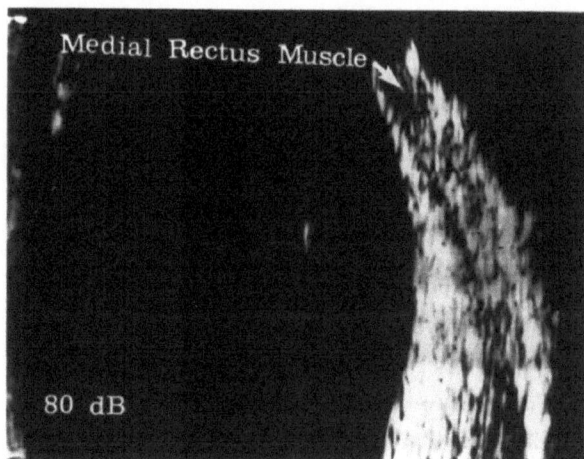

FIGURE 11.1

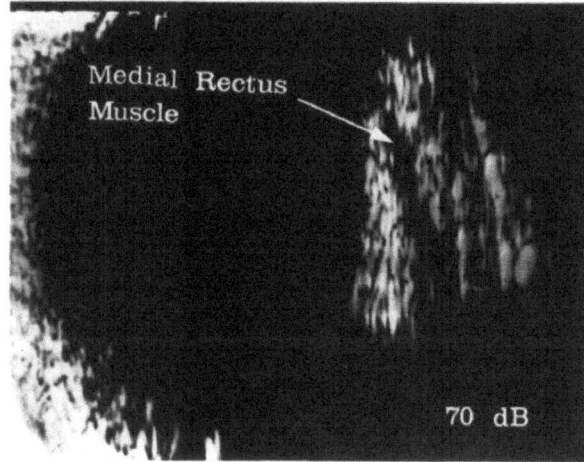

FIGURE 11.2

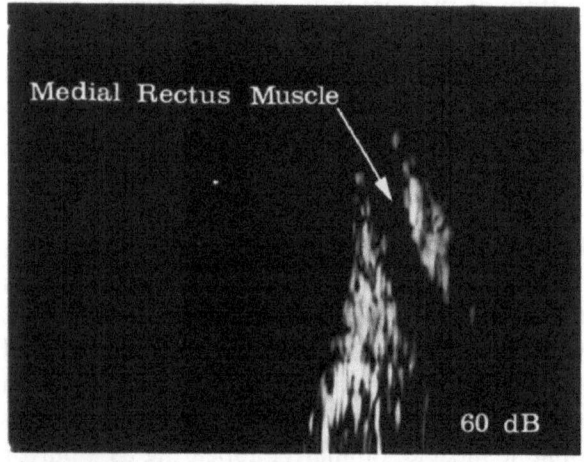

FIGURE 11.3

FIGURE 11.1
The medial rectus muscle at 80 dB is echogenic and extends along the superior aspect of the monitor.

FIGURE 11.2
As the sensitivity is decreased to 70 dB the echo pattern of the muscle becomes echo-poor. This setting is optimal for contrasting the muscles with the orbital fat.

FIGURE 11.3
At 60 dB gain setting the orbital fat echo pattern is greatly diminished in area and the muscle is echo-free.

rectus muscle. Again, care must be taken not to confuse the more proximal superior oblique muscle with the more distal superior rectus muscle. The scans obtained on the superior and inferior rectus muscles are labelled as LOS–S and LOS–I.

This manner of sequential rectus muscle imaging and immediate labelling of each polaroid has proven of enormous value in the geographic localization of lesions of the orbit and muscle cone.

RECTI MUSCLES

The appearance of the muscles of the eye may demonstrate a wide variety of patterns by ultrasonography in the healthy and the diseased state. The changes noted by the sonographer depend upon the scan plane of the transducer, the gaze of the patient and the severity of the pathological process. The muscle pattern varies markedly with the gain setting.

The medial rectus muscle of the normal eye may appear echogenic in lateral gaze extending along the superior aspect of the monitor at 80 dB (Figure 11.1).

When the sensitivity is reduced to 70 dB, the muscle appears less echogenic (Figure 11.2) and the muscle is usually echo-free at the 60 dB gain setting (Figure 11.3).

The recti muscles are usually evaluated at the 70 dB setting since this generally optimally outlines most of the muscular structures against the white orbital fat echo pattern providing the best contrast for dynamic imaging. Also, at 70 dB the

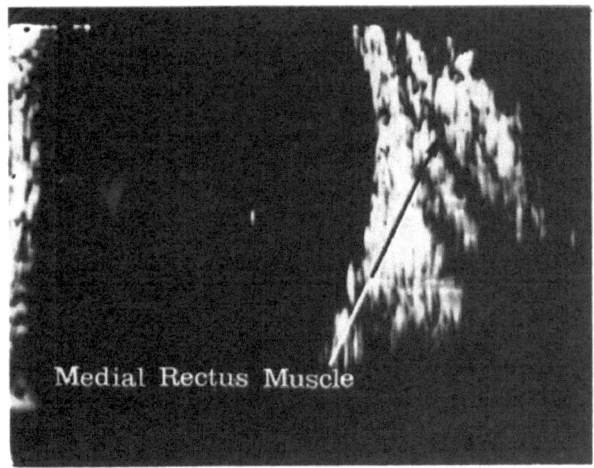

FIGURE 11.4a

FIGURE 11.4a
Scan at 70 dB of the medial rectus muscle demonstrates a linear echogenic band passing superiorly.

FIGURE 11.4b
Same eye shows the lateral rectus muscle to be less echogenic at the same gain setting demonstrating a normal variation in the muscular echo pattern.

FIGURE 11.5
The medial and lateral rectus muscles may be imaged simultaneously producing a V-shaped echo pattern in the orbital fat.

FIGURE 11.6
Extreme angulation of the transducer shows the muscle to lie parallel to the highly echogenic bony orbital wall.

normal muscle is usually echo-poor, this sensitivity setting serves as a rough standard with which to compare the echo pattern of normal variants and diseased muscles. Occasionally we note that the medial rectus muscle may be moderately echogenic while the lateral rectus muscle of the same eye may be echo-poor (Figure 11.4a and b).

The medial and lateral recti muscles imaged in the same scan plane appear as a V-shaped echo pattern within the distal aspect of the orbital fat echoes (Figure 11.5). Extreme angulation of the transducer may scan the medial rectus in the plane of the bony orbital wall producing an image of the muscle running parallel with the echogenic orbital wall distally and parallel to the transducer head (Figure 11.6). At 70 dB the nor-

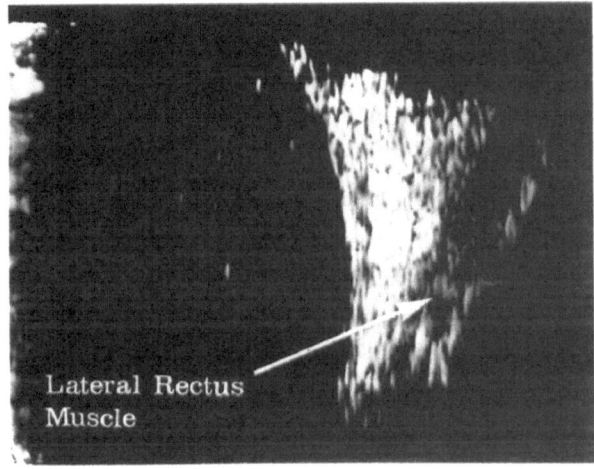

FIGURE 11.4b

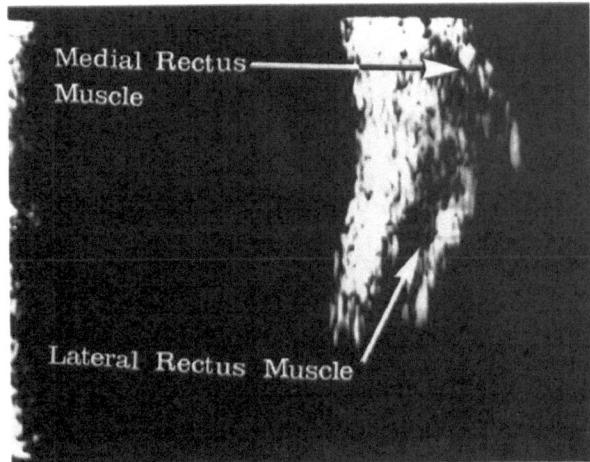

FIGURE 11.5

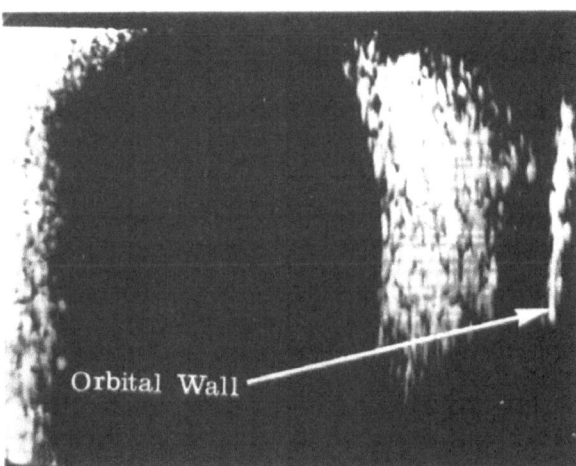

FIGURE 11.6

143

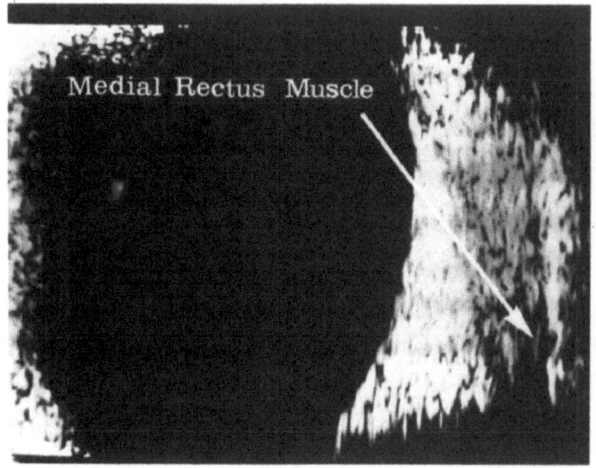

FIGURE 11.7

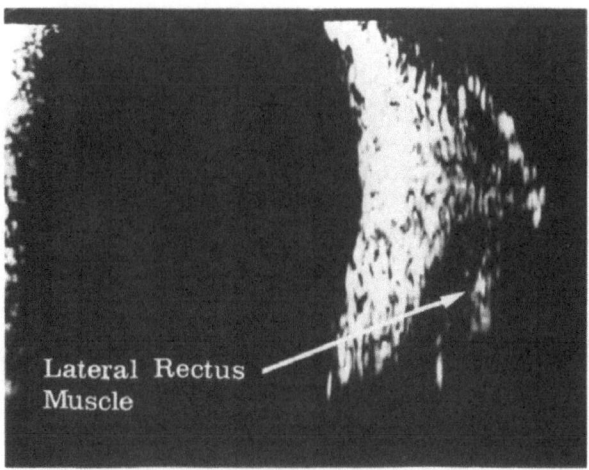

FIGURE 11.9a

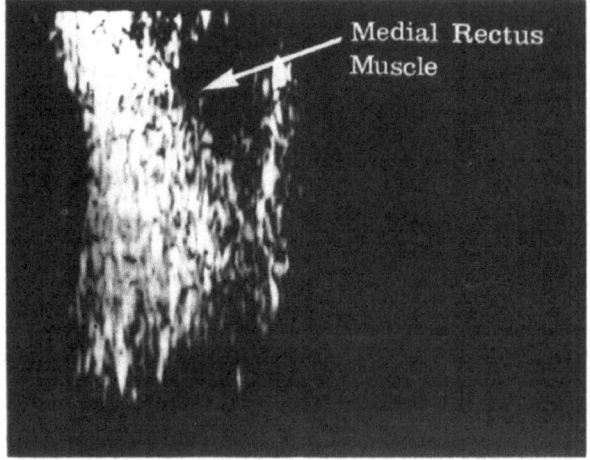

FIGURE 11.8

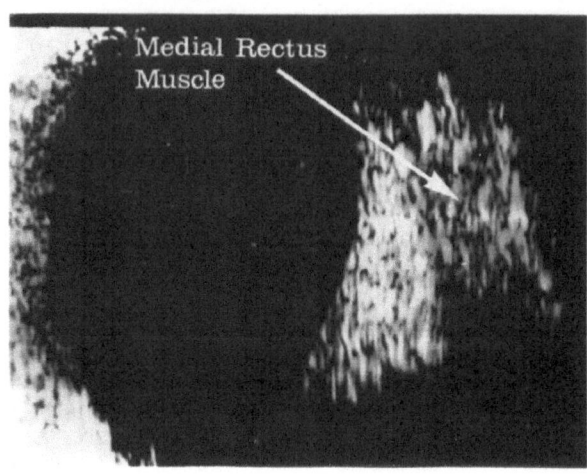

FIGURE 11.9b

FIGURE 11.7
At the standard 70 dB gain setting for examining the muscles, a normal variant may be highly echogenic.

FIGURE 11.8
Echo-poor medial rectus muscle may be imaged at 70 dB which is practically echo-free.

FIGURE 11.9a
Hypertrophy of the medial rectus is one of the first signs in thyroid disease. This muscle is echo-free at the 70 dB gain setting.

FIGURE 11.9b
At 70 dB the enlarged medial rectus is echo-poor.

FIGURE 11.9c
At 70 dB the enlarged medial rectus is echogenic. This appearance is unusual in thyroid disease and may represent chronic changes.

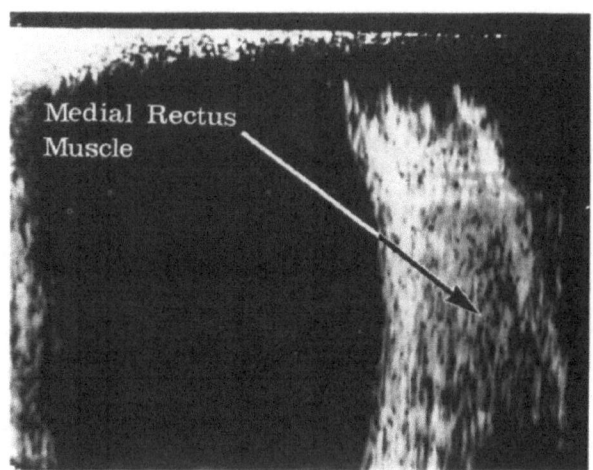

FIGURE 11.9c

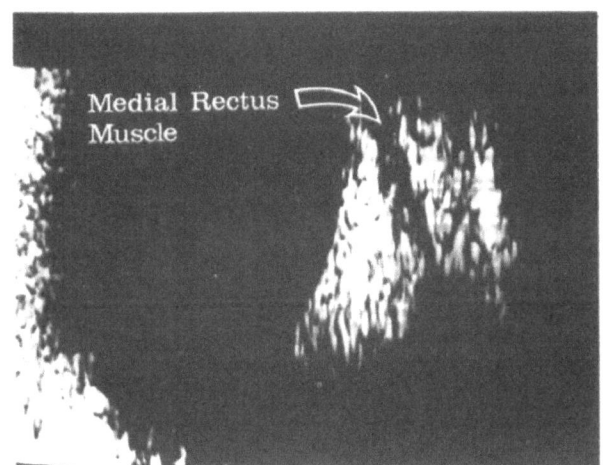

FIGURE 11.10a

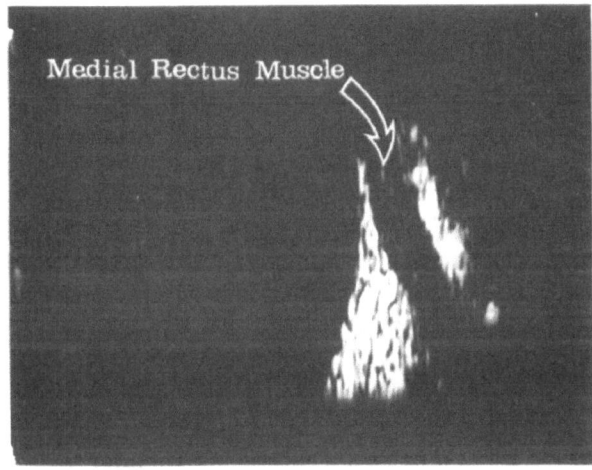

FIGURE 11.10b

FIGURE 11.10a
Pseudohypertrophy. The normally echo-poor medial rectus muscle is of normal size.

FIGURE 11.10b
Oblique scanning enlarges the outline of the muscle and decreases the echogenicity.

FIGURE 11.11a
Gaze position. Frontal scan showing echo-poor and short segment of the lateral rectus muscle.

FIGURE 11.11b
Extreme gaze demonstrates the same muscle to be elongated and of greater echogenicity.

mal muscle may be highly echogenic (Figure 11.7), or almost echo-free (Figure 11.8). The medial rectus muscle is one of the first muscles to become enlarged in thyroid disorders. Hypertrophy of the medial rectus muscle may be echo-poor (Figure 11.9a), echogenic (Figure 11.9b), or echo dense (Figure 11.9c). Pseudoenlargement of the medial rectus may occur when the muscle is scanned in an oblique manner with the scan beam traversing the muscle over a longer diameter and with less perpendicularity of the sound waves to the structure. The slightly echogenic muscle becomes echo-poor and wider (Figure 11.10a and b). This is often accompanied by a decrease in the echo return from the orbital fat creating a smaller orbital fat echo complex.

The lateral rectus muscle occupies the infero-posterior region of the monitor and is imaged in

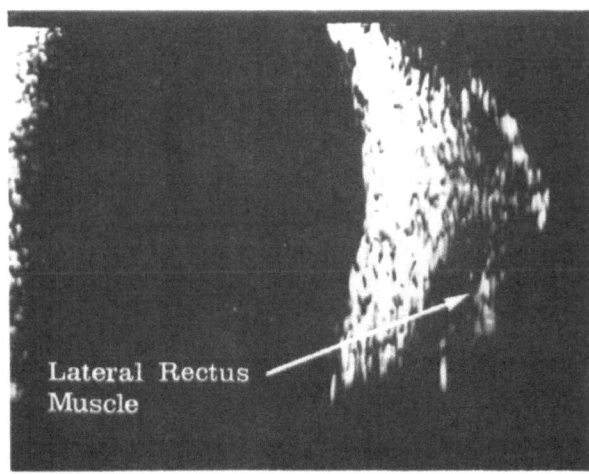

-FIGURE 11.11a

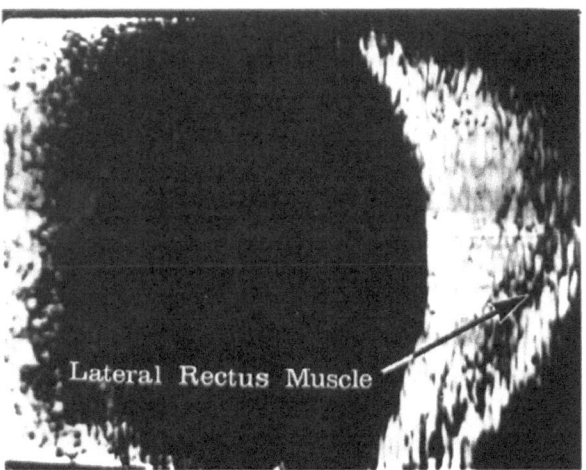

FIGURE 11.11b

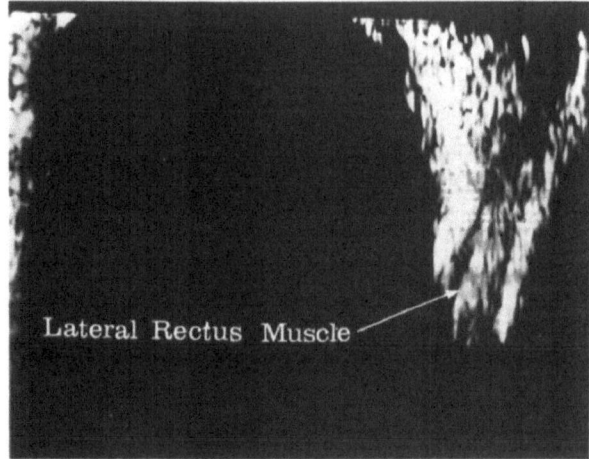

FIGURE 11.12a

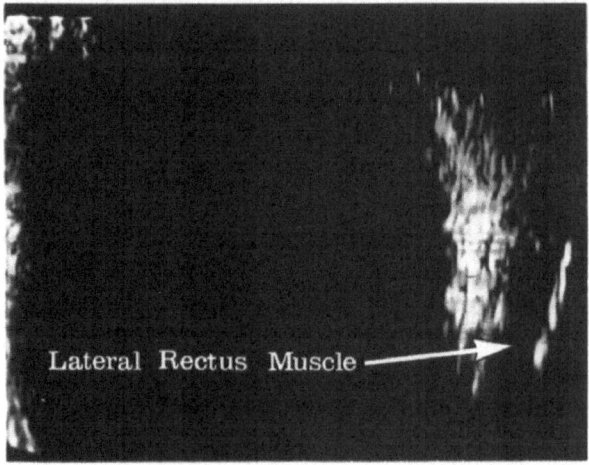

FIGURE 11.12b

FIGURE 11.12a
Normal lateral rectus muscle. The linear band-like echo passing inferiorly may be echogenic at 70 dB.

FIGURE 11.12b
At 70 dB the lateral rectus muscle may be echo-poor.

FIGURE 11.13a
Thyroid disease. Echogenic lateral rectus may be due to fibrotic changes and is not common.

FIGURE 11.13b
Echo-poor lateral rectus muscle noted in acute Grave's disease.

the previously described manner. At 70 dB it appears slightly echogenic. The echogenicity of the recti muscles depends not only on the gain setting and the transducer angulation, but also on the gaze of the patient. As the gaze deviates to the maximal stretch of the muscle, the muscle becomes elongated in the scan and slightly more echogenic as it assumes a position more normal to the interrogating sound beam (Figure 11.11a and b). Normal variations include the lateral rectus muscle being echogenic (Figure 11.12a) and almost echo-free at the 70 dB gain setting (Figure 11.12b). Hypertrophy of the lateral rectus muscle occurs in thyroid conditions and the muscle may be echogenic (Figure 11.13a), but it is most often echo-poor or echo-free (Figure 11.13b). When an enlarged muscle is noted in cross section, it may simulate an orbital tumor if the sonographer does not produce an accurate

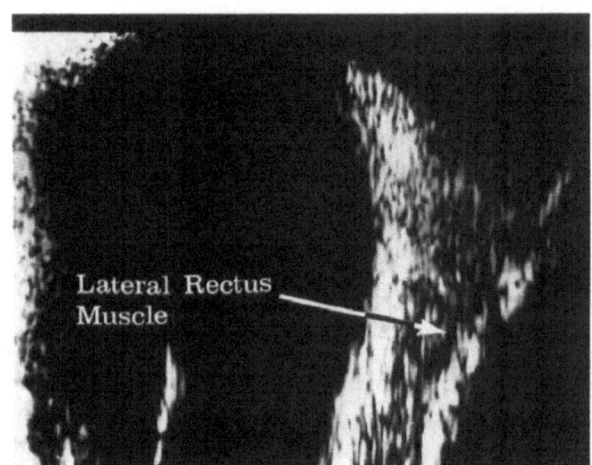

FIGURE 11.13a

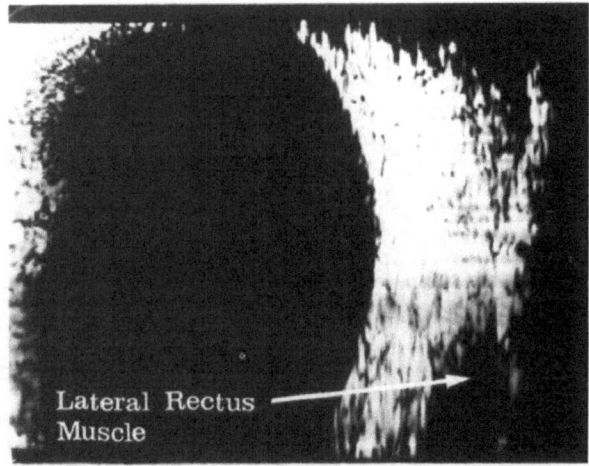

FIGURE 11.13b

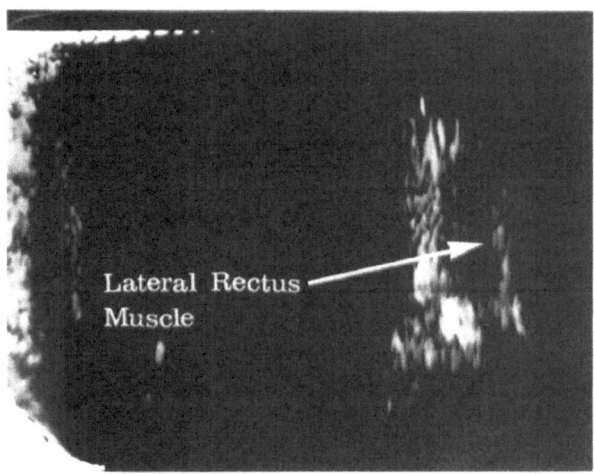

FIGURE 11.13c

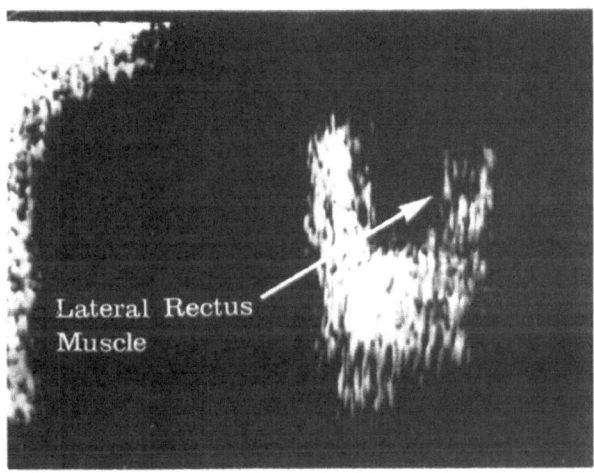

FIGURE 11.13d

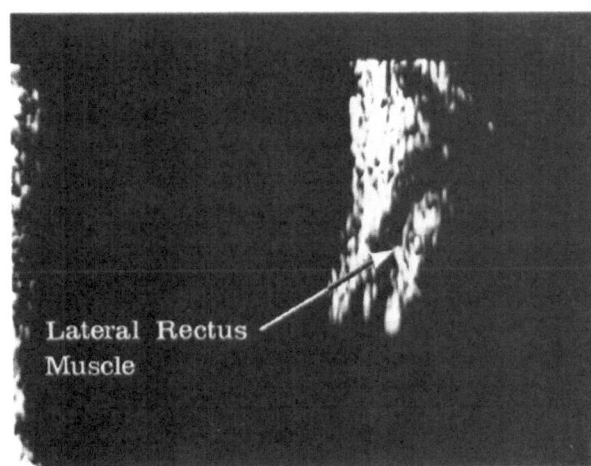

FIGURE 11.14

FIGURE 11.13c
Cross section of 11.13a demonstrates slightly echogenic area simulating orbital tumor.

FIGURE 11.13d
Cross section of 11.13b shows echo-poor area displacing the orbital fat echoes. Three-dimensional scanning is necessary to demonstrate that this is not a lesion.

FIGURE 11.14
Echo-poor zone occurs at the junction of the proximal portions of the medial and lateral rectus muscles. This is to be recognized as a normal variant.

three-dimensional representation of this entity (Figure 11.13c and d). At the junction of the medial and lateral rectus muscles an echo-free zone may be produced demarcating the apex of the muscle cone. This echo-poor or echo-free region should not be confused with a pathological condition (Figure 11.14).

Similarly, the superior rectus and inferior rectus muscles appear at the corresponding upper and lower parts of the television monitor when scanning (Figure 11.15a and b) and may exhibit the same changes described for the other muscles.

The muscles may be so enlarged that they cannot be adequately imaged in the usual scan depth of 1–3 cm and the unit is then switched to the 1.5–4.5 depth setting which provides better delineation of these structures. When evaluating the muscles of the orbit at the medium range depth setting, their size, shape, position, and echo pattern are noted as well as their through-transmission characteristics. This latter parameter, through-transmission, cannot be studied at the near field setting since the sonographer relies on the change in the echo pattern of structures distal to the area under investigation for assessment of through-transmission pattern (Figure 11.16a b, and c).

Rectus muscles may have a flame shape (Figure 11.17a) or a wedge shape (Figure 11.17b). These oddly shaped rectus muscles that are enlarged must not be mistaken for a true tumor of the orbit (Figure 11.17c). However, tumors of the orbit often have other characteristics that distinguish them from anomalous muscular structures. The echoes of the muscles may merge with those

147

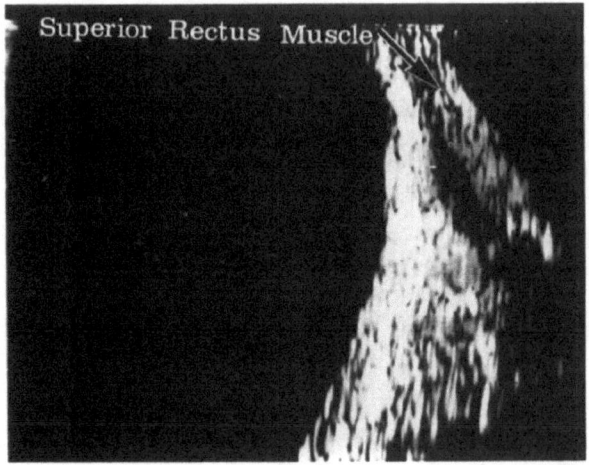

FIGURE 11.15a

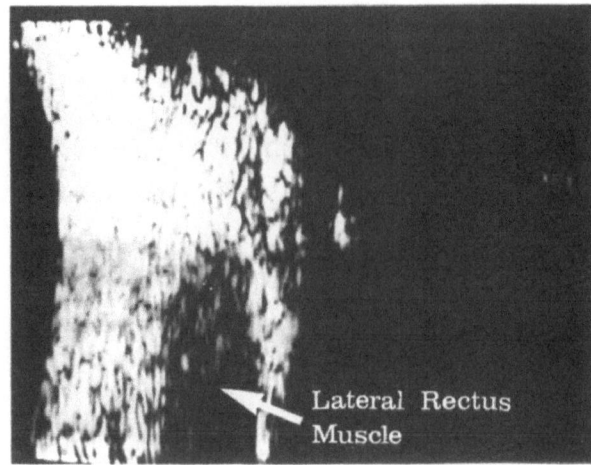

FIGURE 11.16a

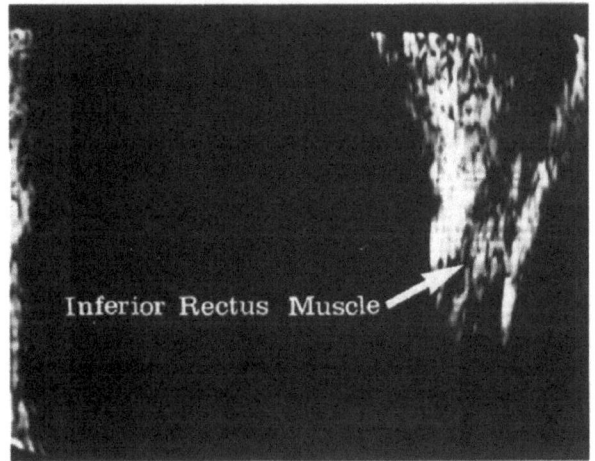

FIGURE 11.15b

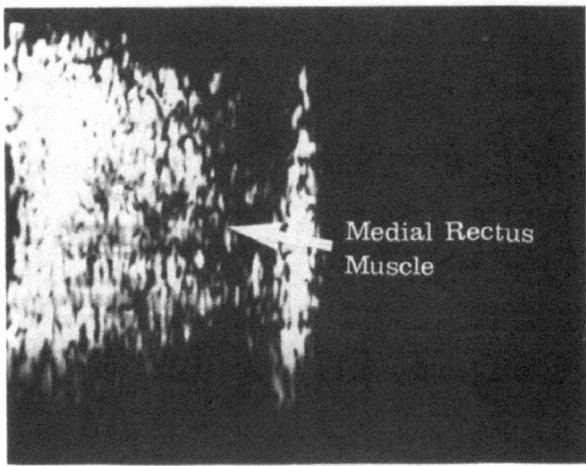

FIGURE 11.16b

FIGURE 11.15a
Superior rectus muscle. Echo-poor band runs superiorly across the monitor.

FIGURE 11.15b
Inferior rectus muscle. Slightly echogenic linear zone passes inferiorly on the scan.

FIGURE 11.16a
Hypertrophic rectus muscle. Enlarged lateral rectus muscle is well imaged at the 1.5–4.5 cm scan depth.

FIGURE 11.16b
Superior rectus muscle is echo-poor with decreased through-transmission.

FIGURE 11.16c
Medial rectus muscle is massively enlarged having high through-transmission and an irregular echo pattern.

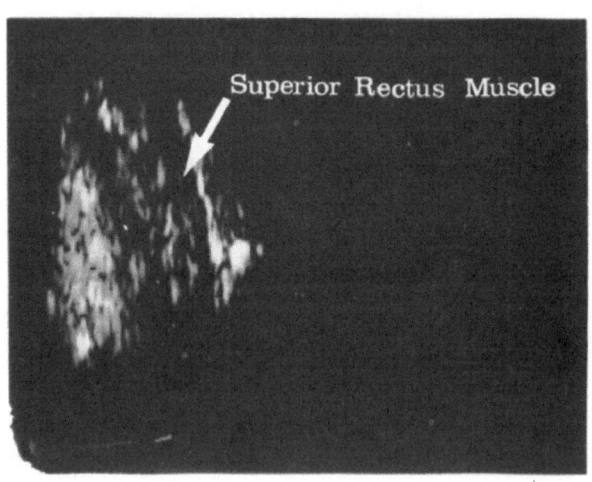

FIGURE 11.16c

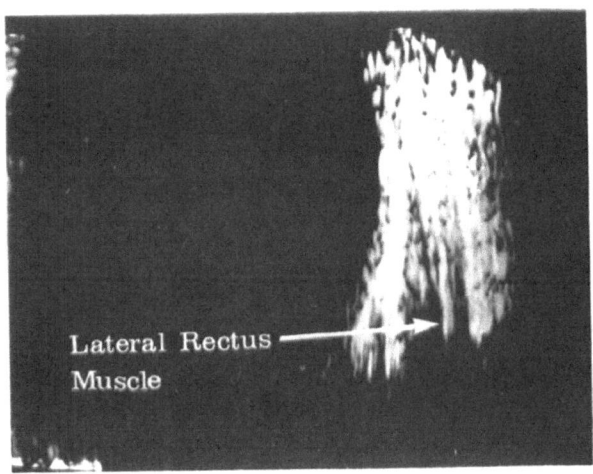

FIGURE 11.17a

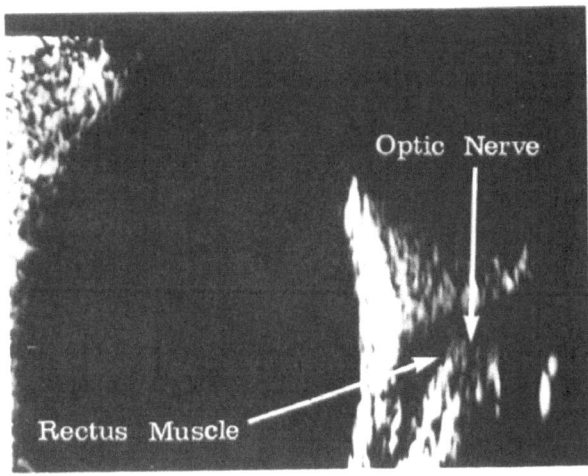

FIGURE 11.18a

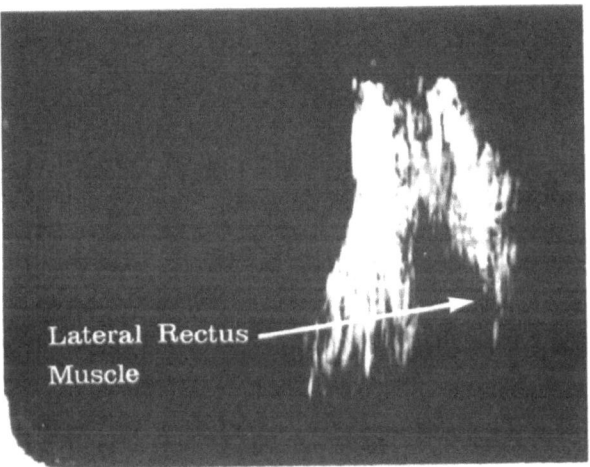

FIGURE 11.17b

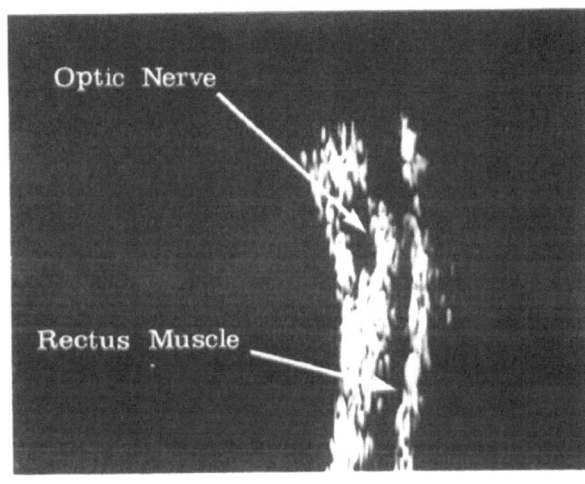

FIGURE 11.18b

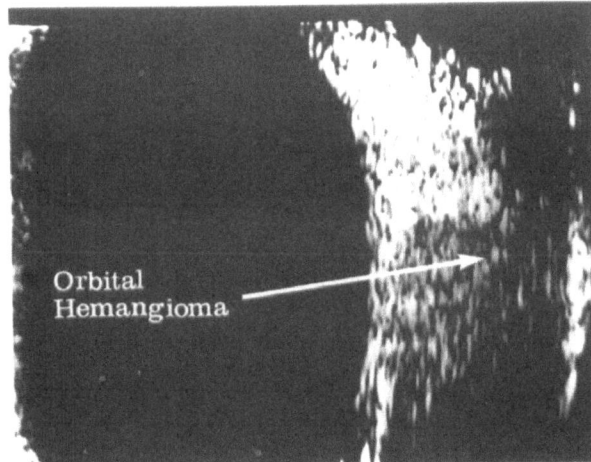

FIGURE 11.17c

FIGURE 11.17a
Flame-shaped muscle. The lateral rectus insertion into the orbital fat echo pattern appears serrated.

FIGURE 11.17b
Lateral rectus has a wedge-shaped appearance.

FIGURE 11.17c
Orbital hemangioma simulating rectus muscle enlargement. Compression revealed the lesion to decrease in size and increase in echo density.

FIGURE 11.18a
The rectus muscle may have its echo-free pattern merge with the echo free optic nerve in oblique scan plane.

FIGURE 11.18b
Cross-section scan demonstrates optic nerve to appear as a cystic lesion anterior to the muscle.

149

of the optic nerve head producing a confusing picture on the frontal scan (Figure 11.18a) or be posterior to a sharply marginated lesion which may simulate an orbital cystic lesion, but simply be the normal optic nerve seen in cross section (Figure 11.18b).

EXOPHTHALMOS

This term refers to the forward protrusion of the globe from the orbit and is measured in terms of the antero-posterior distance from the lateral bony orbital rim to the corneal apex. This distance is normally less than 18 mm and the difference between the two eyes is not greater than 2.5 mm. These measurements are obtained with an exophthalmometer.

CAUSES OF EXOPHTHALMOS

There are systemic and local disorders producing exophthalmos. The most common condition resulting in bilateral and unilateral exophthalmos is thyroid disease. Thyroid disorders are divided into the thyrotropic and thyrotoxic categories. Thyrotropic thyroid disease produces orbital infiltration with inflammatory cells, fat, and edema fluid. There is venous engorgement with lid edema. Extraocular muscle paralysis results in diplopia. Thyroid function may be normal or even depressed. Thyrotoxic exophthalmos is associated with signs of hyperthyroidism. There is normal orbital pressure, minimal edema, and venous congestion. Paresis of the extraocular muscles is not expected.

Exophthalmos which is produced by an orbital tumor is unilateral. Neoplasms may be primary in the orbit, such as hemangioma, dermoid, lymphoma, pseudotumor, lipoma, lacrimal gland tumor, or neurofibroma. The tumor may be invasive from adjacent organs. This is found in carcinoma of the sinus, intracranial meningioma, and ocular melanoma. Metastatic tumors may be from any site. In the pediatric age group, this is classically from an adrenal neuroblastoma.

Extension of ethmoidal sinusitis causes orbital cellulitis which appears as exophthalmos, muscular paralysis, and conjunctival edema. Penetrating wounds may also produce this entity. Orbital contusions may be accompanied by edema and hemorrhage in the retrobulbar space. Pulsating exophthalmos is seen in carotid cavernous arteriovenous fistula which occurs following trauma.

SONOGRAPHY OF EXOPHTHALMOS

If exophthalmos is due to thyroid disease, it is easily detected by sonography. Hypertrophy of the orbital muscle is due to infiltration during the course of thyroid dysfunction and when it is significant, produces exophthalmos. For proper evaluation, the sensitivity should be changed from 80 dB to 70 dB. Recognition of the muscles needs extensive experience and good orientation to the anatomical position of the eye muscles. It should be kept in mind that previous exposure to specific patterns of the appearance of the muscle is essential to a good study. The evaluation of muscle enlargement is usually a gross qualitative estimate rather than a specific measurement at the present time. We have started a measurement protocol, but our experience so far has not been conclusive.

The medial recti muscles are the easiest to examine. The patient is instructed to look in an extreme lateral gaze. The transducer is transverse and angled down towards the medial orbital wall. The eye is rotated towards the transducer. The sensitivity is set at 80 dB. According to the identification system previously discussed, the medial rectus muscle appears as a linear echogenic band extending towards the top of the screen and anteriorly from posteriorly and inferiorly. This appearance is true for both eyes. Note that in the study of the recti muscles a scan at 70 dB may show that the lateral rectus muscle appears echo-poor and band-like between the orbital fat and the orbital wall (Figure 11.19a). The medial rectus in the same eye may have an echogenic center and runs in the orbital fat in the opposite direction (Figure 11.19b). The medial rectus muscle at mid-lateral gaze is also studied during this examination. The muscle band is less stretched and appears thinner. The muscle body

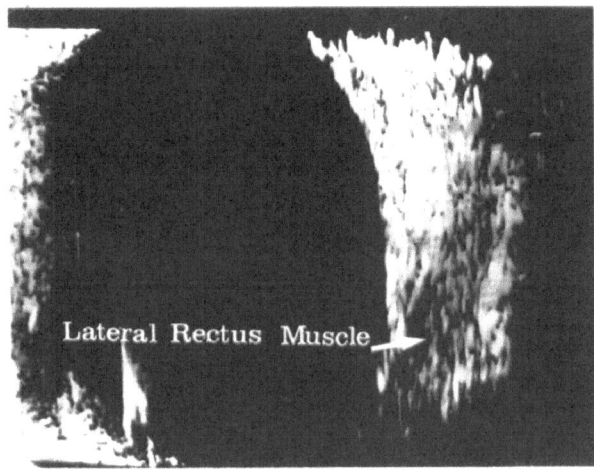

FIGURE 11.19a

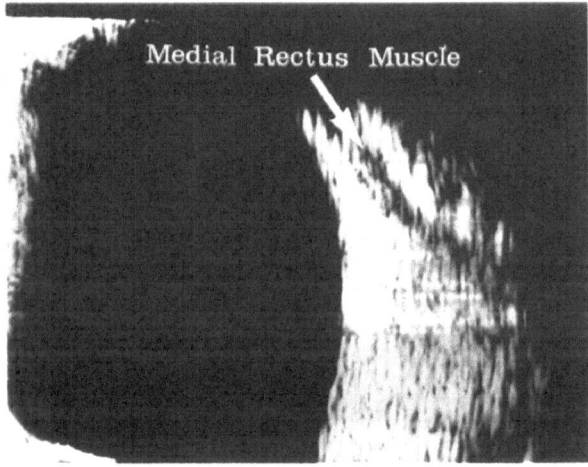

FIGURE 11.19b

FIGURE 11.19a
Echo-poor lateral rectus muscle due to oblique scanning position.

FIGURE 11.19b
Medial rectus muscle with echogenic pattern in same eye.

is less echogenic at 70 dB than at 80 dB. The medial and lateral recti muscles may be studied together on one scan. In certain instances, both the medial and lateral recti muscles may be simultaneously imaged forming a V-shape near the posterior aspect of the screen. The medial rectus muscle is easier to examine. If orbital infiltration is severe, an infiltrated pattern will be seen sonographically. If the orbit is swollen with fluid, it produces a loculated, echo-poor zone in all quadrants. When exophthalmos is due to infiltration of the recti muscles, if possible, each rectus muscle should be scanned in sequence (Figure 11.20a and b).

PSEUDOPROPTOSIS

This term is applied when one globe is congenitally larger than the other. By axial length measurement, the difference may be easily evaluated. If the ultrasonic examination is unremarkable other than increased axial length and the history compatible with the physical finding, no further investigation is necessary.

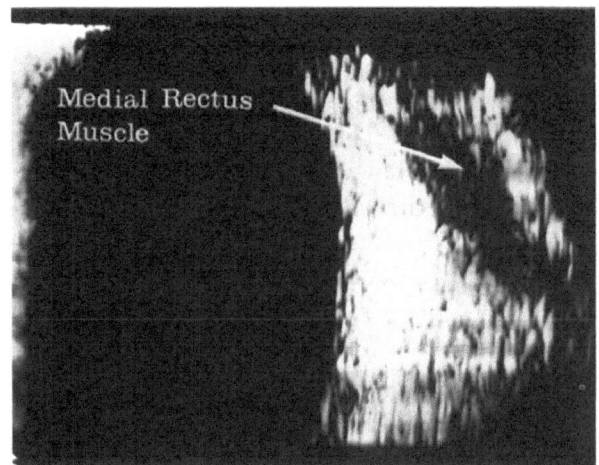

FIGURE 11.20a
Exophthalmos. Hypertrophied medial rectus muscle is echo-poor with moderate through-transmission.

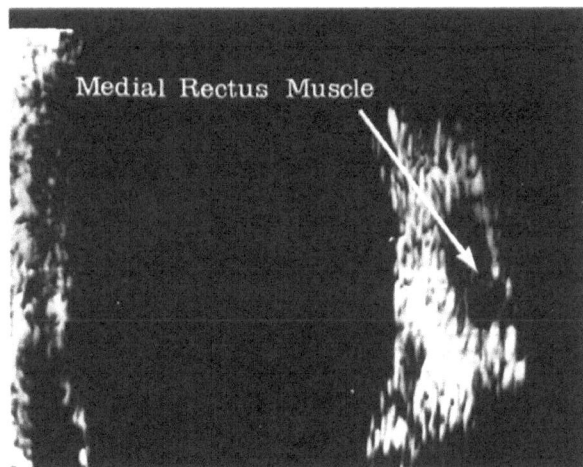

FIGURE 11.20b
Cross-section scan of medial rectus demonstrates increased antero-posterior diameter of muscle.

151

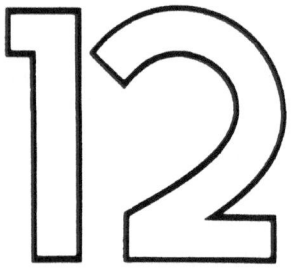

sonography of ophthalmic tumors

GENERAL INTRODUCTION

Tumors of the eye occur in every portion and are composed of all conceivable types of tissue. While the ultrasonographer of today works primarily with diagnostic tools of high prowess in the vitreous, posterior ocular wall, and orbit, the rapidly advancing technical achievements of sonographic equipment will soon permit scanning of lesions heretofore not easily imaged. Tumors of the lid, conjunctiva, cornea, lacrimal sac, and sinuses may now be partially investigated with A-mode using 10, 15, 20, and 25 MHz transducers. A-mode analysis may currently give useful information on the biologic nature of superficial tumors. The sonographer should be aware of the clinical and pathologic nature of all types of eye tumors so that he will be immediately able to apply the more sophisticated scanners of the future to lesions of the globe, orbit, and regional anatomic structures.

CLINICAL PRESENTATION

Most tumors affecting the lids are benign. A variety of lesions occur here since skin, mucous membrane, and glands are present. Carcinomas of the eyelid are generally of the basal cell and squamous cell types. These are curable if treated early. Lesions are elevated and infiltrate the skin. Benign keratoses may simulate carcinomas clinically. Hordeolum is an acute pyogenic infection of the glands. Chalazion is a granulomatous enlargement of a meibomain gland. These are clinically distinguishable from other tumors. The conjunctiva may be the site of carcinoma and papilloma, which may be clinically indistinguishable. The cancerous lesion is white and elevated, while the papilloma is often cauliflower-like. A host of ectasias of the vascular and lymphatic system may occur as separated or mixed lesions. The benign nevus is the most frequent conjunctival tumor and may be either flat or elevated. Malignant transformations may occur in a nevus or malignant melanoma and may arise spontaneously. They appear as an elevated mass of dilated vessels. Pinguecula is a localized elevated yellowish area nasally near the limbus which should not be mistaken for malignant disease. Dermoid or simple cysts may occur. Tumors of the lacrimal apparatus are epithelial in nature. These are locally destructive and produce symptoms of epiphora (tearing) early.

Tumors of the uvea include lesions of the iris, ciliary body, and choroid. Cysts of the iris and the ciliary body may become large enough to obstruct vision and are usually filled with clear fluid. Benign nevi of the iris are usually discrete and small lesions. Most malignant melanomas of the iris arise from pre-existing tumors, possibly focal or diffuse. Adenomatous hyperplasia and degenerative disorders of the choroid may produce symptomatic masses in the eye. Neurofibromas of the uvea occur in the systemic von Recklinghausen's disease or neurofibromatosis. Acute leukemic disease produces infiltrates generally of the posterior choroid. Tumors of the retinal pigment epithelium such as medulloepithelioma (diktyoma) and adenocarcinoma may produce bulky masses.

Nevi of the choroid are often located in the posterior third of this layer with a majority between 2.5 and 5.5 mm in diameter. They are flat lesions but 67% exceed the thickness of the adjacent choroid. There is a tendency to induce overlying drusen formation.

Benign choroidal nevi may transform into malignant melanomas years after the discovery of the original melanotic area. This tumor is preponderant in the caucasian group and unusual in the black race. The median age is 55 years. Clinically, a mass will be found routinely during an examination or blurred vision may bring a patient to the ophthalmologist as extension of the tumor over the macula causes early symptoms. Vitreous hemorrhage, central serous retinopathy, and ocular inflammation occur later.

Malignant melanoma of the ciliary body may produce decreased intraocular pressure and episcleral vascular injection. The tumor is usually solid and composed of a mixed cellular pattern. A small percentage are internally necrotic with conversion of the body of the tumor into a large cystic space. This is of importance since sonic shadowing is a characteristic of malignant melanoma and may not always be present in the 7% of tumors that degenerate. The shape of the tumor depends on whether it has invaded Bruch's membrane. When the membrane is intact, the tumor is limited and assumes an oval form. The tumor that has broken through Bruch's membrane is usually collar-button or mushroom shaped, since the elastic membrane acts as a constricting tourniquet around the base of the tumor and impairs the venous return. Vascular engorgement and pressure necrosis lead to intra-vitreal hemorrhage.

A retinal detachment is present in most cases although this is usually localized rather than total. The sclera and extraocular structures are directly involved by tumor invasion in a small percentage of patients. The presence of orbital extension of the tumor is associated with an 18% recurrence rate of orbital tumor. About 12% of proven melanomas are clinically unsuspected and discovered at operation.

Inflammatory pseudotumor is a non-neoplastic space occupying lesion of the orbit clinically presenting as a neoplasm. This may be associated with chronic granulomatous reaction due to foreign body, fat necrosis, sarcoidosis, chronic granulomatous inflammation, or reactive lymphoid hyperplasia.

Tumors of the reticuloendothelieal system include the reticuloendothelioses of eosinophilic granuloma, Hand-Schuller-Christian disease, and Letterer-Siwe disease which affect younger patients with lytic bony lesions of the orbit and skull as well as histiocystic infiltration of the orbit.

Lacrimal gland tumors usually cause a down and in proptosis. They are locally expansile and usually of mixed cell type. The tumor may infiltrate its own pseudocapsule to involve adjacent periostium. About one half are epithelial tumors and the other half are lymphoid tumors and inflammatory pseudotumors.

SONOPATHOLOGY OF OPHTHALMIC TUMORS

In our experience with B-contact real-time scanners, this is diagnostically an excellent method to detect intraocular tumors. However, for more data we refer these patients for fluorescein evaluation, trans-illumination and radioactive P3 study. To complete the work up, we perform angiography. The collected information is then coupled with the results of the B-scanner. The ultrasonic studies yield information regarding tissue signature, shape, and acoustic density of the tumor. Some tumors have characteristic ultrasonic patterns while others do not. If it is at all possible, and the media is not opaque, visual correlation is performed. The following steps are necessary for establishing an accurate diagnosis:

1. Geographic localization of the mass.

2. Study of the sonic gray-scale characteristics.

3. Evaluation of the size, shape, and configuration.

4. Orientation of the mass and construction of a three-dimensional representation of the mass from a series of two-dimensional echo patterns.

5. The relative distance of the mass from certain known structures such as the iris-lens diaphragm, insertion of the recti muscle, and optic nerve.

6. Maximum attempt should be exerted to avoid lens artifact. Practically, the lens is moved out of the sonic beam path.

7. As the final step, registration of the mass either by polaroid film or videotape.

There are several notations from our experience which deserve to be mentioned. One of them is to avoid interpreting any picture from the top or bottom of the screen, because these areas suffer from major drawbacks due to resolution artifacts. The first attempt should be directed towards sonographically localizing the bony orbit boundaries (Figure 12.1). The bony structures produce a strongly echogenic linear band at the extreme portion of the orbital fat echoes. No sound passes beyond this point. This appearance is due to the sound beam striking the medial or lateral orbital wall in a perpendicular direction.

Usually at maximum sensitivity setting (80 dB), the anterior tumor border echoes are very strong. This is because of a sudden change in acoustical impedance from the normal vitreous to the tumor tissue. The next step is the evaluation of the echo characteristics of the tumor. By reducing the sensitivity from 80 dB to 70 dB, the mass lesion usually is better delineated and may be more readily distinguished from the echo-free vitreous. The internal architecture of a solid mass produces a multiple echo reflection pattern which is due to changes of acoustical impedance detected by the sonic beam. A compact mass absorbs a large amount of low energy ultrasonic waves. This absorption of the echoes is noticeable on the T.V. monitor. Attenuation of the sonic beam is due to the fact that absorption diminishes the echo strength and the number of echoes. As a result, the orbital fat and other tissues located behind the tumor are sometimes not clearly seen. Extra orbital extension of the tumor or a tumor in the vicinity of the orbit can sometimes be identified.

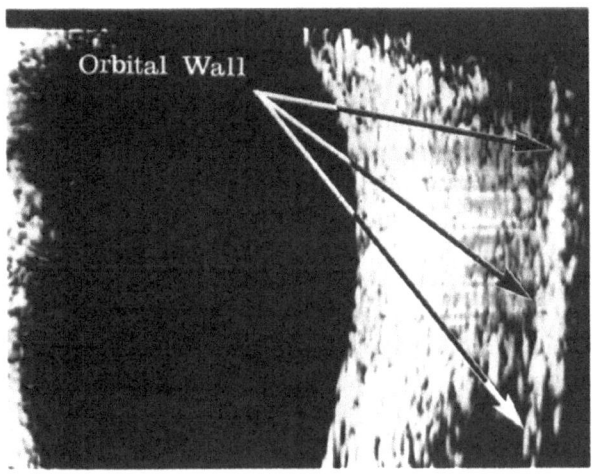

FIGURE 12.1

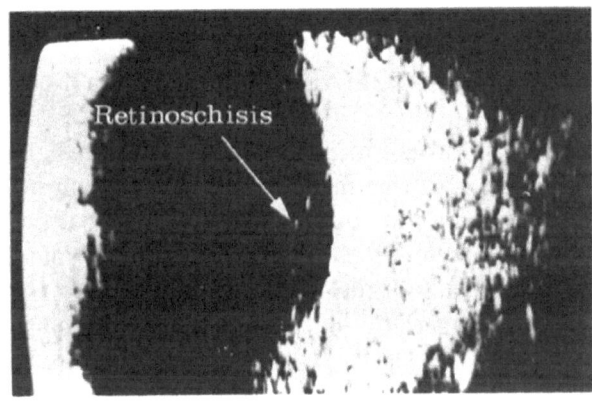

FIGURE 12.2a

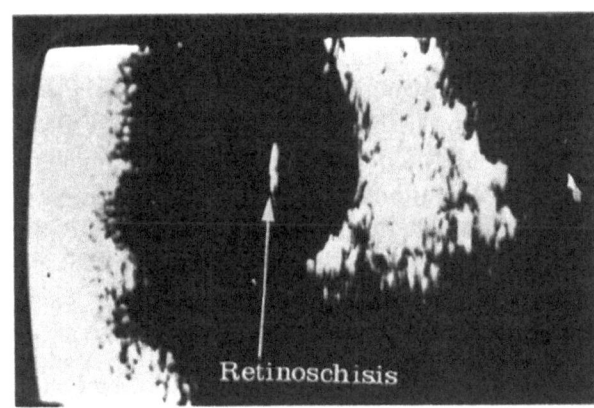

FIGURE 12.2b

TUMORS OF THE RETINA

Tumors of the retina must be distinguished from the many degenerative lesions producing elevated lesions. Retinoschisis is often found in the over 40 age group, and is due to a splitting of the retinal tissue. It is usually found inferotemporally. This may simulate a localized retinal detachment or tumor. In the following case, the echo-free area is confined by the membrane bowing anteriorly. The membrane is moderately echogenic and bulges in the opposite direction to the usual retinal detachment. Retinoschisis (Figure 12.2a and b) presents as linear or curved sheet-like echoes along the posterior ocular wall usually without insertion into the optic nerve head. This is due to degenerative changes in the retina.

RETINOBLASTOMA

Statistically, retinoblastoma is the most common intraocular neoplasm of children. It ranks behind uveal melanoma and metastatic carcinoma as the third most common intraocular malignancy. Bilaterality is common. The condition is inherited through a dominant autosomal gene in a small percentage of familial cases.

Necrosis is present in most tumors. Calcification is frequent and is a radiographically and ultrasonically important diagnostic feature. The tumor may be multifocal, bilateral, and endophytic

FIGURE 12.1
Orbital wall. Sonofluoroscopy of the orbit involves imaging the bony orbital walls which appear in special scan planes as linear strongly echogenic areas distal to the region of the orbital fat and muscular structures. The orbit wall blocks further sound transmission.

FIGURE 12.2a
Retinoschisis. Degenerative changes in the retina produce a splitting of the retina which bows into the vitreous producing an arc-like echo. The membrane is echo-poor and interrupted due to tangential scanning.

FIGURE 12.2b
The curvilinear membrane of the split retina is imaged perpendicularly and may simulate a partial retinal detachment.

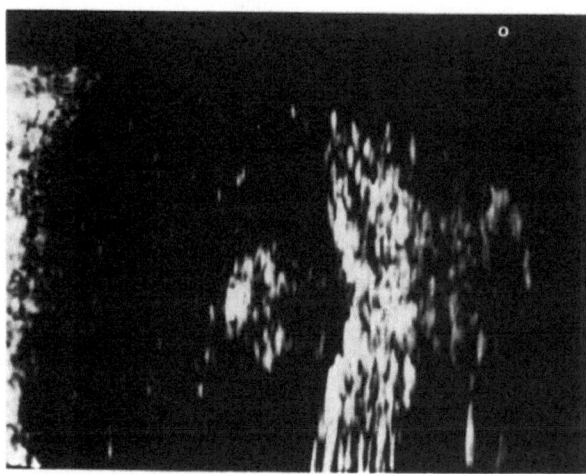

FIGURE 12.3
Retinoblastoma. Scan at 60 dB reveals a highly echogenic mushroom-shaped mass extending anteriorly from the posterior ocular wall. Areas of high amplitude echoes persisted to 40 dB at the surface of the tumor. Incidentally noted in the vitreous are low amplitude echoes of recent hemorrhage.

or exophytic. When it grows into the vitreous the retina is usually intact. Extension into the subretinal space produces a non-rhegmatogenous type retinal detachment. Most tumors have both endophytic and exophytic components. The tumor may seed anteriorly into the vitreous and aqueous, grow into the subarachnoid space or enter the systemic circulation through choroidal invasion.

Pseudoglioma is a term designating a group of entities that may simulate retinoblastoma or "glioma" clinically. Pseudoglioma may present itself with leukokoria (a white retrolental mass seen with retinoblastoma) and may be due to persistent hyperplastic primary vitreous (PHPV), retinal dysplasia, metastatic uveitis, and a host of inflammatory conditions.

ULTRASONOGRAPHY OF RETINOBLASTOMA

Optimal information is obtained by white light examination of this most common malignant intraocular tumor encountered in childhood. If the lens is opaque or there is a retrolental mass producing leukokoria (white pupil), evaluation of this tumor by white light is not possible. Sonography is of great help in these common situations.

In ultrasonography, this tumor appears as an echogenic mass arising from the ocular wall. Neither the location of the mass nor the shape of the tumor specifically differentiates retinoblastoma from other tumors. As a result, clinical data and other factors must be taken into consideration. However, a few ultrasonic criteria may be of extreme help, such as calcification. Calcification is very common in retinoblastoma and these calcifications are excellent reflectors of sonic beam. The tumor may still be detected by reducing the sensitivity even down to 40 dB (Figure 12.3).

Axial length measurement also is important in helping to determine retinoblastoma. The axial length usually does not change and is normal in comparison with the opposite eye.

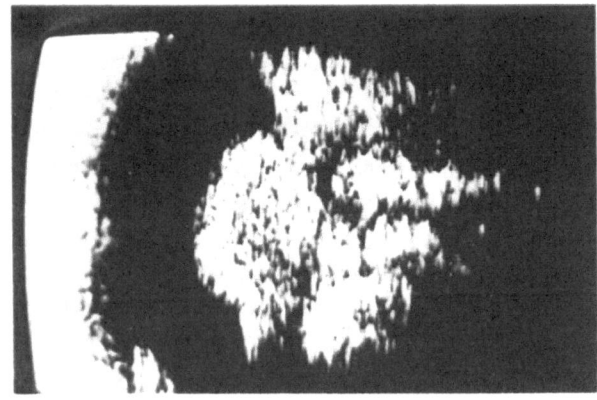

FIGURE 12.4a
Retinal dysplasia. Persistent hyperplastic primary vitreous (PHPV) may simulate a retinoblastoma extending into the vitreous. The differential factor is the decreased axial length associated with retinal dysplasias.

The other factor which deserves to be mentioned is the presence of more than one lesion. It is suggestive rather than conclusive evidence of retinoblastoma.

The definitive differentiation of this tumor from a number of pathological conditions (pseudoglioma) is not entirely possible by ultrasound. A careful clinical evaluation with highly specialized tests is often required. The presence of persistent hyperplastic primary vitreous (PHPV), a uni-ocular maldevelopment of the eye, may be mistaken for this condition. This entity, however, is associated with a small globe. The axial length is significantly decreased in these microphthalmic eyes. The changes associated with uveitis, toxocara granuloma, retrolental fibroplasia, and other developmental disorders are usually distinguished by their clinical features.

TUMORS OF THE CHOROID

MALIGNANT MELANOMA

Malignant melanoma of the eye appears as an elevated rounded mass located deep in the retina (Figure 12.4a). It contains visible nutrient vessels and is associated with some overlying retinal atrophy. There is often a serous, gravity dependent fluid secreted by the tumor. The liquid together with the tumor mass produces a retinal detachment (Figure 12.4b). Unlike the rhegmatogenous retinal detachment, the non-rhegmatogenous retinal detachment associated with this shifting fluid moves with gravitational maneuvers. The dependent part of the detached retina bulges forward when the patient is moved from the supine to the erect position. This may be noted ophthalmoscopically and ultrasonically. Melanomas of the macula are uncommon. Sonographically, the malignant melanoma has a sharp border. This is due to a sudden change in the interface from the vitreous area to the tumoral mass of high acoustical impedance. The tumor is echogenic and, as a result, appears white on the screen. Lesions located at the posterior ocular interface may extend near the optic nerve and associated with a retinal detachment emanating

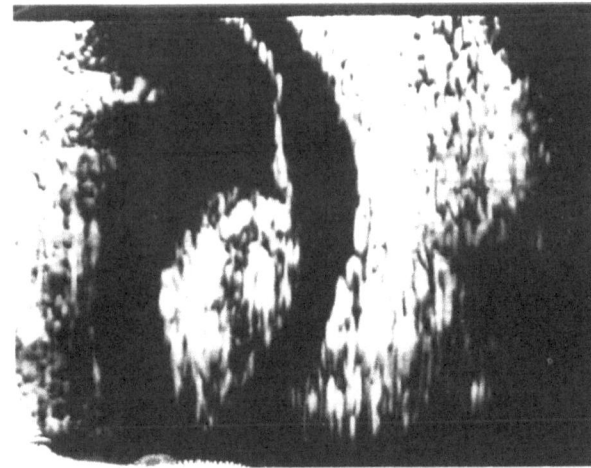

FIGURE 12.4b
Malignant melanoma. A large irregular tumor mass produces a faint sonic shadow in the posterior orbital fat echo pattern. From the lesion a sheet-like membrane extends along the curvature of the posterior ocular wall. Retinal detachment associated with malignant melanoma.

157

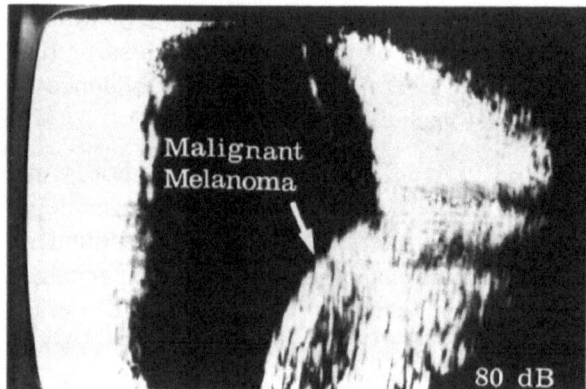

FIGURE 12.5a

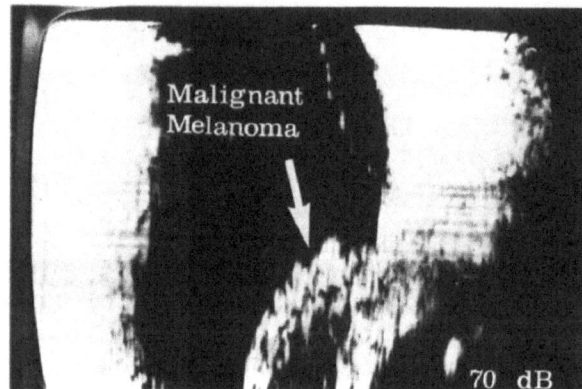

FIGURE 12.5b

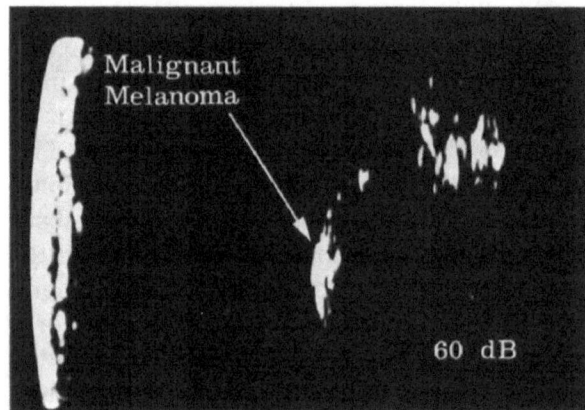

FIGURE 12.5c

from the optic nerve head (Figure 12.5a,b, and c). Sensitivity study of the echo pattern at 70 dB shows that the lower amplitude central echoes disappear within the tumor.

Marked sonic shadowing is noted distally to the tumor mass at 60 dB gain settings (Figure 12.5c). If there is not an associated retinal detachment, the retina is pushed anteriorly by the choroidal tumor mass. Benign macular lesions simulating malignant melanomas are macular choroiditis and disciform macular degeneration. The differential diagnosis is vital since the latter diseases are treated conservatively and malignant melanoma requires enucleation of the eye.

On occasion, the commonly occurring posterior pole tumors may be difficult to distinguish visually. Of course, in the eye with opaque media, there is no way to appreciate the presence of these lesions. Thus, malignant melanoma, metastatic carcinoma, hemangioma, and subretinal hemorrhage may appear clinically and ophthalmoscopically similar in certain instances. Ultrasonography may aid the clinician in localizing the mass and assessing its tissue characteristics.

As mentioned, malignant melanoma often shows internal low amplitude echoes producing a sonic shadow with frequency. Metastatic carcinoma to the choroid occurs most commonly from carcinoma of the breast (Figure 12.6), gastrointestinal tract, and lung although this vascular layer may be the site of lodging of any tumor tissue type. This seeding occurs generally late in the clinical course of the malignant process and the pathologic picture is generally clinically obvious. Since this type of metastasis is blood born, it is most often bilateral and presents in the richly

FIGURE 12.5a
Malignant melanoma. Scan at 80 dB demonstrates choroidal tumor with low amplitude internal echoes and associated linear membrane representing associated retinal detachment.

FIGURE 12.5b
Scan at 70 dB shows marked loss of internal tumor echoes.

FIGURE 12.5c
At 60 dB only the anterior echogenic margin of the tumor and the sonic shadow sign are noted.

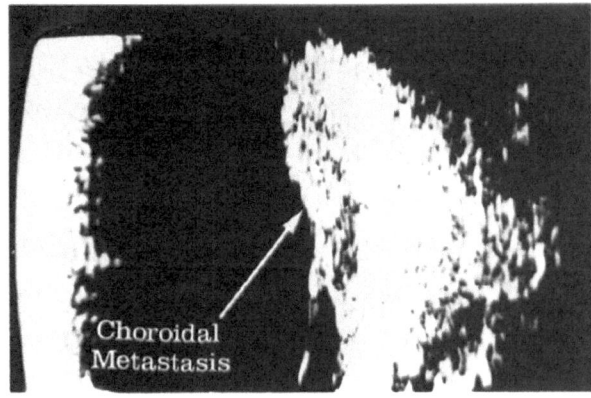

FIGURE 12.6
Metastatic carcinoma. Choroidal metastases are typically echogenic and flatter than melanomas. The linear band adjacent to the flat tumor is the frequently associated retinal detachment.

vascular choroid layer in the posterior pole. The tumor generally appears flatter than malignant melanoma and the lesion occurs late in the course of the malignancy.

The lesion is often sharply limited and is accompanied by a retinal detachment which may show shifting fluid with gravitational maneuvers. The lesions are generally echogenic. The presence of other tumors in the eye under study or the fellow eye lends further support to the diagnosis of a metastatic process.

Hemangiomas of the choroid are rare tumors that may be part of the clinical spectrum of Sturge-Weber syndrome. These tumors often vary in size from 1 to 10 mm in thickness and up to 10 disc diameters in greatest diameter. The tumor may be located anywhere in the choroid layer but is often noted ultrasonically in the region of the posterior pole near the optic nerve head. These lesions are echogenic. They have been described to vary in echo pattern from low amplitude internal echoes to high amplitude internal echoes. Our limited experience with this entity shows medium amplitude echoes internally and an absence of hollowing of the central portion of the tumor resulting from the many reflecting interfaces of blood vessel nests which comprise this tumor. Through-transmission is high. Compression of the globe does not produce the change in size and appearance of the tumor as may be noted in the orbital hemangiomas (Figure 12.7)

Subretinal hemorrhage is usually red, freely mobile, and unclotted. Similar to blood in other portions of the eye, this is ultrasonographically characterized by visible motion with command eye movements and disappearance of the returning echoes of the hemorrhagic contents as the sensitivity control is lowered from 80 dB to 70 dB (Figure 12.8).

A nevus must not be confused with a malignant melanoma. A benign melanotic plaque appears in our experience as a slightly elevated, smoothly marginated lesion with an echo-poor center and an echogenic outer border (Figure 12.9a,b, and c). At 70 dB there is significant

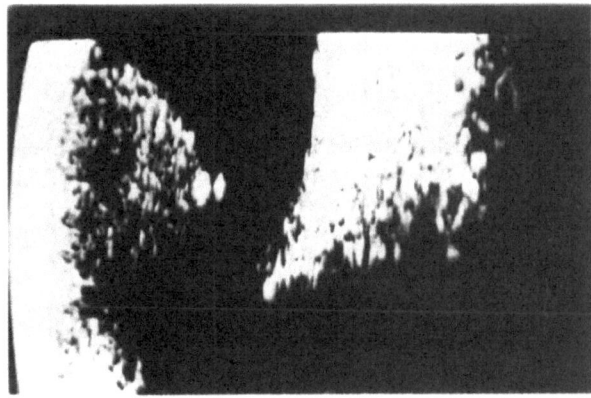

FIGURE 12.7
Choroidal hemangioma. This rare lesion noted in the equator on this oblique scan has medium amplitude internal echoes with high through-transmission. There is no associated retinal detachment.

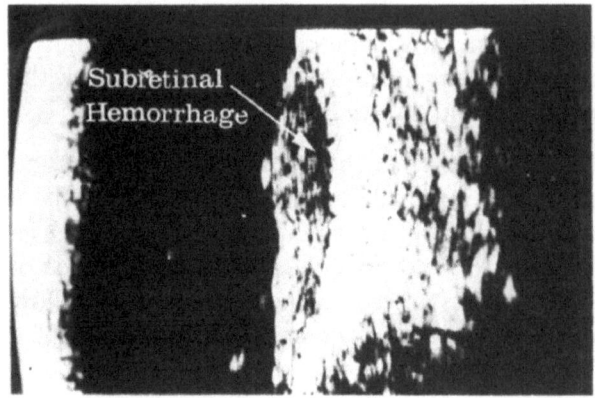

FIGURE 12.8

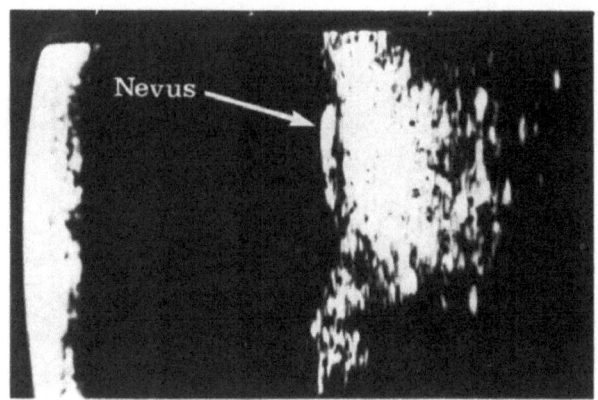

FIGURE 12.9c

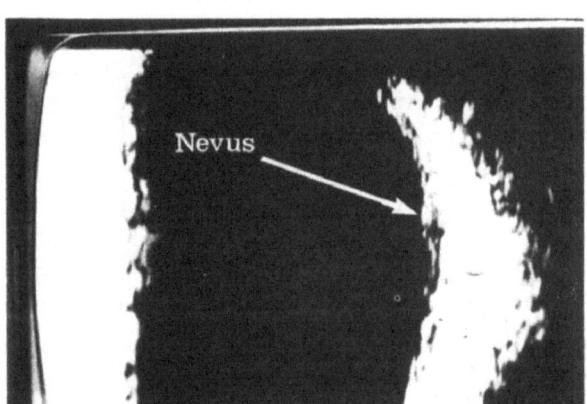

FIGURE 12.9a

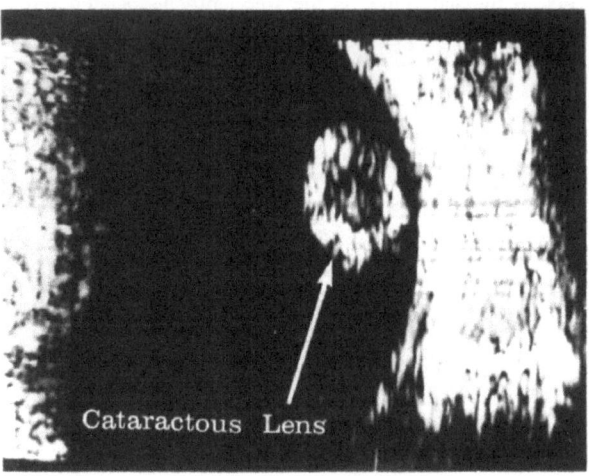

FIGURE 12.10

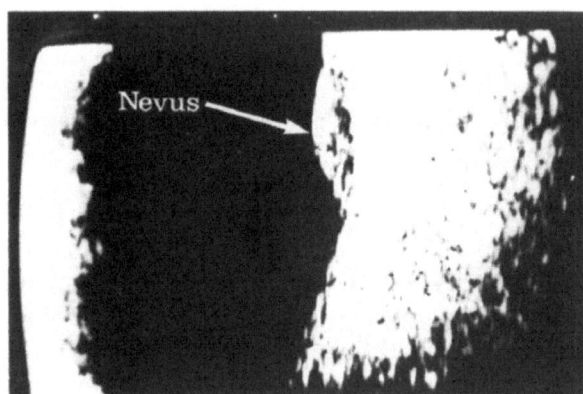

FIGURE 12.9b

FIGURE 12.8
Subretinal hemorrhage. The blood usually is unclotted and the red cells lie in the dependent portion of the subretinal space producing an echogenic inferior portion and an echo-poor superior region.

FIGURE 12.9a
Choroidal nevus. Benign melanotic plaques are flattened lesions many of which do not exceed the critical size to be defined by the ultrasonic scan. When large, they are usually slightly elevated lesions.

FIGURE 12.9b
The lesions are echogenic at their outer border with an echo-poor center best demonstrated by sensitivity studies.

FIGURE 12.9c
Scan at 70 dB shows echo-free center without sonic shadowing.

FIGURE 12.10
Dislocated lens simulating choroidal tumor. This cataractous lens is dislocated. There was no retinal detachment and this moved away from the posterior ocular wall with eye motion.

hollowing to the center of the lesion, and usually there is an absence of sonic shadowing. Sonic shadowing generally occurs with larger lesions and may be absent with tumors of the small size of a nevus. Choroidal nevi do not change in size over the years.

Similarly, a dislocated lens in an opaque eye may appear button like and simulate a malignant melanoma. Distinction is made by the mobility of the lens with eye movements (Figure 12.10).

In summary, the diagnosis of tumors of the posterior pole is aided by the ultrasonic examination. We have not found any definitive ultrasonic pattern for the more commonly occurring choroidal neoplasms.

TUMORS OF THE OPTIC NERVE

Primary tumors of the optic nerve are usually the juvenile pilocystic astrocytoma or "glioma" of the optic nerve. Most of these neoplasms occur during the first decade of life. Proptosis, often temporal and visual loss are the common presenting signs. The astrocytoma is often located in the orbital portion of the optic nerve. The mass may produce enlargement of the optic foramen, or the secondary meningeal hyperplasia may cause this phenomenon. The tumor may involve both the intraorbital optic nerve and the intracranial optic nerve. Papilledema is present early in the course of this tumor. Later the optic nerve atrophies.

Meningioma may occur in the orbital meninges of the optic nerve. This is noted most often during the third decade of life and presents with exophthalmos and visual loss. This is more common in females. The tumor frequently extends extradurally to invade the orbital tissues.

It is important to recognize that drusen of the optic nerve may present clinically as pseudopapilledema and may easily be distinguished by their characteristic ultrasonic pattern.

Secondary tumors of the optic nerve include retinoblastoma, malignant melanoma, pseudotumors of the retinal pigment epithelium, metastatic carcinoma, and intracranial meningioma.

ORBITAL TUMORS

Orbital tumors not only produce exophthalmos, but cause changes in the appearance of the fundus. The flattening effect of the tumor upon the posterior ocular wall structures gives a wavy, fold-like contour to the retina and must be differentiated from surface wrinkling retinopathy.

The pathological varieties of tumors of the orbital region comprise a wide variety of tissue types. Rhabdomyosarcoma is the most common malignant mesenchymal orbital tumor and is the most common primary malignant orbital tumor in children with an average age of onset of six years. The tumor grows rapidly and may clinically simulate an orbital cellulitis. It is an aggressively malignant tumor with massive bony erosion. A lipoma is a rare tumor of the orbit.

Malignant lymphomas involve the orbit late in the disease process. This fact helps to differentiate benign pseudotumors from lymphoma since histologically it is difficult. Leukemia, in contrast to lymphoma, may occasionally initially present itself with exophthalmos. This is especially true of acute granulocytic or stem cell leukemia, which produces an orbital infiltrate of leukemic cells called a chloroma. In other leukemias, orbital infiltration is common late in the disease.

Secondary tumors of the orbit usually metastasize by direct extension. This is frequent in malignant melanoma and retinoblastoma, eyelid neoplasms, conjunctival tumors, and the paranasal sinus cyst or mucocoele which is a common cause of exophthalmos and is frequently noted in the region of the frontal sinus.

SONOGRAPHY OF ORBITAL TUMORS

Orbital tumors are best characterized ultrasonographically by their morphologic appearance and through-transmission pattern.

Study of the mass with the compression technique, to evaluate the alteration in size, shape, and echo pattern of the lesion as well as the change in configuration of the adjacent posterior ocular wall may be performed. Additionally,

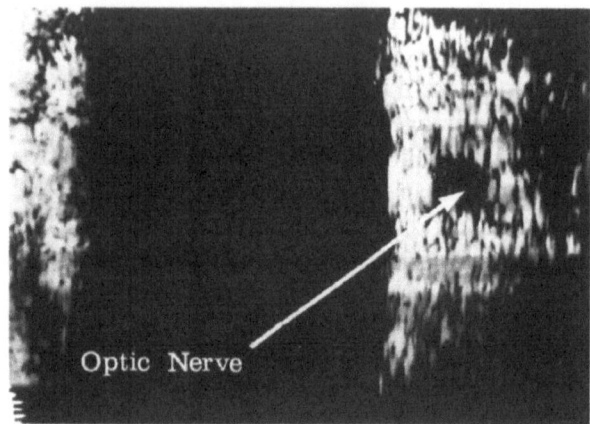

FIGURE 12.11

FIGURE 12.11
Optic nerve simulating orbital tumor. The cross section of the normal optic nerve produces an echo-free or echogenic sharply marginated area in the orbital fat echoes.

FIGURE 12.12a
Cyst of the orbit. Small cystic lesion of the orbit simulates an echo-free optic nerve.

FIGURE 12.12b
Cross-sectional scanning demonstrates that the echo-free lesion is rounded in three dimensions.

FIGURE 12.13
Hypertrophic rectus muscle. Enlargement of the rectus muscle in thyroid disorders may simulate an orbital tumor.

evaluation of the lesion with the eye in motion is routinely done.

Thus, orbital tumors may be subclassified into lesions that are smoothly encapsulated with high through-transmission, smoothly marginated with poor through-transmission, irregularly marginated with high through-transmission and irregularly outlined with poor through-transmission. The sonographer must be aware that the cross section of the normal optic nerve may simulate a small orbital lesion (Figure 12.11). Conversely, small orbital cyst (Figure 12.12a and b) and tumors near the optic nerve must not be mistaken for the nerve. This is accomplished by careful three-dimensional scanning. Also, hypertrophy of the rectus muscles (Figure 12.13) should not be confused with a true orbital tumor.

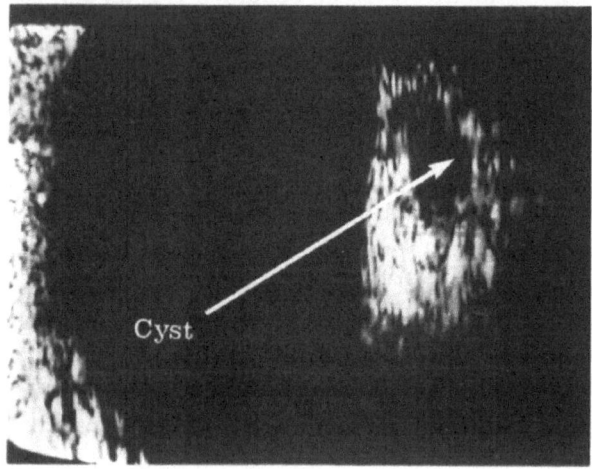

FIGURE 12.12a

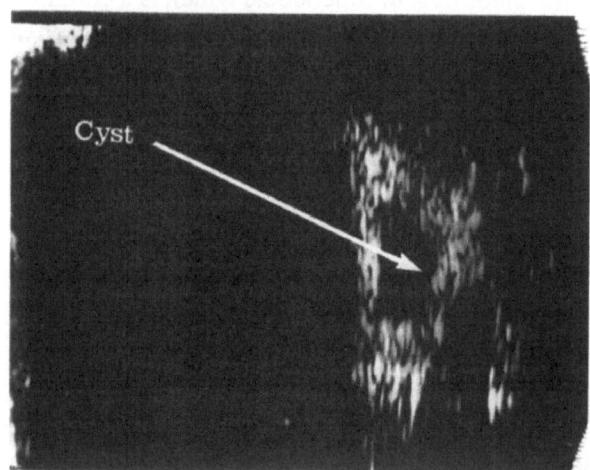

FIGURE 12.12b

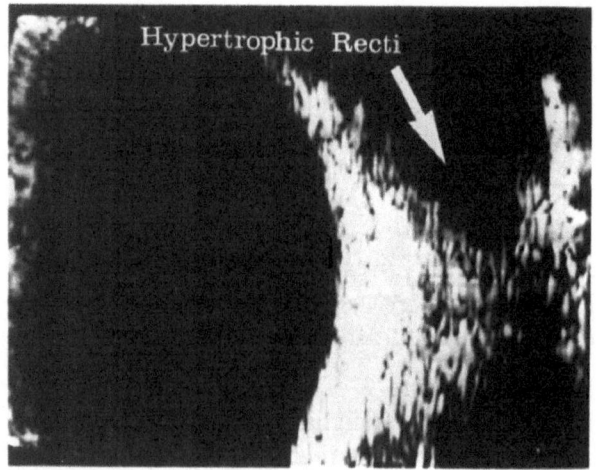

FIGURE 12.13

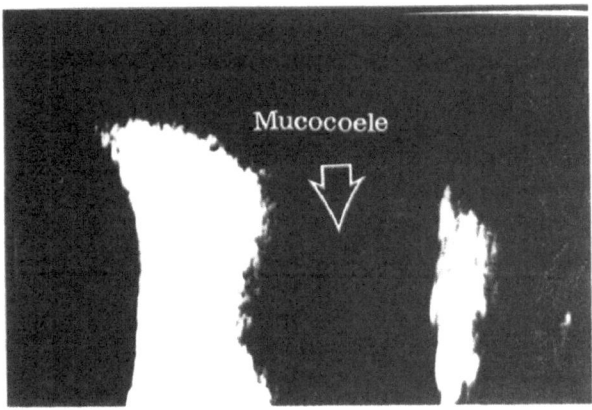

FIGURE 12.14a

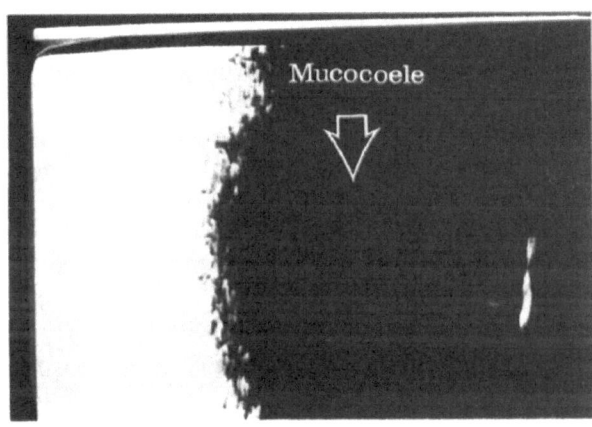

FIGURE 12.14b

FIGURE 12.14a
Mucocoele. Large echo-free cystic lesion even at high gain setting extends from the roof of the orbit typical of a frontal mucocoele.

FIGURE 12.14b
The mucocoele may be scanned transversely through the roof of the orbit. The area of the mucocoele is echo-free but the distal echo is weaker than expected to sonic attenuation by the thinned bony frontal sinus.

FIGURE 12.15a
Cavernous hemangioma. Scan at 1.5–4.5 cm setting shows moderately echogenic lesion that is well circumscribed with high through-transmission.

FIGURE 12.15b
Compression of the lesion produces marked decrease in size of the mass and an increase in the echo density.

Tumors with a round shape and high through-transmission may have no internal echoes or scattered internal echoes of low amplitude. The high transonicity of these lesions allows for strong echo return from the more distally located muscular or bony structures and a highly echogenic surrounding orbital fat echo pattern. These lesions are poorly compressible and show no change in motion if they are outside the muscle cone. Compression may produce an indentation on the posterior ocular wall. Masses frequently falling into this ultrasonic appearance are dermoid cysts, mucocoeles of the frontal sinus (Figure 12.14a and b), cavernous hemangiomas (Figure 12.15a and b), and lipoma (Figure 12.16).

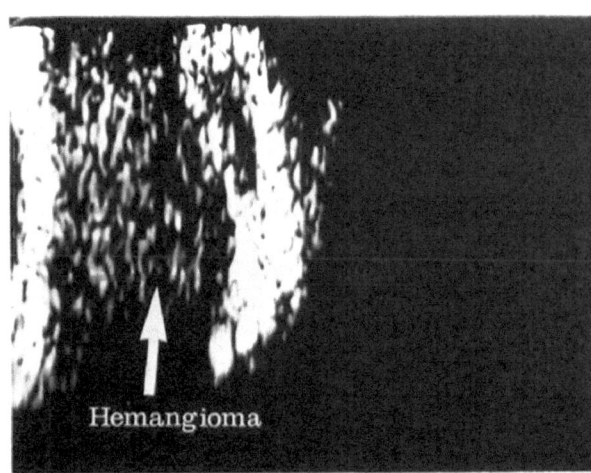

FIGURE 12.15a

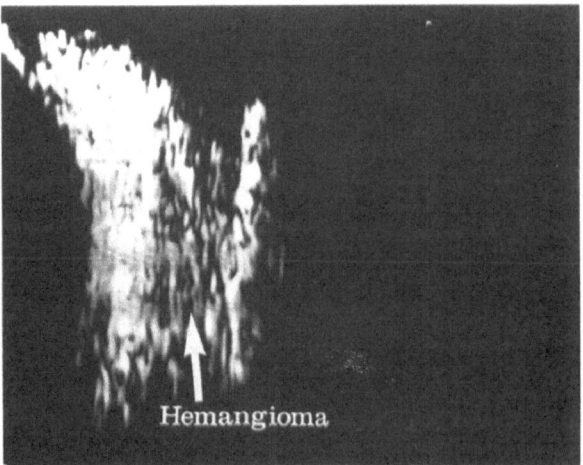

FIGURE 12.15b

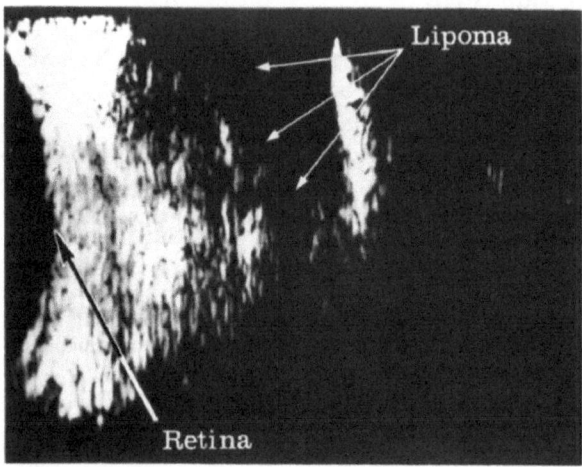

FIGURE 12.16
Lipoma. Moderately well circumscribed, anteriorly echogenic mass with good through-transmission.

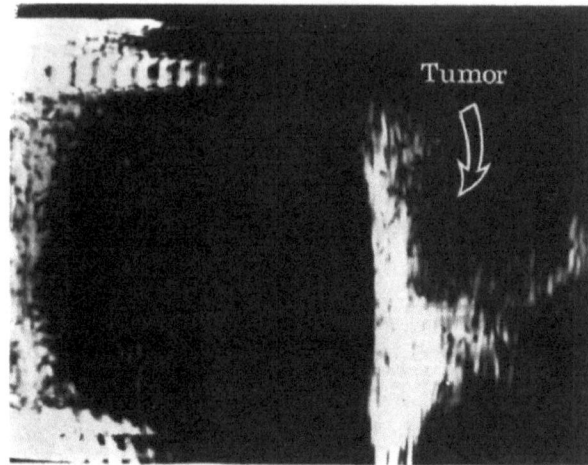

FIGURE 12.17
Orbital tumor at low gain setting shows absence of internal echoes with decreased through-transmission.

Since the mucocoele of the frontal sinus is a common orbital tumor a modification of the examination may be performed. Proptosis is produced when the superior roof of the orbit is pushed inferiorly by the expanding frontal sinus cystic lesion. Sonography may be performed with the transducer directly over the area of the expanding mucocoele in a horizontal position. The tissues of the superior orbit are highly echogenic and rapidly attenuate the sound waves. The mucocoele replaces this tissue and the resulting area becomes highly sonolucent. Through-transmission is high and the lesion is rounded in shape.

After this scan, routine scanning is performed and then the globe is examined in the six o'clock position to evaluate the effects of tumor compressibility. As the eye is pushed posteriorly by the transducer, the mucocoele will not change its size or shape. However, the resulting pressure on the globe may flatten the posterior ocular wall adjacent to the tumor.

Neoplasms with a smooth boundary and poor through-transmission usually have a strongly echogenic anterior boundary with a poorly or irregularly imaged posterior boundary. In some cases, it is not possible to delineate the distal interface in its entirety in spite of multiple scanning maneuvers. These lesions with poor transonicity usually have few internal echoes of low or medium amplitude which are most often noted anteriorly. The echoes in the distal aspect of the mass are often weak or nonexistent. At 70 dB these solid lesions show almost no internal echoes indicating their poor reflectivity (Figure 12.17). Neoplasms of neurogenic origin such as meningioma, neurofibroma, and gliomas frequently produce this ultrasonic appearance. Compression techniques usually do not add further information.

Tumors with an irregular shape and high through-transmission often have a moderately echogenic anterior border which is most likely due to scattering of the interrogating sound beam by the interfaces which do not lie perpendicular to the plane of the scan. The posterior border is

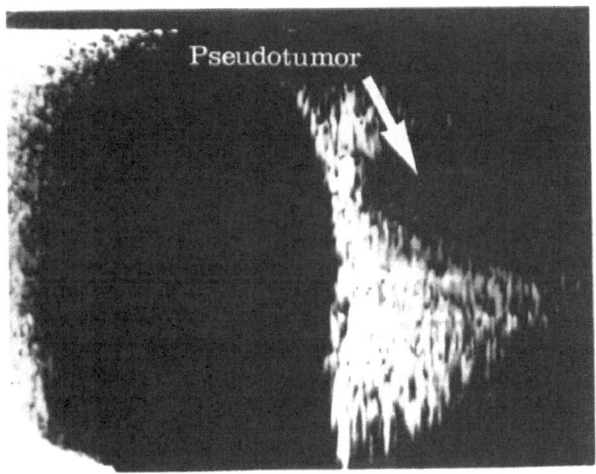

FIGURE 12.18
Lymphoma. Poorly outlined tumor with irregular anterior and no echoes coming from the distal orbit or posterior tumor boundary due to very high attenuation.

similarly irregular with a medium to low amplitude echo pattern. Often multiple high and medium amplitude internal echoes are noted within the substance of the tumor indicative of its strongly reflective nature. Compression and position maneuvers are often useful in these conditions. Since these masses are usually fluid filled, sound transmission is high and changes in the mass with compression are demonstrable. Compression of hemangiomatous (Figure 12.15a and b) or lymphangiomatous tissue in the orbit frequently results in a decrease in size of these lesions. On occasion, there will be actual collapse of the lesion as its anterior and posterior walls are pushed together. A varix of the orbit will increase in size as it assumes a dependent position with respect to the heart and will decrease in size as the eye is elevated above the plane of the heart.

Irregularly outlined tumors with poor through-transmission tend to have an anterior boundary which is interrupted and of medium to low amplitude echoes and a distal border with low amplitude echoes. Not infrequently the anterior and posterior boundary is not definitively imaged. The internal echo pattern is variable with high, medium, and low amplitude echo patterns being observed. Through-transmission is poor resulting in decreased imaging of the muscles, orbital fat, and bony outlines that may be scanned in a location distal to the lesion. The only clue to an orbital lesion of this type may be an ill defined irregularity to the echoes of the normally symmetrical distal aspect of the orbital fat echo pattern. This may produce a finger like appearance to the distal orbital fat as compared with another portion of the orbital fat or the other eye. Extreme expertise is necessary to appreciate these subtle alterations in the orbital fat echo pattern. Tumors producing this ultrasonic appearance are lymphoma, metastatic carcinoma, and pseudotumor (Figure 12.18).

Orbital abscess may simulate an orbital tumor. The patient may be febrile or afebrile. This entity has followed sinus infection, orbital fracture, and systemic infection in our experience. The abscess may appear echo-free with either smooth

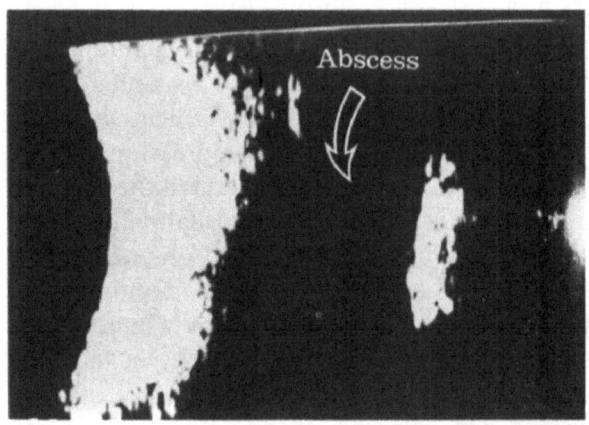

FIGURE 12.19a

or, more commonly, irregular margins. At times, the presence of inflammatory or necrotic debris may produce scattered internal echoes (Figure 12.19a and b).

ADNEXAL TUMORS

Tumors of the lacrimal gland may be evaluated by real-time ophthalmic scanning with a gel type or water bath delay to place the superficial lesion at the 15 mm focal point of the sound beam. Lacrimal gland tumors may be primary as in carcinoma or secondary as in diseases such as lymphoma (Figure 12.20a and b).

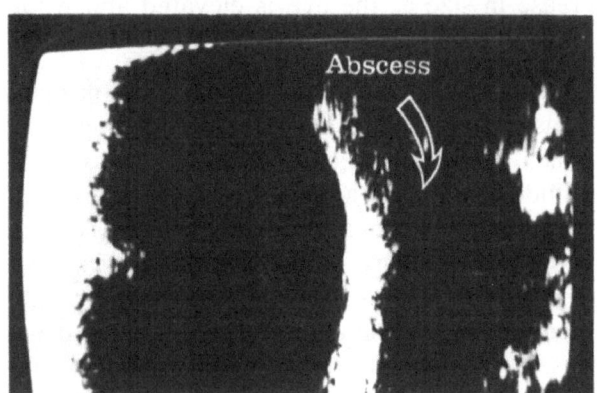

FIGURE 12.19b

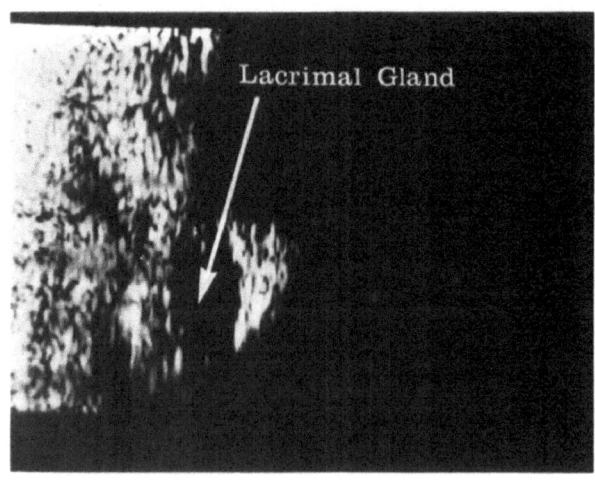

FIGURE 12.20b

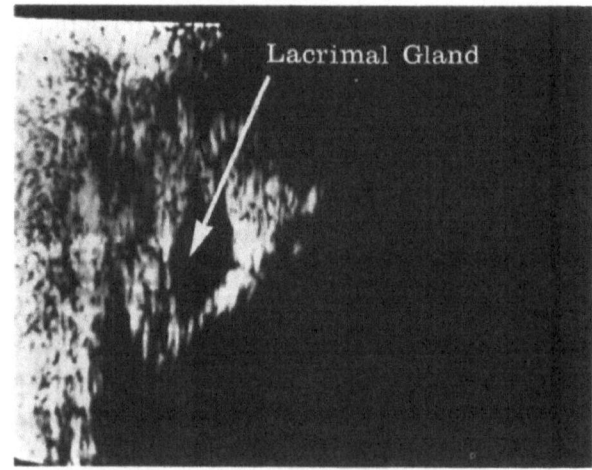

FIGURE 12.20a

FIGURE 12.19a
Orbital abscess. The abscess may be echo-free and smoothly marginated with high through-transmission.

FIGURE 12.19b
The abscess may have irregular walls, scattered internal echoes, and high through-transmission.

FIGURE 12.20a
Carcinoma of the lacrimal gland. The gland is enlarged and echo-poor with very high through-transmission almost simulating a cystic lesion. The borders are still well defined. No bony erosion was noted at this stage.

FIGURE 12.20b
Lymphoma of the lacrimal gland. The gland is enlarged and slightly echogenic with slightly irregular borders. Through-transmission is not as great as the case of carcinoma.

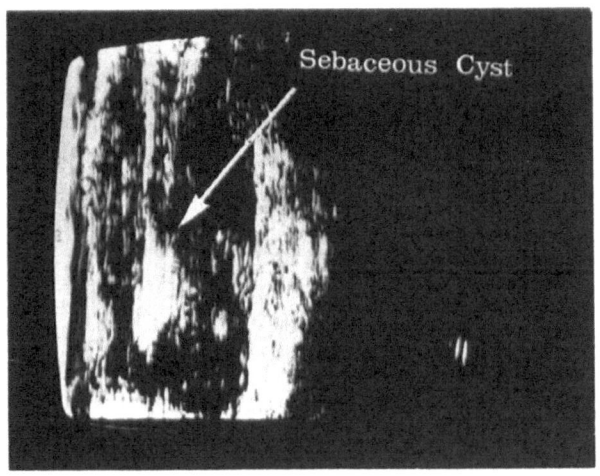

FIGURE 12.21
Sebaceous cyst. The lesion is highly echogenic with coarse
echoes. Through-transmission is decreased.

Lesions of the eyelid and adjacent periocular
soft tissues may also be studied with high frequency ultrasound. Sebaceous cysts are filled
with echogenic material and are poorly transmitting areas (Figure 12.21). Lipomas are echo-poor
and have medium through-transmission. Subcutaneous cysts or hematomas are echo-free and
highly transonic. Even lesions of the skin may be
atraumatically investigated in this manner. Per-
haps higher resolution scanners of the future will
allow the sonographer with an understanding of
dermatologic and subcutaneous disorders to dis-
cover a characteristic echo pattern for malignant
lesions.

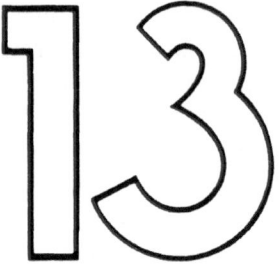

sonography of the eye in systemic disease

INTRODUCTION

Ocular manifestations of systemic diseases may appear as the first sign of a generalized disorder. Careful examination of the eye has been of prime importance to the internist in ferreting out significant diagnostic clues in complex disorders. In numerous instances specific ocular findings and symptoms have lead to the correct diagnosis of a systemic problem.

The eye may be considered the gateway to the discovery of general medical disorders. This one square inch of tissue contains the most concentrated collection of physical findings for the discerning clinician.

Systemic disorders affecting the eye include metabolic disease, collagen and rheumatic disorders, nutritional problems, endocrinopathies, diabetes mellitus, and other vascular diseases. Hematologic conditions of the acute and chronic type are commonly manifested in the eye and orbit. Ocular signs and symptoms may even accompany gastrointestinal and skin diseases. A host of microorganisms are responsible for a

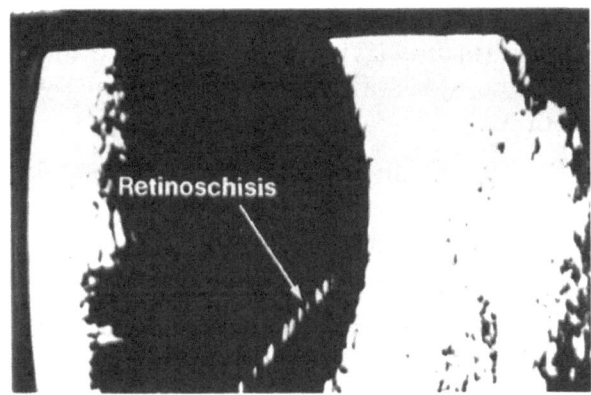

FIGURE 13.1a

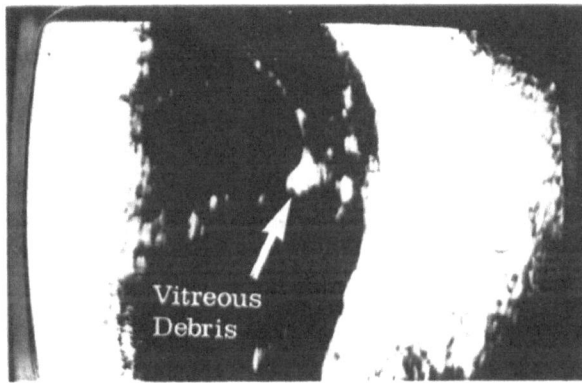

FIGURE 13.1b

variety of ocular inflammatory disorders. The eye is truly a microcosm for the study of systemic diseases and this chapter will emphasize the ultrasonic aspects of special interest to the clinician.

INFLAMMATORY DISORDERS

Ocular and orbital inflammation may be due to specific agents such as bacteria and fungi or to sarcoidosis in which no organisms have been incriminated. The use of the term intraocular inflammation is preferable to the commonly used term "uveitis". In performing sonographic examination for uveitis an associated retinoschisis (Figure 13.1a) may be discovered, in addition to vitreous traction bands and posterior vitreous debris of moderate echogenicity (Figure 13.1b). Retinal detachment often demonstrates a linear

FIGURE 13.1a
Uveitis. Retinoschisis may accompany posterior inflammation and presents as a sheet-like linear echo.

FIGURE 13.1b
Inflammatory debris often appears as floaters echogenic band in the posterior vitreous.

FIGURE 13.1c
Retinal detachment is noted as an irregularly echogenic membrane in this case of chronic inflammation.

FIGURE 13.1d
Focal hemorrhage often occurs adjacent to region of uveitis.

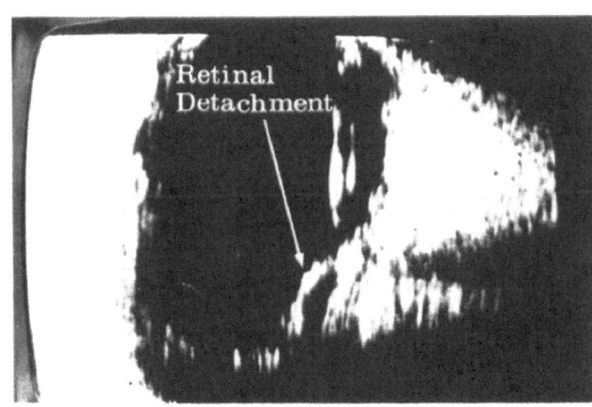

FIGURE 13.1c

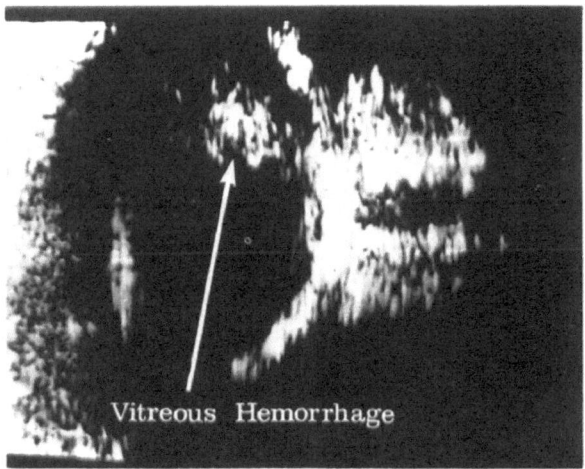

FIGURE 13.1d

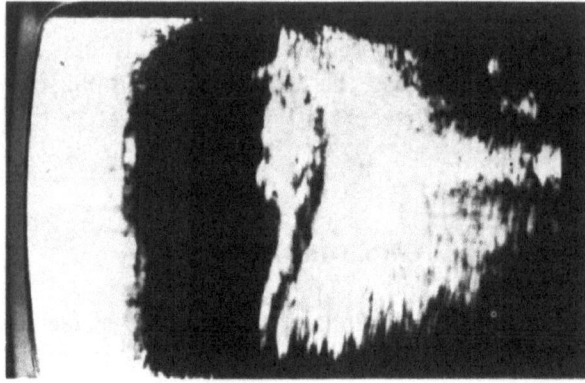

FIGURE 13.2
Phthysis bulbi. Panophthalmitis may destroy the internal architecture of the eye producing axial length shortening and choroidal thickening.

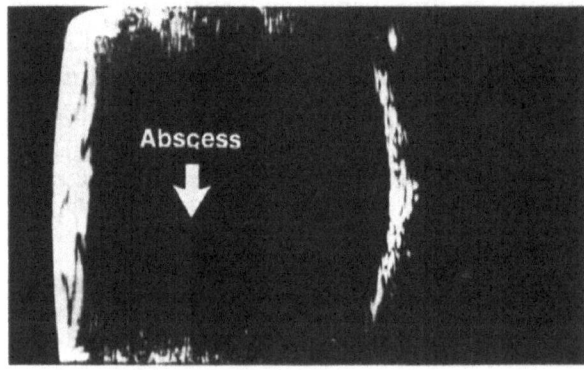

FIGURE 13.3a
Orbital abscess. Horizontal scan through the orbital roof shows echo-free area with sharp distal echo pattern.

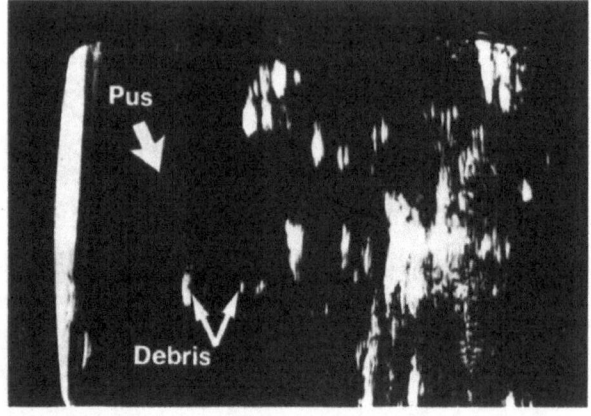

FIGURE 13.3b
Chronic abscess with inflammatory debris shows coarse internal echoes with irregular posterior wall.

membrane of mixed echogenicity in the posterior vitreous (Figure 13.1c), and focal hemorrhage may be noted near the site of inflammation (Figure 13.1d).

Uveitis is generally not limited to the uveal tract and often involves other or all ocular tissues (panophthalmitis) and may result in a phthysical eye (Figure 13.2).

Orbital abscess is rare, and isolation of the agent is difficult. The eye is scanned through the plane of the globe and through the plane of the orbital floor and orbital roof horizontally. The globe is out of the plane of the scan when the orbit is scanned transversely.

The echogenic orbital tissue in the presence of an abscess is replaced with echo-free areas with scattered low or medium amplitude internal echoes. The posterior limiting membrane is often irregular due to areas of pus with necrotic debris (Figure 13.3a and b).

Histoplasmosis is an intracellular mycotic infection common in the south-central United States. This disease has a wide clinical spectrum. Ocular histoplasmosis consists of hemorrhagic or non-hemorrhagic macular disciform lesions, peripheral and peripapillary choroidal atrophic scars. These lesions usually accompany a positive histoplasmin skin test. The organism has never been positively identified in human eyes with these lesions. Macular involvement generally follows years after peripheral choroidal scars have formed.

Visceral larva migrans is a parasitic infestation in man due to Toxocara canis, a common ascarid of dogs. Ocular involvement from parasitism is being increasingly recognized in the past decade due to immigration of peoples from underdeveloped nations to medically sophisticated areas. In the United States, Toxoplasma gondii and Toxocara canis are the ophthalmologist's prime concern although the majority of cases of infection occur from other agents in Asia and Africa. Clinically, Toxocara presents with three discrete forms. A mild infection may produce a peripheral localized granuloma in a quiet eye. More severe involvement may cause a localized granu-

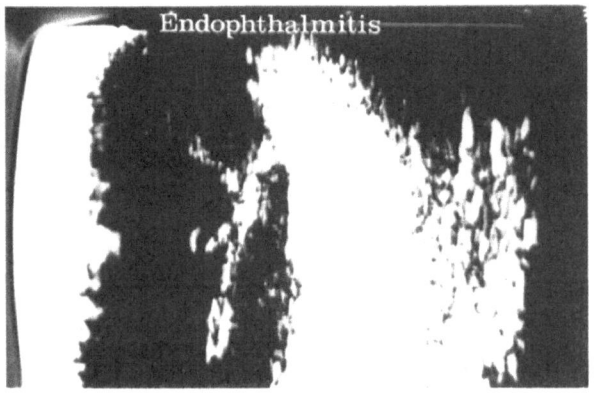

FIGURE 13.4
Endophthalmitis. Axial length shortening in pre-phthysical globe from parasitic infection.

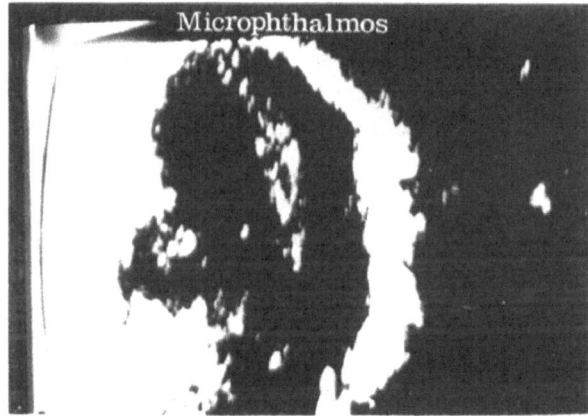

FIGURE 13.5
Congenital rubella. Diffusely disorganized internal structure of the globe in two-month old child.

loma in the posterior pole. Diffuse endophthalmitis results from overwhelming infection (Figure 13.4).

Ocular manifestations of congenital rubella are an integral part of this syndrome. Every part of the eye may be affected by the virus, but the lens, cornea, iris, and ciliary and RPE are primarily involved (Figure 13.5). The virus enters the fetal eye within two weeks of maternal infection. Cataract, corneal haze, glaucoma, retinopathy, and microphthalmos may be produced.

Sarcoidosis is a granulomatous disease of undetermined etiology. Ocular involvement occurs in approximately one quarter of patients with sarcoidosis and may lead to permanent blindness (Figure 13.6). Millet-seed nodules may appear on the external eye or conjunctiva. Iridocyclitis is probably the most common ocular pathology in sarcoidosis. This acute inflammation produces ciliary congestion. Cataractous changes (Figure 13.7), glaucoma secondary to peripheral anterior synechia and gray or yellow retinal lesions called candle-wax drippings may be noted. It may affect the optic nerve but rarely affects the orbital tissues.

Toxoplasmosis is considered with Toxocara canis (visceral larva migrans) to be the most common parasitic ocular infections in the United

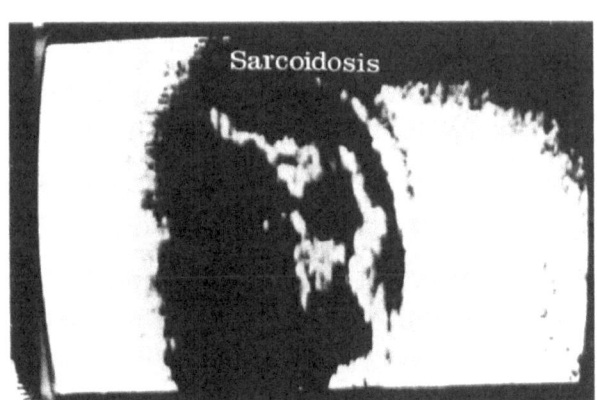

FIGURE 13.6
Sarcoidosis. Vitreous hemorrhage was noted in this globe with advanced changes of chronic inflammation.

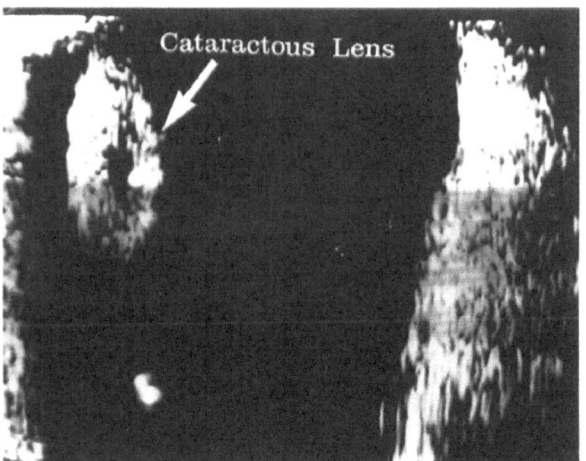

FIGURE 13.7
Cataract formation is a complication of this granulomatous disease process.

171

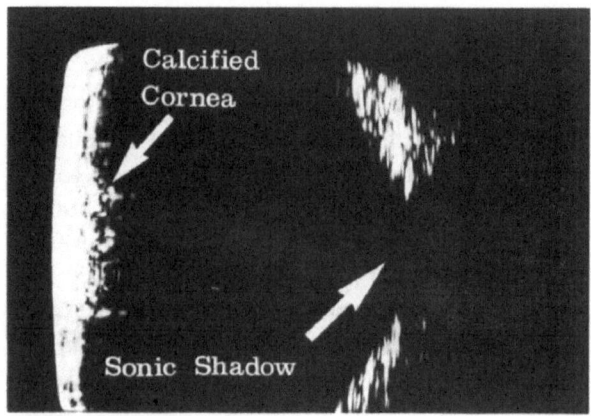

FIGURE 13.8
Calcified cornea. Scattered reverberation echoes are noted anteriorly due to dense calcification from post inflammatory changes which cast a strong sonic shadow.

States. Toxoplasmosis is a common infestation of man and other animals and is caused by Toxoplasma gondii. Infection may be aquired or congenital. Toxoplasmic retinochoroiditis is a frequently diagnosed form of uveitis accounting for up to 50% of cases of uveitis in certain areas. It is not possible to determine whether the ocular disease has been congenital or acquired by the pathologic changes. The organism localizes in the human retina and secondarily involves the choroid, vitreous, and sclera. After the retinal architecture is destroyed, cellular debris and inflammatory exudate spill into the vitreous. The pathologic changes are usually in the posterior pole. In sonographic evaluation of inflammatory disorders we have occasionally found corneal calcification which guided us to the etiology of the disease through further investigation of other parts of the body. The calcified cornea (Figure 13.8), scanned at 80 dB shows a sonic shadow of the posterior ocular wall. The cornea is visually opaque, but parts may be imaged sonographically at 50 dB with strong echoes. X-ray tomography shows a band like corneal calcification. The presence of a sonic shadow without explanation should suggest the presence of anterior chamber calcifications and point to inflammation as a possible etiology.

HEREDITARY METABOLIC DISORDERS

A large percentage of hereditary systemic diseases of metabolism may affect the eye. However, in these inborn errors of metabolism only three may be specifically diagnosed by ocular examination and include albinism, Fabry's disease, and Wilson's disease.

The general nature of metabolic disorders producing ocular lesions are disordered metabolism of lipids, connective tissues, amino acids, carbohydrates, and deficient transport proteins (Wilson's disease). Wilson's disease has the distinctive Kayser-Fleischer ring. Albinism has hyperopia and nystagmus along with other signs and symptoms.

Fabry's disease has corneal dystrophy and star shaped opacities in the posterior lens. Retinal edema and papilledema are usually secondary to the chronic renal disease.

Collagen and rheumatic diseases produce a wide variety of eye disorders. Rheumatoid arthritis causes scleritis and keratoconjunctivitis sicca. The scleritis is usually gradual in onset. Long-standing scleritis may thin and bulge the sclera leading to scleromalacia perforans.

Iridocyclitis is a serious manifestation of juvenile rheumatoid arthritis. Calcific band keratophthy accompanies chronic iridocyclitis in children. Ankylosing spondylitis, like juvenile rheumatoid arthritis, frequently has an associated iridocyclitis as a manifestation. Lupus erythematosus has a retinopathy consisting of soft exudates which is non-specific. Lesions of hypertension are also noted in this disorder. The fundoscopic changes in scleroderma are similar.

Cranial arteritis or giant cell arteritis may produce a true medical emergency for the ophthalmologist. Blindness occurs acutely and is due to ischemic neuritis. The disc is often only slightly elevated. This disorder occurs in patients over the age of 60 and is often effectively treated by steroids. Scanning of the carotid arteries for plaque formation should be performed by the ultrasonographer to rule out embolization as the etiology of the acute blindness.

NUTRITIONAL EYE DISEASE

Malnutrition may produce blindness and is one of the oldest signs of disease recorded in history in the form of night blindness. Vitamin A deficiency is a leading cause of blindness throughout the world in the pediatric age group. Keratomalacia and white dots in the retina may be noted. Vitamin B deficiency can give rise to corneal vascularization and temporal pallor to the optic nerve head.

ENDOCRINE DISEASES

The eye is the target organ for the endocrinopathies of Grave's disease and diabetes mellitus. Involvement of the eye in other endocrine disorders is either less frequent or less significant and will not be discussed in detail. Hypertensive retinopathy is found in pheochromocytoma, Addison's disease, Cushing's syndrome, and primary aldosteronism. Papilledema is noted in hypothalamic tumors and hypoparathyroidism.

THYROID DISORDERS

Ptosis and edema of the lids and periorbital areas are common in hypothyroidism. Rarely are noted abnormalities of the lens, uvea and myotonia of the extraocular muscles. Lenticular opacities are usually small but cretinism may produce a dense cataract.

HYPERTHYROIDISM (GRAVE'S DISEASE)

Grave's disease is poorly understood as to the etiology and pathogenesis of this dramatic ophthalmic disorder. Clinically, the spectrum of ophthalmopathy ranges from asymptomatic to physically devastating. Retraction of the upper lid causes widening of the palpebral fissure and lid lag. About one fifth of the patients exhibit proptosis which is thought to be due to retro-orbital infiltration. Marked retro-orbital changes result in periorbital edema, lid edema, chemosis, ophthalmoplegia, and evidence of pressure or ischemia on the optic nerve producing decreased visual acuity and papilledema. Diplopia is due to infiltration of the extraocular muscles producing edema which is later followed by fibrosis. Optic nerve compression within the orbit is a serious complication of Grave's disease which must be frequently checked clinically. Ophthalmopathy may start before hyperthyroidism is noted, simultaneous with hyperthyroidism, after treatment of hyperthyroidism or be unassociated with the status of the thyroid function. However, once exophthalmos has started to progress, it worsens and finally plateaus. This then subsides over a number of years. Mild exopthalmos may return to normal but severe eye changes seldom completely reverse themselves. Most patients have an autonomous thyroid gland that is non-

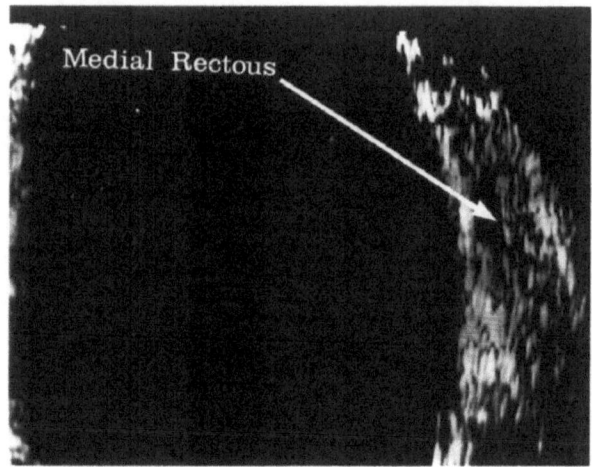

FIGURE 13.9
Grave's disease. Enlarged and echogenic medial rectus muscle may represent fibrotic changes in the muscle tissue due to longstanding process.

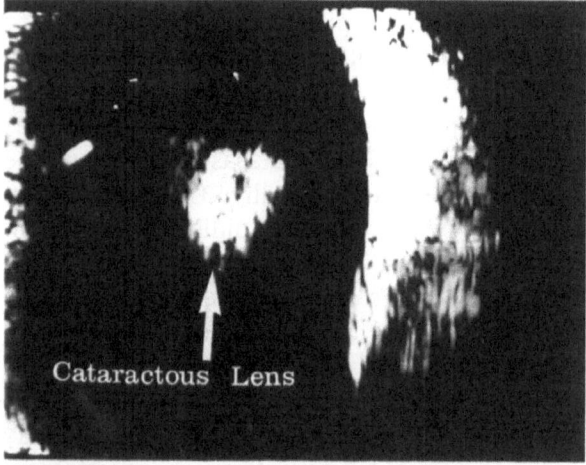

FIGURE 13.10
Dislocated lens. Cataractous lens is a common complication of diabetic oculopathy.

suppressible with thyroid administration. The extraocular muscles may increase in size up to eight times normal and the orbital volume may quadruple. Histologically there is an interstitial inflammatory edema and infiltration with lymphocytes, macrophages, mast cells, and plasma cells. Muscle fibers show loss of striation and perivascular round cell infiltration. The inferior and medial rectus muscles are usually the first to become involved and edema of Tenon's space is noted. Fibrosis follows in the later stages of this myopathy (Figure 13.9).

DIABETES MELLITUS

Few disorders affect the visual apparatus as widely and profoundly as diabetes. Lesions produced may be extraocular or intraocular and involve all portions of the eye and orbit.

Extraocular manifestations of diabetes involve the lids, conjunctiva, extraocular muscles, and orbit. Yellow elevated plaques called xanthelasma may be noted in the lids. Vasoconstriction of the conjunctival vessels and microaneurysms may occur. Extraocular muscle palsies are characteristic of diabetes mellitus. These may be unassociated with other central nervous system manifestations and are often painful. Lateral rectus muscle paralysis due to sixth nerve involvement is more common than the paresis of the muscles innervated by the third nerve. This usually clears spontaneously over several months and the pupil is usually spared in contrast to third nerve palsy from aneurysms or neoplasms. Ischemic neuritis is most likely due to angiopathy of diabetic disease. Orbital infection from mucormycosis is a rare but lethal complication of poorly controlled diabetes. Pain, exophthalmos, and ophthalmoplegia are the usual presenting symptoms.

Intraocular problems associated with diabetes include disorders of the cornea, iris, lens, ciliary body, vitreous, retina, and optic nerve. Wrinkles in the central portion of Descemet's membrane are common. The iris may be covered by a fibrovascular membrane which is secondary to retinitis proliferans and result in anterior cham-

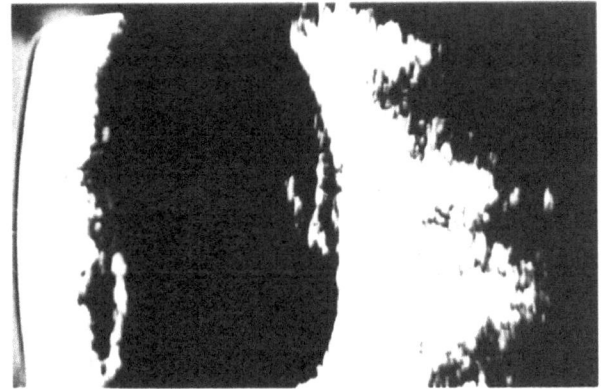

FIGURE 13.11a
Macular disease. Macular edema elevates the area of the macula on the posterior ocular wall.

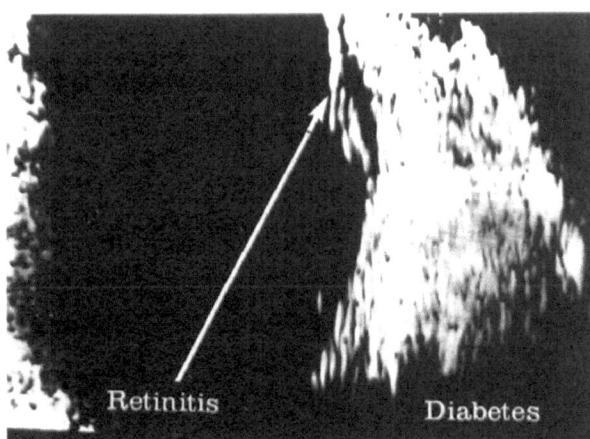

FIGURE 13.11b
Retinopathy with membranes over the macula produces an identical scan picture.

ber angle occlusion with glaucoma. The lens may be involved in dynamic shape alterations due to changes in blood glucose level which causes refractive errors. Cataract formation of the senile type occurs with greater frequency and at an earlier age in diabetics. The cataractous lens of severe diabetes typically shows the distal border of the lens to be echogenic and irregular. The lens may be dislocated (Figure 13.10).

Optic neuritis may accompany this disorder. Retinopathy is the most significant clinical alteration in diabetes. The small vessel angiopathy produces a characteristic picture of retinal microaneurysms at the posterior pole. Retinopathy is usually symmetric and bilateral. The posterior pole is usually involved and the periphery is spared. The disorder is generally progressive but may be somewhat reversible. Dilated and hypercellular arterioles, capillaries, and venules may be noted. Neovascularization may occur within and anterior to the retina and capillary shunts may exist. Macular edema may produce severe visual loss (Figure 13.11a and b). Sometimes the retinopathy in a diabetic may be due to other causes than diabetes. Proper history is essential to prevent mistaking a case of retinal detachment for diabetic retinopathy when frond-like echoes emerge from the optic disc. Mobility is limited in retinal detachment and diabetic vitreous bands are frozen and show no motion with rotational maneuvers (Figure 13.12a,b,c, and d).

Typical retinal hemorrhage and exudates of diabetic retinopathy develop secondary to the vasculopathy. Vitreous hemorrhage may be massive or mild and repetitive or intermittent. The focal shape of diabetic retinal hemorrhage are due to their deep retinal location (Figure 13.13). Bleeding from the proliferating vessels into the posterior vitreous are the cause of vitreous hemorrhage (Figure 13.14).

Vitreous hemorrhage should be differentiated from retinopathy and retinal detachment due to the diabetes. Vitreous hemorrhage simulating a retinal detachment may show a V-shaped or circular shaped moderately echogenic membrane appearing in the vitreous which is highly mobile and disappears at 70 dB. Scattered very low

175

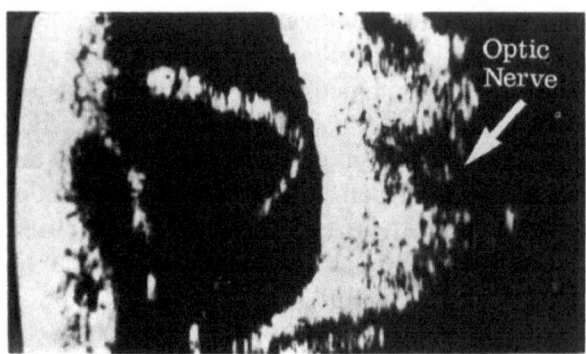

FIGURE 13.12a
Retinal detachment. This often accompanies diabetic disease and appears slightly mobile with eye movements.

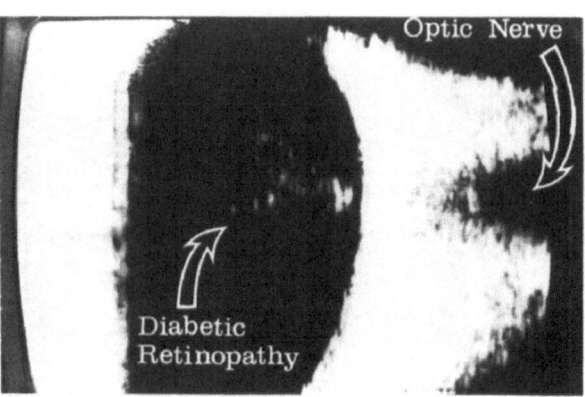

FIGURE 13.12d
Membranes of retinitis proliferans may extend out from the optic nerve head.

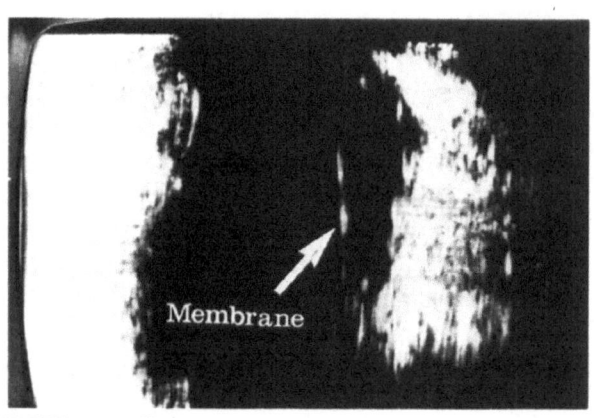

FIGURE 13.12b
Retinitis proliferans. Linear echogenic membrane may simulate part of a retinal detachment.

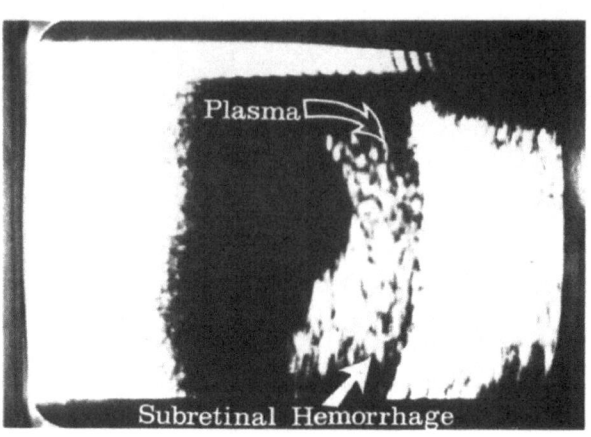

FIGURE 13.13
Subretinal hemorrhage. Longitudinal scan. This localized echogenic area is echo-poor superiorly and echo-dense inferiorly as the blood settles to the dependent portion of this zone limited anteriorly by the retina and the plasma rises superiorly.

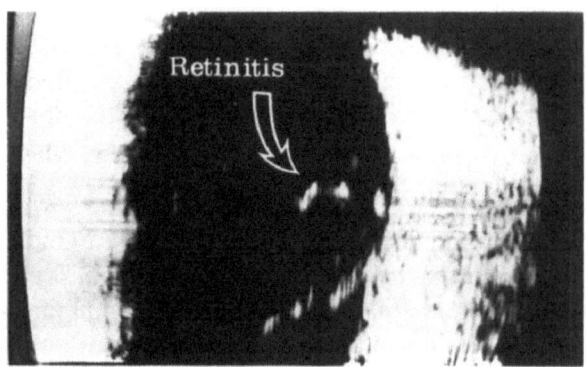

FIGURE 13.12c
Rescanning this area shows typical frond-like immobile echogenic structure.

amplitude echoes may be noted in the midvitreous representing smaller or circular areas of hemorrhage (Figure 13.15).

The development of new blood vessels portends a serious change in the prognosis of diabetic retinopathy. Usually, the vessels arise from a retinal vein at an arteriovenous crossing at the posterior pole. Initially there is a collection of delicate lacelike naked vessels called the rete mirabile. These are extremely permeable and become more fibrous in appearance with connective tissue proliferation surrounding them. These are associated with retinal and vitreous

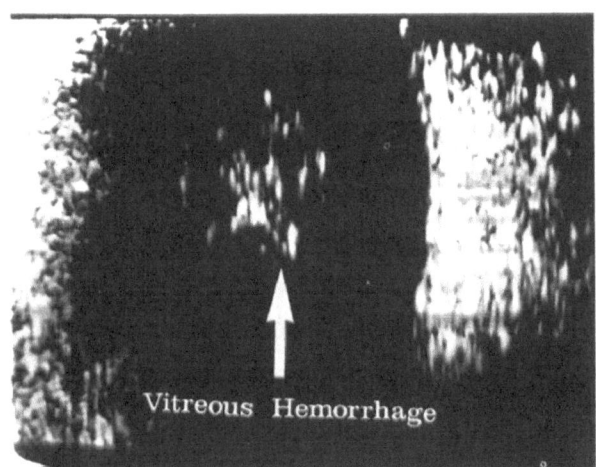

FIGURE 13.14

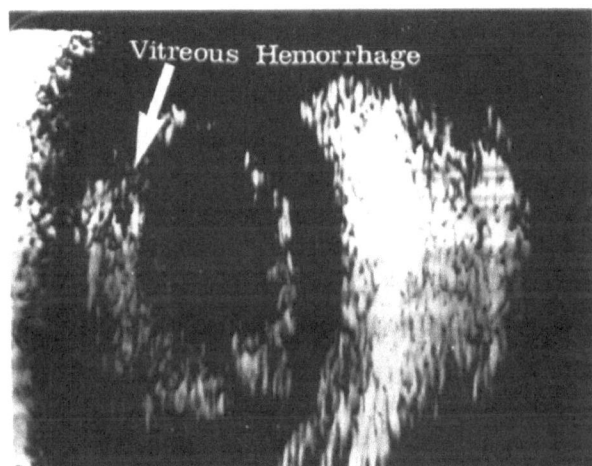

FIGURE 13.15

FIGURE 13.16

hemorrhage. As long as the vitreous remains in contact with the retina, the blood vessels lie flat along the inner retinal surface. If the vitreous body contracts, blood vessels adherent to its posterior face may rupture and cause hemorrhage or drag the retina inward causing retinal detachment. With time the fibrous blood vessels grow into the vitreous gel (Figure 13.16).

HYPERTENSION

The smaller arteries and veins of the body are readily visible with the direct and indirect ophthalmoscope and provide the clinician data on the smaller vessels of the body. The retinal arterial vessels are generally arterioles.

Hypertension produces a variety of changes in the retinal vessels. These include vasconstriction, hemorrhage, exudates, and retinal edema. Generalized and local vasoconstriction occur in acute hypertension and are reversible with therapy of the high blood pressure. Cotton wool patches are soft exudates which represent thickening of the terminal nerve fibers of the retina and are nonspecific findings. Hemorrhages and microaneurysms begin to appear after exudates have formed. Hemorrhages associated with severe hypertensive disease usually occur near the disc in the nerve fiber layer and extend along the nerve fibers parallel to the retinal surface which gives the typical flame shape. These may regress rapidly with appropriate treatment. Papilledema is an ominous sign when occuring from malignant hypertension and often signifies severe renal compromise (Figure 13.17). Arteriosclerotic retinopathy is a diffuse thickening of the small

FIGURE 13.14
Vitreous hemorrhage. Typical moderately echogenic pattern of diffuse echoes within the midvitreous due to diabetes.

FIGURE 13.15
Vitreous hemorrhage with circular shape may simulate a retinal detachment. Echoes are highly mobile and disappear at 70 dB.

FIGURE 13.16
Neovascularity. Blood vessels in chronic diabetes grow from the retinal surface into the vitreous.

177

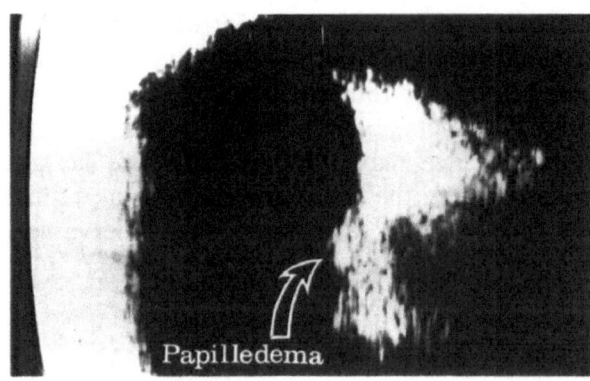

FIGURE 13.17
Papilledema. Echogenic projection from the optic nerve head into the vitreous due to severe hypertension.

vessels, primarily the arterioles. Tortuousity and widening of the light reflex are noted. Later obliteration of the vein on either side of the arteriole will be noted. This is a generalized disorder of all the small vessels of the body and retinal vascular changes may correlate with renal vessel findings.

GASTROENTEROLOGICAL DISEASES

The eye may be affected in a variety of gastroenterological disorders, such as regional enteritis, Whipple's disease, intestinal parasites, and peptic ulcer problems.

In Crohn's disease or regional enteritis, the eye may be involved with conjunctivitis, iridocyclitis, exudative retinal detachment, and chronic retinitis. Whipple's disease is medically treatable and the eye findings are supranuclear type ophthalmoplegia and nonspecific ocular inflammation. Parasites have already been discussed under the heading of infectious disorders. Peptic ulcer disease treated by gastrectomy may produce a vitamin B-12 deficiency syndrome characterized by a central optic neuropathy.

HEMATOLOGIC DISORDERS

Abnormalities in the number of cells, the viscosity of the plasma, or the function of the blood constituents may produce marked ocular pathology.

Ocular lesions of hemoglobinopathies arise from the intravascular changes in the conjunctiva or retinal vessels. Retinal vasculopathy is more marked than conjunctival disease and is located at the periphery of the retina, generally temporally. Arteriolar occlusion is followed by arteriolar-venular anastomoses and aneurysmal dilatations. Neovascularization and fibrous proliferation give rise to vitreous hemorrhage and retinal detachment. This anterior or peripheral neovascularization distinguishes this from diabetic retinopathy. Leukemia produces ophthalmic lesions secondary to tissue infiltration and hemorrhage, especially into the choroid layer. These findings are more common in acute leukemias rather than the chronic forms. Tortuous veins, exudates, superficial and deep retinal hemorrhages may be found.

Findings from multiple myeloma may be due to the neoplasm presenting as an orbital tumor or hyperviscosity changes producing retinal hemorrhages and vascular occlusion. Similarly in Waldenstrom's macroglobulinemia, increased viscosity causes dilated veins, hemorrhage and exudative retinal detachment. Eosinopilic granu-loma usually produces a lytic lesion of the bony orbital tumor. Hand-Schuller-Christian disease, with its reticuloendothelial and histiocytic proliferation, may produce bony lesions and exophthalmos. Exophthalmos results from orbital accumulation of granulomatous tissue. Ocular signs in Letter-Siwe disease are usually secondary to skull involvement in this rapidly fatal pediatric disorder.

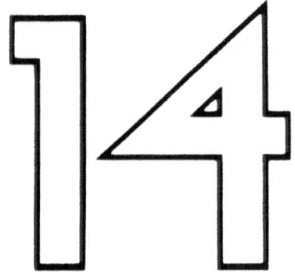

artifacts

A wide variety of mechanical and ultrasonic artifacts occur during real-time scanning of the eye. These problems may be simply annoying to the ultrasonographer or lead to serious misinterpretation of the study. Artifacts must be recognized, their source or sources identified and properly corrected in order to avoid gross errors in the scan interpretation. In this section, we shall only consider the artifacts pertinent to real-time contact B-scanning of the eye which will be discussed below.

LIGHT ARTIFACT

A frequent artifact is the light artifact. The examination is best performed in a fairly dark room. A sufficient supply of film must be available to avoid opening the door to the ultrasonic examining room to obtain more film or other supplies and the scanning assistant must be familiar with the exposure technique and able to replace the exposed film with new film in a dimly lit room. A brightly lit room will produce a

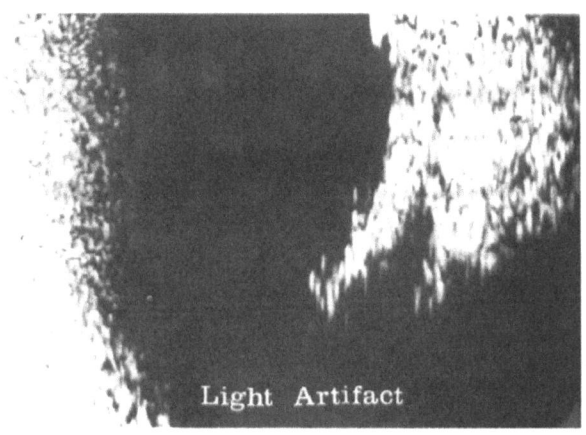

FIGURE 14.1a
Light artifact. The polaroid film was taken in a brightly lit room and appears gray instead of black. This may be mistaken for underdevelopment of the film by opening the polaroid before the recommended developing time.

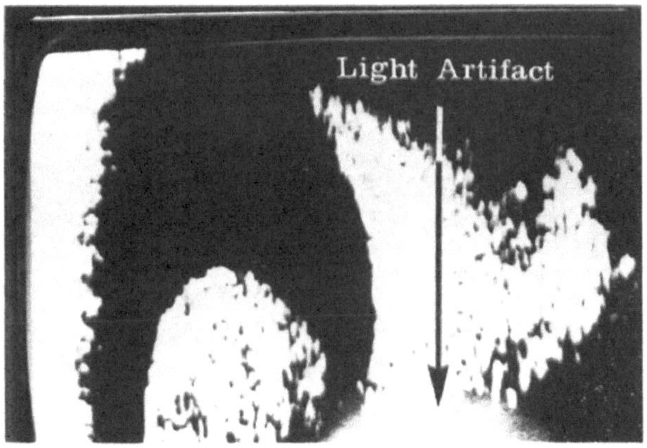

light film that may be mistaken for an underdeveloped polaroid (Figure 14.1a and b).

REFLECTION ARTIFACT

A small room lamp is often used for reduced lighting. This light should be placed far from the scanning area and its beam directed away from the T.V. monitor. Failure to observe this arrangement may result in reflection light artifacts which may be confusing to the ultrasonographer. The presence of a very bright light causing a total reflection of the lamp by the monitor screen is usually obvious; however, many subtle variations may occur and produce diagnostic problems if they fall in the region of the vitreous, retina, or orbit that appears on the television screen face (Figure 14.2a,b,c, and d).

SHUTTER ARTIFACT

The lens shutter of the camera should be checked before examination and adjusted to proper setting which gives maximum information. Prior usage of the unit and changes of the shutter speed may produce difficulty for the next examination on the same unit. The improper setting causes loss of information. The film itself is important. Before the introduction of a new type of polaroid film, ordinary 107 polaroid was used which needed coating. Recently, we use 667 for which there is no need for coating, but occasionally it will roll. On the other hand, better information can be gained by 667 film since more shades of gray can be captured by this emulsion.

CAMERA ARTIFACT

Occasionally another artifact occurs during pulling out of the polaroid film from the camera. If the extraction is improper, the rod passing over the film may spread the emulsion unevenly and produce a typical artifact (Figure 14.3).

FIGURE 14.1b
Reproduction light artifact. Milky artifact is demonstrated at the inferior portion of the polaroid picture. Incidentally noted is a bulky intravitreal extension of a choroidal melanoma.

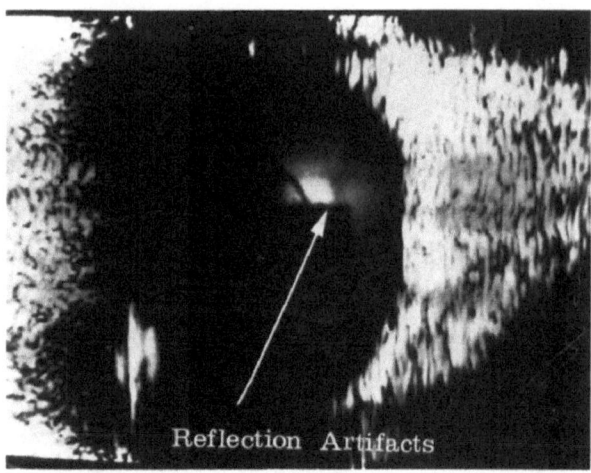

FIGURE 14.2a

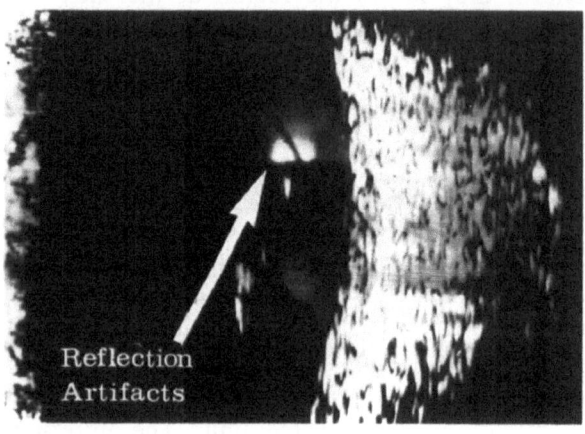

FIGURE 14.2b

FIGURE 14.2a
Reflection artifact. This is due to extraneous light falling on the T.V. monitor. This light gray artifact has a flat inferior border since the top of the polaroid camera blocks the light source.

FIGURE 14.2b
Reflection artifact. This may fall in the vitreous simulating vitreous pathology.

FIGURE 14.2c
Reflection artifact. The light source reflects from the area of the screen on which the retina is imaged. The sonographer should carefully distinguish this from a true lesion.

FIGURE 14.2d
Reflection artifact. Scan at the 1.5–4.5 range demonstrating light artifact to fall in the posterior orbital region.

Development timing is a matter of personal experience, but is often 45 seconds for the 667 type film. If time lapses more than 60–90 seconds, surface artifact may appear on the film.

The other group of artifacts are sonic artifacts. This artifact is related to the properties of ultrasound waves. Ultrasonic waves obey the same rules as light waves such as reflection, diffraction, refraction, and absorption. A number of artifacts may occur as a result of the above phenomena.

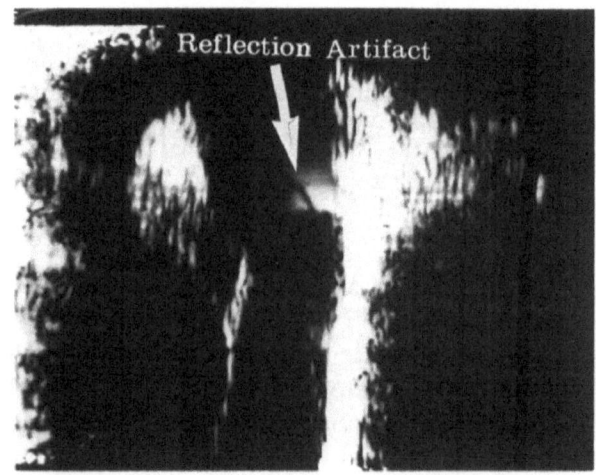

FIGURE 14.2c

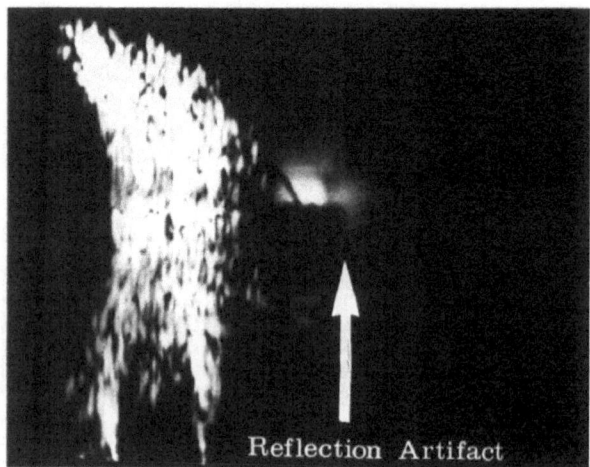

FIGURE 14.2d

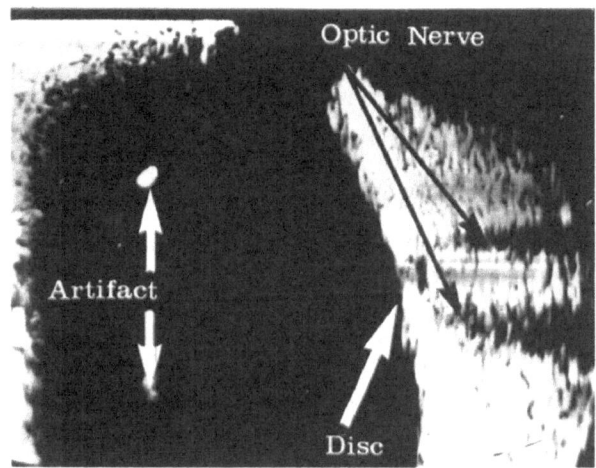

FIGURE 14.3

FIGURE 14.3
Camera artifact. Irregularity of the smooth rollers through which the film passes produced these artifacts simulating vitreous floaters. This disappeared after cleaning of the rollers.

FIGURE 14.4a
Reverberation artifact. Multiple linear echoes of decreasing size and strength occur as the sound beam bounces back and forth from the interface and the transducer head.

FIGURE 14.4b
Reverberation artifact simulating orbital tumor. Scan at 1.5–4.5 cm depth shows an echo-free space separating the orbital fat from a far distal moderately strong echo. This should not be confused with an extra ocular tumor.

REVERBERATION ARTIFACT

In one category which is called false echo artifact, there is no relationship between the organ structure and the final photo. They are usually produced by multiple internal reflections between two interfaces or from the transducer head, which may be secondary to a non-perpendicular position of the transducer or poor crystal placement. This is actually a reverberation type of distortion (Figure 14.4a and b). If these artifacts are produced by multiple internal reflections, usually they are serial with each echo weaker than the primary echo, having an image of diminishing size. In scanning the eye with real-time B-contact scanner, this phenomenon is most apparent when the sonic beam passes through the lens.

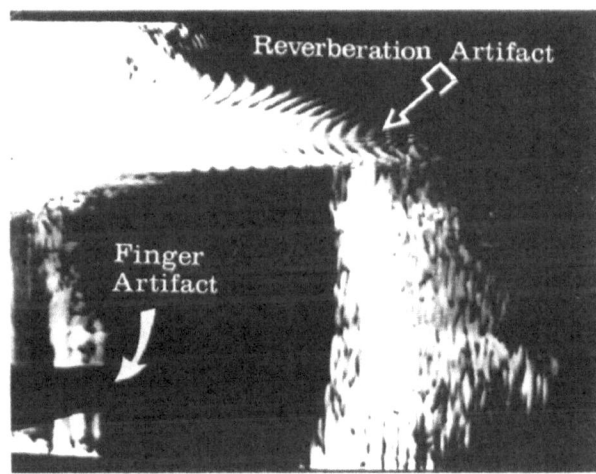

FIGURE 14.4a

LENS ARTIFACT

The lens is a major source of sonic artifact within the eye. Those portions of the sonic beam which pass through the edges of the lens strike the side of the eyeball instead of continuing in a straight line to the posterior portion of the eye. This is the result of the convexity of the lens and deflection of the beam at the edge of the lens. As a result, a lens artifact appears. The increased velocity of sound in the lens tissue causes a forward displacement of structure behind the center of the lens. The path of the sonic beam to

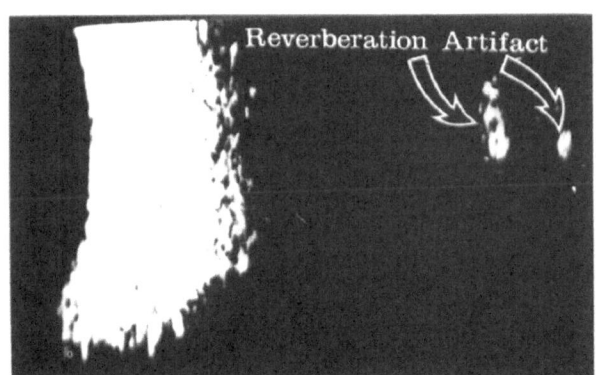

FIGURE 14.4b

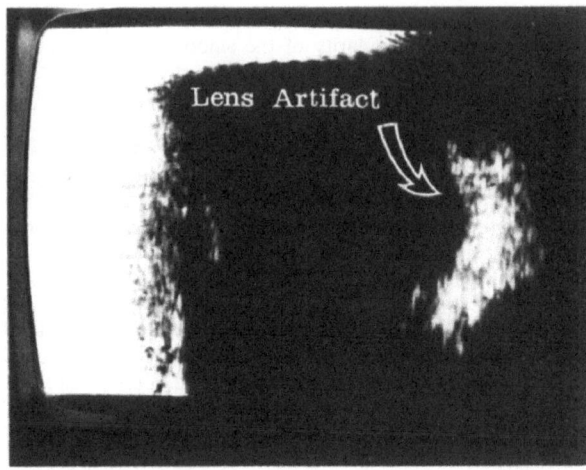

FIGURE 14.5a

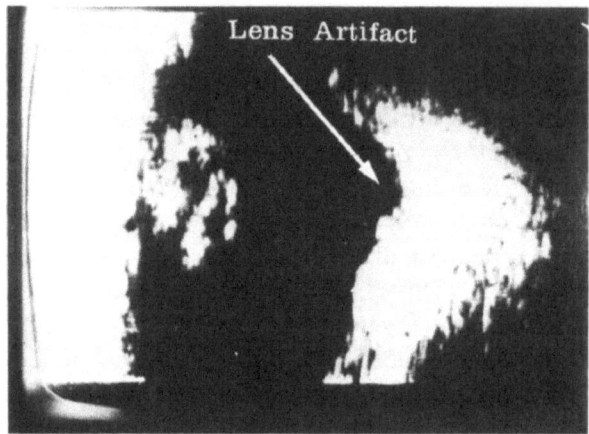

FIGURE 14.5b

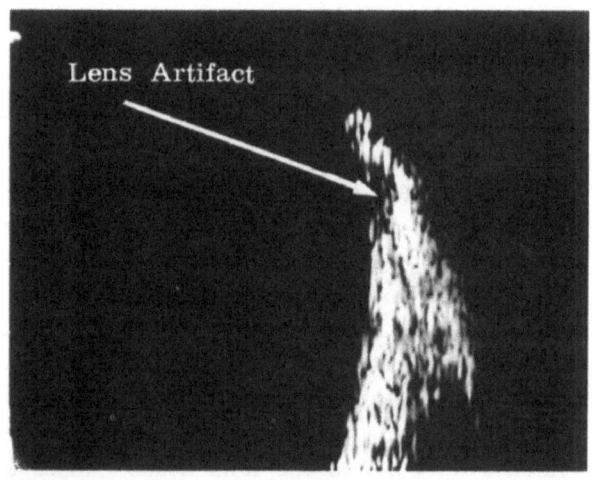

FIGURE 14.5c

FIGURE 14.5a
Lens artifact. Anteriorly the lens is faintly imaged since it is only partially in the scan beam. Distal to this is a depression in the posterior ocular wall which is an artifact produced by the normal lens.

FIGURE 14.5b
Lens artifact. Cataractous lens produces a greater posterior indentation of the posterior ocular wall than the normal lens artifact.

FIGURE 14.5c
Lens artifact. Peripherally located lens artifact presents as a scalloped area on the posterior ocular wall due to an oblique scanning plane.

the side of the eyeball is shorter than the path to the posterior wall of the eyeball. This phenomenon causes an anterior step which results in lens artifact.

When the eye is looking straight ahead, the lens artifact appears as an increased convexity of the central portion of the retina with a sharp anterior projection which corresponds to the edge of the lens. One edge or both edges may disappear and only outward bowing may be seen. A number of variations exist which depend on the lens, gaze, position of the transducer, and lenticular disorders which are discussed elsewhere in the text.

This false lens induced displacement of the posterior ocular wall depends on the distance between the lens and the retina and is smaller as the lens is closer to the posterior ocular wall as in the condition of a dislocated lens. The lens artifact is more pronounced when the lens is cataractous and at times a sonic shadow may be produced (Figure 14.5a,b, and c).

COUPLING ARTIFACT

Air bubbles may occur in the gel stand off used to image the anterior structures of the eye and may even produce a sonic shadow sign (Figure 14.6). Air bubbles within the transducer housing are common but usually produce a weak sonic output. This artifact must be entertained when the orbital fat echoes do not appear as bright as usual.

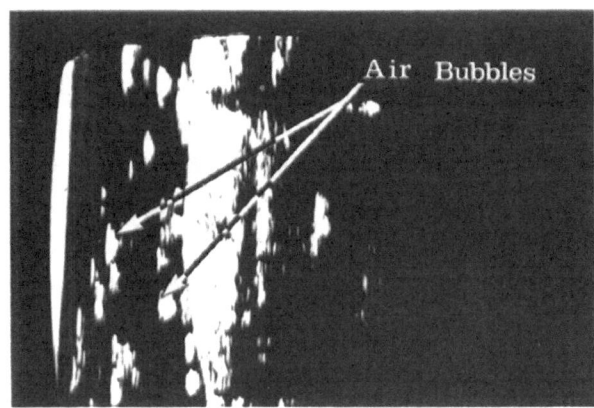

FIGURE 14.6

Another coupling artifact is due to the "dead zone" in the near field which obscures information from anterior structures such as the cornea and anterior portion of the lens. This is due to continued oscillation of the crystal during the receiving phase.

INTERFERENCE ARTIFACT

Electromagnetic waves from external sources may produce a variety of small lines or dots on the T.V. monitor. These may remain stationary or move depending upon the nature of the electromagnetic source (Figure 14.7).

SONIC SHADOW SIGN ARTIFACT

The sonic shadow is produced by absorption of sound waves by structures with high sound attenuation or high reflection qualities. If the absorption of the sound beam is complete, there is a total sonic shadow sign and no information can be obtained distally. If attenuation is partial, some of the sonic beam will pass through, and limited scan data will return. Even though the sonic shadow is troublesome and causes difficulties in interpretation in many areas of ultrasonography, it may be of great help in the detection of tumors with calcifications, air in the tissues, and foreign bodies (Figure 14.8).

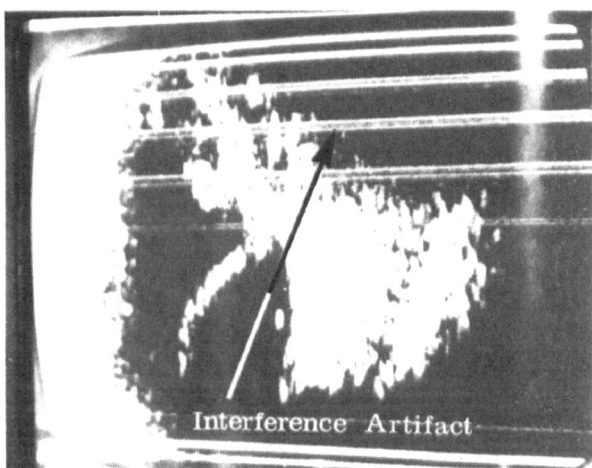

FIGURE 14.7

FIGURE 14.6
Coupling artifact. Air bubbles in the thick layer of methylcellulose used to stand off the sonic beam to examine the anterior segment of the eye are numerous in this field and the larger bubbles produce a partial sonic shadow sign.

FIGURE 14.7
Interference artifact. Scan through a globe with a retinal detachment is marred by parallel electronic echo pattern produced by electrical interference with the scanning unit.

FIGURE 14.8
Sonic shadow artifact. The presence of a sonic shadow in the posterior orbital fat echoes must alert the sonographer to the presence of anterior pathology. In this case there is a dislocated and cataractous lens which is absorbing the sonic beam.

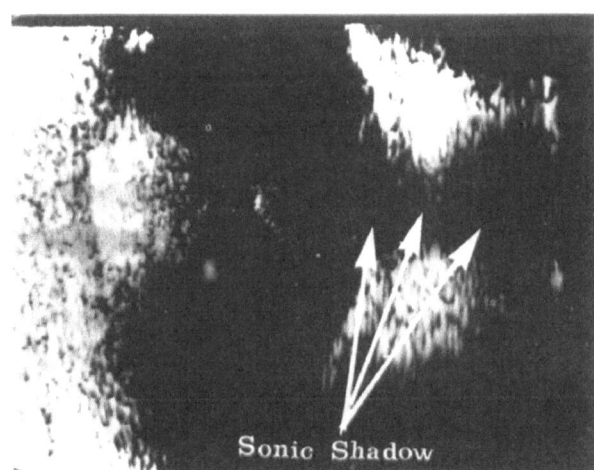

FIGURE 14.8

In conclusion, although artifacts may cause serious problems in diagnostic interpretation, a continuing awareness of these entities and their varying appearances will prevent most difficulties. The sonographer should consciously examine all lesions with the lens outside of the scanning plane. Lesions should be examined in the center of the screen to prevent beam width distortion at the edges of the field scanned. The artifacts of the sonic shadow and multiple reverberation type may guide the examiner to unsuspected lesions such as a calcified structure or a foreign body.

glossary

ABNORMAL (ANOMALOUS) RETINAL CORRESPONDENCE

Condition in which corresponding points on the two retinas do not have the same relative direction in space.

ACCOMMODATIVE ESOTROPIA

Inward deviation of the eyes characteristically more marked for near than far gaze and increased by ciliary muscle contraction in accomodation

ACCOMMODATIVE EXOTROPIA

Outward deviation of the eyes, usually secondary to uncorrected myopia

AMAUROSIS

Nearly obsolete term indicating loss of vision

ANGIOID STREAKS

Abnormality of the elastic layer of Bruch's membrane giving rise to pigmented striations of the ocular fundus; associated with a variety of systemic diseases such as pseudo-xanthoma elasticum, sickle cell disease, and osteitis deformans (Paget's disease) and a variety of generalized diseases affecting the elastic lamina of blood vessels

ANGLE-CLOSURE GLAUCOMA

Ocular abnormality in which the intraocular pressure increases, often quickly, because the anterior aqueous humor is mechanically prevented from reaching the trabecular meshwork

ANIRIDIA

Absence of iris, usually incomplete with iris root present

ANISOCORIA

Condition in which the pupils of the two eyes are of unequal size

ANKYLOBLEPHARON

Condition in which the margins of the eyelids are fused together

ANOPHTHALMOS

Absence of the eye

APHAKIA

Absence of the crystalline lens of the eye

AQUEOUS HUMOR

Fluid that fills the posterior and anterior chambers

ARCUATE SCOTOMA

Area of blindness in the field of vision of characteristic arc shape caused by interruption of a nerve fiber bundle in the retina; usually seen in glaucoma

ASTEROID HYALOSIS

Fixed opacities composed of a calcium lipid complex that occur in otherwise normal vitreous body; there are no symptoms

BAND KERATOPATHY

Deposition of calcium in the cornea most marked in horizontal meridian; occurs in degenerating eyes, hypercalcemia, hypophosphatemia, and juvenile arthritis (of Still)

BEDEWING OF CORNEA

Subepithelial cornea edema, often associated with sudden prolonged increase in intraocular pressure or wearing of contact lenses for an excessively long period (Sattler's veil)

BELL'S PALSY

Peripheral paralysis of the facial nerve

BELL'S PHENOMENON

Upward and outward deviation of the eyes occurring with forcible closure of the eyelids or sleep

BLINDNESS

Inability to see; defined by the internal revenue service as reduction of best visual acuity to 20/200 (6/60) or less in the better eye or restriction of the visual field to 20° or less

BLOWOUT FRACTURE OF ORBIT

Fracture of the roof of the maxillary sinus with prolapse of the intraorbital contents into the antrum. There is enophthalmos, blepharoptosis, inability to turn the eye upward, and usually infraorbital anesthesia.

BLUE SCLERA

Abnormality in which the sclera is thin and has a blue appearance arising from the underlying pigmented choroid

BUPHTHALMOS

Enlargement of the eye, usually occurring as a result of congenital glaucoma

CAROTID-CAVERNOUS FISTULA

Rupture of a carotid aneurysm into the cavernous sinus (infrasellar) that causes an increased venous pressure in the sinus. Also occurs with dural shunt

CATARACT

An opacity of the lens; the opacity arises from either denatured protein or imbibition of fluid

CENTRAL ANGIOSPASTIC RETINOPATHY

Condition characterized by separation of the neural retina from the pigment epithelium in the macular area by a serous fluid

CENTROCECAL SCOTOMA

Area of blindness in the field of vision involving both the fixation point and the blind spot (cecum); characterizes toxic amblyopias

CHERRY-RED SPOT

Ophthalmoscopic appearance of the fovea centralis (which contains only the outer layers of the retina adjacent to the choroid) when surrounded by either edematous or lipid-filled inner layers of the retina, as occurs in occlusion of the central retinal artery, in amaurotic familial idiocy, and in Niemann-Pick disease

CHOROIDEREMIA

X-chromosome linked abnormality characterized by atrophy of the choriocapillaris and degeneration of the retinal pigment epithelium

CHOROIDITIS

Inflammation of the choroid

CERCINATE RETINOPATHY

Rare monocular disorder, mainly of elderly women, characterized by an oval zone of small, discrete, coalescing white spots engirdling the macular area

CLOSED ANGLE GLAUCOMA

Arising because apposition of iris to peripheral cornea prevents aqueous humor from draining through the trabecular meshwork

COLOBOMA

Congenital fissure of a part of the eye

COMMOTIO RETINA

Traumatic lesion of the posterior pole with edema and hemorrhage following contusion of the anterior ocular segment

CONGRUOUS FIELD DEFECTS

Visual field defects that are exactly the same in extent and intensity in both eyes; characterizes lesions in the optic radiation and occipital cortex

CONJUNCTIVITIS

Inflammation of the conjunctiva

CONSENSUAL LIGHT REFLEX

Constriction of the pupil in the fellow eye when the retina is stimulated by light

CONTACT LENS

Worn beneath the eyelids

CORTICAL BLINDNESS

Caused by a lesion in the cortical visual center

COTTON WOOL SPOTS

A microinfarct causing acute edema of nerve fiber layer of retina (cytoid body)

CRYSTALLINE LENS

Transparent biconvex tissue located behind the pupil and in front of the vitreous

CYANOSIS RETINEA

Old term for vascular dilation in hyperviscosity of blood syndromes

CYCLOPLEGIA

Paralysis of the ciliary muscle giving rise to paralysis of accomodation

DACRYOADENITIS

Inflammation of the lacrimal gland, often chronic and due to a granulomatous disease; acute dacryoadenitis occurs with mumps and infectious mononucleosis

DETACHMENT, RETINAL

Separation of the sensory retina from the retinal pigment epithelium

DIOPTER

Unit of measurement of the refractive power of lenses equal to the reciprocal focal length of the lens expressed in meters

DIPLOPIA

Double vision; simultaneous perception of two grossly dissimilar images

DISCIFORM DEGENERATION OF MACULA

Secondary type of macular degeneration, often arising from abnormalities in the elastic layer of the lamina vitrea

DISCIFORM DETACHMENT OF THE RETINA

Term commonly applied to separations of the retina in the macular region arising because blood or serous fluid separates the sensory retina from the retinal pigment epithelium

DISCIFORM KERATITIS

Stromal type of corneal inflammation, roughly circular in shape, often seen as secondary stromal involvement to herpes simplex keratitis

DISHARMONIOUS

Angle of abnormality is less than the angle of strabismus

DISLOCATION OF LENS

Condition in which the crystaline lens is completely unsupported by the zonular fibers so that the lens is free, either in the vitreous body or the anterior chamber

DRUSEN

Hyaline excrescences of the retinal pigment epithelium

DYSMETRIA

Abnormality of ocular movements in which there is an overshoot of the eyes on attempt to fixate an object

ECTASIA OF SCLERA

Localized bulging of the sclera lined with uveal tissue; a staphyloma

ELECTRORETINOGRAM

Action potential that follows stimulation of the retina

ENDOGENOUS UVEITIS

Inflammation of the uveal tract arising from causes within the body in contrast to that introduced from outside the body as in injuries (exogenous)

ENDOPHTHALMITIS

Purulent inflammation of the intraocular contents

ENUCLEATION

Removal of the eye

EPIPHORA

Tearing in which faulty drainage of tears permits their overflow

EROSION

A recurrent loss of corneal epithelium that may follow minor injury

EVISCERATION

In ophthalmology, the surgical procedure in which the intraocular contents are removed, retaining the cornea (sometimes) and the sclera

EXCITING EYE

Initially injured eye that gives rise to sympathetic ophthalmia for the fellow eye, the sympathizing eye

EXENTERATION, ORBITAL

Removal of all the orbital tissues, including the eye and its nervous, vascular, and muscular connections

EXOPHTHALMOS

Protrusion of the eyes

EXOPHTHALMOS (ENDOCRINE)

Associated with abnormalities of the thyroid

EXOPHTHALMOS (OPHTHALMOPLEGIC)

Inability to move the eye because of exophthalmos

EXOPHTHALMOS (PULSATING)

Associated with a carotid cavernous fistula

FLOATER

Object seen in the field of vision that originates in the vitreous body; the most common floaters are muscae volitantes, minute residues of the hyaloid vasculature seen in bright, uniform illumination

FLUORESCEIN ANGIOGRAPHY

Serial photography of ocular fundus following intravenous administration of fluorescein solution

GONIOSCOPE

Special instrument for studying the angle of the anterior chamber of the eye

GONIOTOMY

Operation for congenital glaucoma in which the trabecular meshwork in the region of Schlemm's canal in incised

HETEROPHORIA

Condition in which there is a latent tendency of the eyes to deviate that is prevented by fusion

HOLE, RETINAL

Break in the continuity of the sensory retina so that there is a communication between the vitreous cavity and the potential space between the sensory retina and the retina pigment epithelium

HOMONYMOUS

In ophthalmology, having the same side of the field of vision; thus a right homonymous hemianopsia is right half-blindness and arises from a defect involving the nasal fibers of the right eye that decussate and the non-crossing fibers of the left eye; the lesion is on the left side, posterior to the optic chiasma

HYDROPHTHALMOS

Buphthalmos or the distended eye that occurs in infantile glaucoma

HYPERTELORISM

Excessive width between two organs; in ocular hypertelorism there is an increased distance between the eyes that is often associated with mental deficiency and exotropia

HYPHEMA

Blood in the anterior chamber

HYPOPYON

Pus in the anterior chamber

HYPOTONY, OCULAR

Diminished ocular pressure

IRIDECTOMY

Cutting out of part of the iris

IRIDENCLEISIS

Surgical procedure for glaucoma in which an incision is made at the corneoscleral limbus and the iris is incarcerated in the wound to create a filtering wick between the anterior chamber and subjunctival space

IRIDOCYCLITIS

Separation of the base of the iris from the ciliary body; main cause is blunt trauma to the eye

IRIDODONESIS

Tremulousness of the iris as occurs following loss of support after lens removal

IRIS BOMBE

Condition in which the pupil is adherent to the lens so that aqueous humor accumulates in the posterior chamber; iris tends to balloon forward peripherally and it may close the angle with secondary glaucoma

IRIS COLOBOMA

Defects of the iris that follow iridectomy or occurs as a congenital abnormality

IRITIS

Inflammation of the iris

KERATITIS

Inflammation of the cornea

LENS

Glass or other transparent material used optically to modify the path of light

MACULA LUTEA

Yellow spot; the ill defined retinal area surrounding the fovea centralis

MICROANEURYSMS

Capillary outpouching of the retina in diabetes mellitus, pulseless disease, hypertension

MICROPHAKIA

Anomaly in which the crystalline lens is abnormally small

MICROPHTHALMIA

Condition in which the eyeball is abnormally small

MICROPSIA

Disturbance in visual perception in which objects appear smaller than their true size

MIOSIS

Condition in which the pupil is constricted

MIOTIC

Pertaining to or characterized by constriction of the pupil

MORGAGNIAN CATARACT

Hypermature cataract in which the cortex is liquified, permitting the lens nucleus to float within the capsule

MUSCAE VOLITANTES

Flitting flecks darting about in the field of vision caused by the opacities in the vitreous humor (floaters)

MYDRIASIS

Dilation of the pupil

MYOPIA

Optical condition in which parallel rays of light come to focus in front of the retina

MYOPIA (AXIAL)

Caused by abnormal length of antero-posterior diameter of the eye

MYOPIA (DEGENERATIVE)

Associated with conus of optic disk and retinal abnormalities

MYOPIA (REFRACTIVE)

Caused by increased index of refraction of lens as occurs in nuclear sclerosis

NARROW-ANGLE GLAUCOMA

Glaucoma arising because of apposition of the iris to the peripheral cornea (closed-angle preferred)

NEBULA OF CORNEA

Minor opacity of the cornea

NIGHT BLINDNESS

Inefficient dark adaptation so that vision is markedly reduced in reduced illumination

OPEN-ANGLE GLAUCOMA

That form of increased intraocular pressure in which the aqueous humor has access to the trabecular meshwork

OPHTHALMOPLEGIA

Paralysis of the ocular muscles

OPHTHALMOSCOPE

Instrument for examining the interior of the eye

OPHTHALMOSCOPE, DIRECT

Convex lens is held in front of the eye and an inverted image is observed; provides a magnification of about four times, but allows examination of a more peripheral portion of the fundus than direct ophthalmoscopy

OPTIC ATROPHY

Atrophy of the optic nerve

PAPILLEDEMA

Passive edema of the optic disc

PAPILLITIS

Inflammation of the optic disc or optic neuritis

PHAKOMATOSES

Group of hereditary diseases characterized by the presence of spots, tumors, and cysts in various parts of the body; types recognized as associated with ocular findings are tuberous sclerosis, Lindau-von Hippel disease, Recklinghasen's disease, Bourneville's disease, and Louis-Bar syndrome

PHOTOPHOBIA

Ocular discomfort induced by bright lights

PHOTOPSIA

Subjective sensation of sparks or flashes that occur in some pathologic conditions of the optic nerve, retina, and brain

PHTHISIS BULBI

Degenerative shrinkage of the eye

PRESBYOPIA

Refractive condition in which there is a diminished power of accomodation arising from impaired elasticity of the crystalline lens, as occurs with aging

PSEUDOPAPILLITIS

Blurring of optic disc margins in hyperopia

PUPIL

Aperture of the iris of the eye for the passage of light

PUPIL (ADIE'S ABNORMALITY)

Abnormality in the reaction of the pupil to light and associated with hypotonic deep reflexes

PUPIL (ARGYLL-ROBERTSON)

Pupil that does not constrict to light, but constricts to accommodation; pupils are small, unequal in size, and irregular seen mainly in tabes dorsalis

PUPIL (CAT'S EYE)

Pupil with a white reflex when light is directed into it; most commonly associated with retinoblastoma

RED EYE

Lay term applied to any condition with dilation of conjunctival or ciliary blood vessels

REFLEX

Involuntary, adaptive response to a stimulus

REFLEX, ACCOMMODATION

Constriction of the pupils when the eyes converge for near vision; and associated reaction and not a reflex

REFLEX, CONJUNCTIVAL (LID)

Closure of the eyelids induced by touching the conjunctiva (also called corneal reflex)

REFLEX, CONSENSUAL LIGHT (CROSSED)

Constriction of the pupil when the opposite retina is stimulated by light

REFLEX, DIRECT LIGHT

Contraction of the sphincter pupillae induced by stimulation of retina with light (also called pupillary reflex)

REFLEX, RED

Red glow of light seen to emerge from the pupil when the interior of the eye is illuminated

RETINITIS

Inflammation of the retina

RETINOBLASTOMA

Common autosomal dominant malignant retinal tumor of infancy

RETINOPATHY

Any disease condition of the retina

RETINOPEXY

Surgical procedure to correct retinal detachment by means of diathermy

RETINOSCHISIS

Retinal abnormality in which the neural retina splits at the level of the bipolar layer

RETINOSCOPY

Objective method of determining the refraction of the eye by observing the movements of the reflection of light from the eye (skiascopy)

RETROBULBAR NEURITIS

Inflammation of the optic nerve occurring without involvement of the optic disc

RETROLENTAL FIBROPLASIA

Condition of cicatricial neovascularization of the retina that occurs predominantly in infants who weigh less than 1,500 grams at birth and who require oxygen at an excessively high concentration for a long period

RUBEOSIS IRIDIS

Neovascularization of the iris as in diabetes mellitus and after central vein closure

SCLERITIS

Inflammation of the sclera

SCOTOMA

Area of blindness in the field of vision

SEROUS CHORIORETINOPATHY

Term applied to limited separation of the sensory layer of the retina from the pigment epithelium layer by fluid

SIDEROSIS

Chronic inflammation of the eye caused by a retained iron foreign body within the eye

SNOW BLINDNESS

Inability to open eyes to see; secondary to ultraviolet keratitis

STAPHYLOMA

Ectasia of the wall of the eye that is lined with uveal tract

SUBCONJUNCTIVAL HEMORRHAGE

Bleeding beneath the conjunctiva, often occurring spontaneously

SUBHYALOID HEMORRHAGE

Hemorrhage between the vitreous face and the neural retina

SUBLUXATION OF THE LENS

A condition of the lens when a portion of the supporting zonule is absent and the lens lacks support in one or more quadrants

SUPPRESSION

Physiologic mental process whereby the retinal image transmitted by one eye is ignored

SYMPATHETIC OPHTHALMIA

Granulomatous uveitis that follows in the opposite eye when there are penetrating injuries of one eye; the eye secondarily affected is called the sympathizing eye, while the injured eye is called the exciting or activating eye

SYNCHYSIS SCINTILLANS

Cholesterol crystals in liquified vitreous

SYNDROME

Group of symptoms and signs that occur together; disease or definite morbid process having characteristic sequence of symptoms; may affect the whole body or any of its parts

(Axenfeld anomaly)
Posterior corneal arcus, glaucoma, and hypertelorism

(Batten-Mayou)
Juvenile form of amaurotic familial idiocy with macular degeneration and optic atrophy

(Bechet aphthous ulcers) (canker sores)
Of mouth and genitalia combined with uveitis, iritis, and hypopyon

(Berlin's disease)
Perimacular retinal edema following trauma (commotio retina)

(Best's disease)
Hereditary type of vitelliruptive macular degeneration characterized by a macular lesion having an ophthalmoscopic appearance of an egg fried "sunny side up" and associated in this stage

with good vision; when the egg is "scrambled", vision deteriorates

(Bourneville's disease)
Mental deficiency, tuberous sclerosis, and adenoma sebaceum; glaucoma, conjunctival, and retinal tumors may occur

(Cavernous sinus)
Thrombosus of the cavernous sinus with third, fourth, and sixth cranial nerve palsy and edema of the face and eyelids and infection

(Doyne)
Familial drusen of retinal pigment epithelium

(Eale's disease)
Vasculitis of the retinal vessels characterized by inflammation, occlusion, neo-vascularization and recurrent retinal hemorrhages, occurring particularly in young men

(Ehlers-Danlos)
Widespread systemic disorder with overextensibility of the skin, fragility of the skin, and pseudotumors following trauma; there may be epicanthal folds, esotropia, blue sclera, glaucoma, ectopic lens, proliferating retinopathy, and acanthocytosis

(Foster-Kennedy)
Optic atrophy on the side of the lesion and papilledema on the opposite side that occurs in tumors of the frontal lobe of the brain

(Francois)
Dyscephaly, micro-ophthalmia, and cataract

(Fuch's)
Unilateral heterochromia, inflammation of the iris and ciliary body, and secondary cataract

(Grave's disease)
Hyperthyroidism, goiter, and exophthalmos (Basedow, Parry)

(Grönblad-Strandberg)
Angiod streaks of the fundus and pseudoxanthoma elasticum of the skin

(Hallerman-Streiff)
Mandibulofacial dysostosis with microphthalmia and congenital cataract (Francois)

(Hand-Schüller-Christian disease)
Insidious and progressive abnormality of children characterized by exophthalmos, diabetes insipidus, and softened areas in the bones, particularly in femurs and those of the skull, shoulder, and pelvic girdle

(Harada)
Vogt-Koyanagi syndrome combined with retinal detachment

(Hepatolenticular degeneration) (Wilson)
Abnormality of copper metabolism associated with progressive degeneration of the liver and lentate nucleus, mental retardation, in a brownish ring (Kayser-Fleischer) composed of copper at the periphery of the cornea

(Horner)
Sympathetic nerve paralysis with miosis, blepharoptosis, and anhydrosis of the face

(Jensen's disease)
Chorioretinitis adjacent to the optic disc (juxtapapillary)

(Kimmelstiel-Wilson)
Hypertension, retinopathy, and intercapillary glomerulosclerosis in diabetes mellitus

(Lindau's disease)
Angioma of the central nervous system, particularly in the cerebellum, and associated Lindau-von Hippel disease with angioma of the cerebellum, retina, pancreas, and kidney

(Marfan)
Spider fingers and toes (arachnodactyly), ectopia lentis, cardiovascular defects, and widespread defects of elastic tissue

(Paget's disease)
Bone thickening and thinning sometimes with angioid streaks

(Purtscher's disease)
Traumatic angiopathy of the retina

(Recklinghausen's disease)
Autosomal dominant neurofibromatosis

(Rollet)
Orbital apex syndrome with involvement of II, III, IV, V, and sympathetic nerves

(Roth's spot)
Retinal hemorrhage with white center in sub-acute bacterial endocarditis

(Stargart's disease)
Type of fundus flavimaculatus with macular degeneration at onset

(Stilling-Duane-Turk)
A fibroadhesive syndrome with absence of abduction and with adduction retraction of globe and blepharoptosis

(Stock-Spielmeyer-Vogt) (Batten Mayou)
Juvenile amaurotic familial idiocy; a retinal cerebral degeneration, apparently not a sphingolipidosis

(Sturge-Weber-Dimitri disease)
Nevus flammeus (port wine), often associated with glaucoma

(Vogt-Spielmeyer)
Juvenile amaurotic familial idiocy

(Weber)
Paralysis of the oculomoter nerve (N III) on the same side as the lesion and spastic hemiplegia on the side opposite the lesion with increased reflexes and loss of superficial reflexes

(Weill-Marchesani)
Short fingers and toes, compact body, glaucoma, small lens, dislocated lens (inverted Marfan)

(Wilson's)
Autosomal recessive deficiency ceruloplasmin with cirrhosis of the liver, lenticular degenera-tion, and deposition of copper in periphery of Descemet's membrane (Kayser-Fleischer ring)

SYNECHIAE
Adhesion between the iris and adjacent structures

SYNECHIAE, ANTERIOR
Between the iris and the cornea

SYNECHIAE, PERIPHERAL ANTERIOR
Occurs with unrelieved attacks of angle closure glaucoma when the iris remains in contact with the cornea for a long period; may occur following injury or surgery when the anterior chamber does not form

SYNECHIAE, POSTERIOR
Adhesion between the iris and the lens as occurs commonly with uveitis

TEMPORAL ARTERITIS
Giant cell arteritis

TONOGRAPHY TEST
Test by means of which the amount of fluid forced from the eye by a constant pressure during a constant period is determined

TONOMETER
Instrument for measuring ocular tension

UVEITIS
Inflammation of the uveal tract

VISION, BINOCULAR
Faculty of using both eyes synchronously, with dyplopia

VISION, COLOR
Ability to distinguish subjectively a large variety of wavelengths of light in the visible spectrum

VISION, PHOTOPIC
Vision in bright illumination

VISION, SCOTOPIC

Vision in dim illumination or vision following the biochemical or neurologic changes occurring in dark adaptation

VISUAL ANGLE

Angle that an object or detail subtends at the point of observation; usually measured in minutes of arc

VISUAL FIELD

Locus of objects of points in space that can be perceived when the head and eyes are kept fixed; the field may be monocular or binocular

bibliography

1. Alajmo, A, DeConcilis N. On the applications of ultrasonics in ophthalmological diagnosis III. Possibilities of ultrasonics in the detection of endo-ocular foreign bodies. *Riv Infort Mal Prof 47*:956, 1960.
2. Alekseev BN, Shirshikov IUK. Echographic study of the ciliary body and choroid detachment following antiglaucomatous operations. *Vestn Oftalmol 4*:33, 1976.
3. Apple DJ, Rabb MF. *Clinicopathology correlation of ocular disease.* St Louis, CV Mosby, 1974.
4. Araki M. Studies on reflective elements of the human eye by ultrasonic waves I. Accuracy of the measurement of ocular axial length by ultrasonic echography. *J Clin Ophthalmol* (Tokyo) *15*:111, 1961.
5. Arentsen JJ, Rodriguez MM, Laibson PR et al. Corneal opacification occurring after phacoemulsification. *J Am Ophthalmol 83*:794, 1977.
6. Aronson SB, Elliot JH. *Ocular Inflammation.* St Louis, CV Mosby, 1972.
7. Baum G. Ultrasonics in orbital diagnosis: B-mode. *Int. Ophthalmol Clin 9*:585, 1969.
8. Baum G. Ultrasonography in clinical ophthalmology. *Trans Am Acad Ophthal Otolaryngol 68*:265–276, 1964.
9. Baum G, Greenwood J. I. Orbital lesions; localization by three dimensional ultrasonography. *NY State J Med 61*:414, 1961.
10. Baum G, Greenwood J. I. The application of ultrasonic locating techniques to ophthalmology. II. Ultrasonic slit lamp in the ultra-

sonic visualization of soft tissues. *Arch Ophthalmol* 60:263–279, 1958.

11. Baum G, Greenwood J. I. Ultrasound in ophthalmology. *Am J Ophthalmol* 49:249, 1960.

12. Belkin M, Levinson A. Ultrasonographic refraction of aphakic infants and children. *Doc Ophthalmol* 43:147, 1977.

13. Belle H. Extreme antepartum fetal tachycardia. *Zentralbl Gynaekol* 98:998, 1976.

14. Bellone G. Ultrasonographic study in the vitreous. In *Simposio Internazionale Sulla Diagnostica Ultrasonica in Oftalmologia*. Torino, Documenta Italseber, 1970, 1968.

15. Bellone G, Gallenga PE. Ultrasonic features of changes in the vitreous body caused by degenerative, inflammatory, vascular and deforming diseases of the eye. In Boeck J, Ossoinig K (eds): *Ultrasonographia medica Verlag Wiener Med Akad* 2:229, 1971.

16. Bertenyi A. Localization of intraocular and intraorbital foreign bodies of means of A-scan ultrasonography. *Ultrasonics* 14:183, 1976.

17. Bigar F, Bosshard CT. Combined A- and B-scan echography of the eye. *Klin Monatsbl Augenheilk* 170:24, 1977.

18. Boeck, J, Ossoinig K. Fundamentals of nontraumatic tissue differentiation by ultrasound. Part III. Histological structures and ultrasonograms. In Boeck J, Ossoinig K (eds): *Ultrasonographia medica Verlag Wiener Med Akad* 1:411, 1971.

19. Bonink M. *Ocular and Adnexal Tumors*. St Louis, CV Mosby, 1964.

20. Bronson NR. Development of a simple B-scan ultrasonoscope. *Trans Am Ophthalmol Soc* 70:365–408, 1972.

21. Bronson NR. Foreign body management. *Int Ophthalmol Clin* 9:685, 1969.

22. Bronson NR. Nonmagnetic foreign body localization and extraction. *Am J Ophthalmol* 58:133, 1964.

23. Bronson NR, Fisher YL, Tragnor EM, Pickering EM. *Contact B-Scan Ophthalmic Sonography*, Westport, Connecticut, Intercontinental, 1976.

24. Bronson NR, Turner FT. Standardization of A-mode ultrasound equipment. In Boeck J, Ossoinig K, (eds). *Ultrasonographia medica Verlag Weiner Med Akad* 2:55, 1971.

25. Buschmann W, Linnert D. Peripheral retinal detachment, ultrasonic diagnosis and therapeutic consequences. *Ber Dtsch Ophthalmol Ges* 74:345, 1977.

26. Buschmann W, Linnert D. Visualization of orbital tissues using various echographic techniques. *Ultrasound Med Biol* 2:295, 1977.

27. Cherniavski GIA, Fridman FE, Mogilevskaia FIA et al. Surgical treatment of glaucoma with the use of ultrasonic knife. *Oftalmol Zh* 31:24, 1976.

28. Cohen JS, Stone RD, Hetherington J Jr et al. Glaucomatous cupping of the optic disk by ultrasonography. *Am J Ophthalmol* 82:24, 1976.

29. Coleman DJ. Orbital scanning using combined A and B scan techniques. In Boeck J, Ossoinig K, (eds): *Ultrasonographia medica Verlag Wiener Med Akad* 2:403, 1971.

30. Coleman DJ. Reliability of ocular and orbital diagnosis with B-scan ultrasound II. Orbital Diagnosis. *Am J Ophthalmol* 74:704–718, 1972.

31. Coleman DJ. Ultrasonic evaluation of the vitreous. In Gitter KA (ed). *Current Concepts of the Vitreous Including Vitrectomy*. St Louis, CV Mosby, 1976, pp 129–141.

32. Coleman DJ. Ultrasound in vitreous surgery. *Trans Am Ophthalmol Otolaryngol* 76:467–479, 1972.

33. Coleman DJ, Carlin B. A new system for visual axis measurements in the human eye using ultrasound. *Arch Ophthalmol* 77:124, 1967.

34. Coleman DJ, Carrol FD. Evaluation of optic neuropathy with B-scan ultrasonography. *Am J Ophthalmol* 74:915–920, 1972.

35. Coleman DJ, Jack RL. B-scan ultrasonography of the retina and vitreous. *Int Ophthalmol Clin* 16:31, 1976.

36. Coleman DJ, Jack RL, Cardonna H. Ultrasonic evaluation of eyes with keratoprostheses. *Am J Ophthalmol* 74:543–554, 1972.

37. Coleman DJ, Jack RL, Franzen LA. High resolution B-scan ultrasonography of the orbit I. The normal orbit. *Arch Ophthalmol* 88:358–367, 1972.

38. Coleman DJ, Jack RL, Franzen LA et al. High resolution B-scan ultrasonography of the orbit V. Changes of Graves Disease. *Arch. Ophthalmol* 88:465–471, 1972.

39. Coleman DJ, Jack RL, Jones IS et al. High resolution B-scan ultrasonography of the orbit IV. Pseudotumors of the orbit. *Arch Ophthalmol* 88:472–480, 1972.

40. Coleman DJ, Konig WF, Katz L. A hand operated ultrasound scan system for ophthalmic evaluation. *Am J Ophthalmol* 68:256, 1969.

41. Coleman DJ, Lizzi FL, Jack RL. *Ultrasonography of the Eye and Orbit*. Philadelphia, Lea and Febiger, 1977.

42. Dadd M, Kossoff G, Hughes H. An unusual flat interface in orbital ultrasonic examinations. *Ultrasound Med Biol* 2:213, 1976.

43. Dallow RL, Momose KJ, Weber AL et al. Comparison of ultrasonography computerized tomography (EMI scan) and radiographic techniques in evaluation of exophthalmos. *Trans Am Acad Ophthalmol Otolaryngol* 81:305, 1976.

44. Dominguez A. Ultrasonic control of ocular dimensions and surgical indentations in retinal detachment. *Mod Probl Ophthalmol 18*:77, 1977.

45. Dyszynsks-Rosciszewska B, Szreterowa M, Mianowicz J. Intraocular foreign bodies in ultrasound investigations. *Klin Oczna 47*:263, 1977.

46. Eliseeva OI, Fridman FE, Pleshanov PG. Experimental echographic characteristics of intraocular fragments. *Vestn Oftalmol 6*:61, 1976.

47. Everett WG, Hurite FG, Sorr EM. Retinal detachment following cataract extraction by phacoemulsification. *Mod Probl Ophthalmol 18*:503, 1977.

48. Filipczynski L, Etienne J, Lypacewicz G, Rosciszewska B. Ultrasonic problems of the diagnostic equipment for eye examinations. *Acta Fac Med Univ Brunen 35*:27, 1968.

49. Flament J. Echographic aspects of scleral sacs. Experimental study preliminary note. *Bull Soc Ophthalmol Franc 70*:165, 1970.

50. Fledelius H. Diagnostic ultrasound in orbital diseases. Proceedings. *Acta Ophthalmol Suppl 125*:6, 1975.

51. Forrester JV, Sutherland GR, McDougall IR. Dysthyroid ophthalmopathy: orbital evaluation with B-scan ultrasonography. *J Clin Endocrinol Metab 45*:221, 1977.

52. Francois J. Ultrasonics in the diagnosis of eye diseases. Possibilities and limitations of the examinations. *Bull Soc Belge Ophthalmol 150*:600, 1968.

53. Francois J, Goes F. A-mode echography and unilateral exophthalmos. *Bull Soc Belge Ophthalmol 155*:475, 1970.

54. Freyler H. It is possible to successfully operate cases of ablatio, despite dense clouding of the media, using echography. *Klin Monatsbl Augenheilkd 158*:75, 1971.

55. Freyler H, Arnfelser H, Weiss H. Experimental ultrasonography of the rabbit eye. *Albrecht von Graefes Arch Klin Ophthalmol 199*:267, 1976.

56. Freyler H, Egerer I. Echography and histological studies in various eye conditions. *Arch Ophthalmol 95*:1387, 1977.

57. Freyler H, Goes F. A-mode echography and unilateral exophthalmos. *Bull Soc Belge Ophthalmol 155*:475, 1970.

58. Freyler H, Kutschera E. Echooculometry in retinal detachment surgery without subretinal drainage. *Klin Monatsbl Augenheilkd 169*:442, 1976.

59. Fridman FE, Khvatova AV, Timakova VI, et al. New possibilities of echographic diagnosis of retinoblastomas. *Vestn Ophthalmol 1*:65, 1977.

60. Fridman FE, Kruzhkova GV, Kirillova LI. Ultrasonic attenuation in orbital tumors as a diagnostic test. *Vestn Ophthalmol 2*:46, 1977.

61. Fuller DG, Laqua H, Machemer R. Triangle retinal detachment. Ultrasonic identification of massive periretinal proliferation in eyes with opaque media. *Mod Probl Ophthalmol 18*:68, 1977.

62. Fuller DG, Laqua H, Machmer R. Ultrasonographic diagnosis of massive periretinal proliferation in eyes with opaque media (triangular retinal detachment). *Am J Ophthalmol 83*:460, 1977.

63. Gaertner J, Loepping B. Vitreous body in systemic connective tissue changes. Studies using ultrasonics. *Ber Dtsch Ophthalmol Ges 68*:40, 1968.

64. Gallenga R. The importance of ultrasonic diagnostics in ophthalmology for clinical routine work. In Boeck J, Ossoinig K, (eds): *Ultrasonographia medica Verlag Wiener Med Akad 2*:313, 1971.

65. Gernet H. Basic values in clinical oculometry. *Bull Mem Soc Franc Ophthalmol 83*:379, 1970.

66. Gernet H. On the axis length and refraction of the emmetropic living eye. *Graefe Arch Ophthalmol 166*:424, 1964.

67. Gernet H, Juergens V. Echographic findings in primary chronic glaucoma. *Graefe Arch Ophthalmol 168*:419, 1965.

68. Giglio EJ, Ludlam WM, Wittenberg S. Improvement in the measurement of intraocular distances using ultrasound. *J Acoust Soc Amer 44*:1359, 1968.

69. Giglio EJ, Meyers RR. An automatic probe transport to the eye for ultrasound. *Am J Ophthalmol 46*:275, 1969.

70. Gitter KA, Keeney AH, Sarin LK, Meyer D (eds): *Ophthalmic Ultrasound*. St Louis, CV Mosby, 1969.

71. Gitter KA, Meyer D, Sarin LK. Limitations and misinterpretations of time amplitude ultrasonography. In Gitter KA, Keeney AH, Sarin LK, Meyer D (eds): *Ophthalmic Ultrasound*. St Louis, CV Mosby, 1969, p 237.

72. Gitter KA, Meyer D, Sarin LK. Ultrasound to evaluate eyes with opaque media. *Am J Ophthalmol 64*:100, 1967.

73. Gitter KA, Meyer D, White RH Jr. Ultrasonic aid in the evaluation of leukocoria. *Am J Ophthalmol 65*:190, 1969.

74. Goldberg RE, Sarin LK, Meyer D. Applications of ultrasonography in Ophthalmology. *Trans Am Acad Ophthalmol Otolaryngd 71*:880, 1967.

75. Graymore CN. *Biochemistry of the Eye*. London, Academic Press, 1976.

76. Grignolo A, Rivara A, Altieri GG. The localization of the equator of the globe with the help of ultrasonography and its value for retinal surgery. In Boeck J, Ossoinig K (eds): *Ultrasonographia medica Verlag Wiener Med Akad 2*:123, 1971.

77. Haddad HM. *Metabolic Eye Disease.* Springfield, Ill, CC Thomas, 1974.

78. Hagreh SS. *Anterior Ischemic Optic Neuropathy.* New York, Springer-Verlag, 1975.

79. Hamard H, Bregeat P. Orbital echo-tomography. *Arch Ophthalmol 31*:137, 1971.

80. Henderson, JW. *Orbital Tumors.* Philadelphia, WB Saunders, 1973.

81. Hilal SK, Trokel SL, Coleman DJ. High resolution computerized tomography and B-scan ultrasonography of the orbits. *Trans Am Acad Ophthalmol Otolaryngol 81*:607, 1976.

82. Hodes BL, Choromokos E. Standardized A-scan echographic diagnosis of choroidal malignant melanomas. *Arch Ophthalmol 95*:593, 1977.

83. Hodes BL, Stern G. Phacoanaphylactic endophthalmitis, echographic diagnosis of phacoanaphylactic endophthalmitis. *Ophthalmic Surg 7*:60. 1976.

84. Hodes BL, Weinberg PA. A combined approach for the diagnosis of orbital disease. Computed tomography and standardized A-scan echography. *Arch Ophthalmol 95*:781, 1977.

85. Holasek E, Sokollu A. Direct contact hand held scanner. In *Proceedings of the Institute of Electronic and Electrical Engineering Ultrasonics Symposium.* Boston Institute of Electrical and Electronics Engineers Inc. October, 1972, pp 38–43.

86. Jack RL, Coleman DJ. Detection of retinal detachment secondary to choroidal melanoma with B-scan ultrasonography. *Am J Ophthalmol 174*:1057–1065, 1972.

87. Jansson F. Determination of the axis length of the eye roentgenologically and by ultrasound. *Acta Ophthalmol 41*:236, 1963.

88. Janula J, Preisova J, Stavratjev M. Thermography and ultrasonography in ophthalmology. *Cesk Oftalmol 32*:415, 1976.

89. Jungschaffer OH and Fritch CD. Phacoemulsification and retinal detachment. *Mod Probl Ophthalmol 18*:508, 1977.

90. Kaneko A. A high quality ultrasonic apparatus for the ophthalmological diagnosis using manual compound scanning. *Acta Soc Ophthalmol Jpn 80*:1101, 1976.

91. Kaneko A, Shigeyama S, Uchida R. A new ultrasonic apparatus for ophthalmology using manual compound scanning. *Doc Ophthalmol 43*:137, 1977.

92. Kawabata H, Uchida H. Clinical echography in ophthalmology. *Folia Ophthalmol Jpn 18*:941, 1967.

93. Koretskaia IUM, Mozerenkov VP, Ukhaneva GL. Table for determining the volume of the vitreous body based on echographic biometry data. *Vestn Oftalmol 6*:63, 1976.

94. Kossoff G, Robinson BE. The CAL ultrasonic echoscope for ophthalmological investigations. *J Coll Radiol Aust 9*:168, 1965.

95. Krill AE. *Hereditary Retinal and Choroidal Diseases.* New York, Harper and Row, 1972.

96. Kulikova IA, Nechaev IUA. Method of stabilization of acoustic contact during ultrasonic diagnosis in ophthalmology. *Med Tekh 6*:38, 1975.

97. Leary GA. Ophthalmological biometrics. *Ultrasonics 7*:138, 1969.

98. Lerman S. *Cataracts.* Springfield, Ill. CC Thomas, 1964.

99. Levchenko OG, Drukman AB. Ultrasonic biometry of children's eyes with different refraction. *Vestn Oftalmol 5*:47, 1976.

100. Machmer R. *Vitrectomy.* New York, Grune and Stratton, 1975.

101. Mallek DR, Oliver M. The use of contact B-mode ultrasound in pediatric ophthalmology. *J Pediatr Ophthalmol 13*:45, 1976.

102. Marmur RK, Gavrilov LR, Dumbrova NE et al. Cytochemical and ultrastructural changes of the retina under the effect of low frequency ultrasonics. *Oftalmol Zh 31*:459, 1976.

103. Massin M, Poujol J. Differential diagnosis between idiopathic symptomatic retinal detachment using echography. *Bull Soc Franc Ophthalmol 66*:1225, 1966.

104. Metz GA, Bronson NR. Ultrasonic appearance of senile lens changes. In Gitter KA, Keeney AH, Sarin LK et al (eds): *Ophthalmic Ultrasound.* St Louis, CV Mosby, 1969, pp 218–223.

105. Moore WS, Bean B, Burton R et al. The use of ophthalmosonometry in the diagnosis of carotid artery stenosis. *Surgery 82*:107, 1977.

106. Moses RA. *Adler's Physiology of the Eye.* 5th edition. St Louis, CV Mosby, 1970.

107. Mozherenkov VP, Mitkokh DI, Shirshikov IUK. Echobiometry of eye changes depending on the refraction in opaque media. *Oftalmol Zh 31*:596, 1976.

108. Mundt GH, Hughes WF Jr. Ultrasonics in ocular diagnosis. *Am J Ophthalmol 41*:488, 1956.

109. Nover A. Clinical studies with retinal detachment and intraocular tumors. *Klin Monatsbl Augenheilkd 142*:176, 1963.

110. Nover A. *Ocular Fundus.* Philadelphia, Lea and Febiger, 1966.

111. Nover A, Kunde G. Ultrasonic studies of the vitreous body of healthy and diseased eyes. *Klin Monatsbl Augenheilkd 152*:639, 1968.

112. Nover A, Stallkamp H. Experimental studies with ultrasonics on eyes with intraocular foreign bodies. *Graefe Arch Ophthalmol 164*:157, 1962.

113. Oksala A. About selective echography in some eye diseases. *Acta Ophthalmol* (Kobenhaven) *40*:466, 1962.

114. Oksala A. A-mode diagnosis of intraocular diseases. *Int Ophthalmol Clin 9*:543, 1969.

115. Oksala A. Experimental and clinical observations on the echograms in vitreous hemorrhages. *Br J Ophthalmol 47*:65, 1963.

116. Oksala A. Experimental investigations of the effect of various parts of the eye on the sound field in the ultrasonic method. *Acta Ophthalmol* (Kobenhaven) *48*:1157, 1970.

117. Oksala A. Ten years experience in clinical ultrasound investigation. *Acta Ophthalmol* (Kobenhaven) *45*:489, 1967.

118. Oksala A. The benefits and limits of ultrasound diagnosis in ophthalmology. Proceedings. *Acta Ophthalmol Suppl 125*:5, 1975.

119. Oksala A. The pathway of ultrasound in the eye and its clinical aspects. *Klin Monatsbl Augenheilkd 150*:408, 1967.

120. Oksala A. Ultrasonic diagnosis of the diseased eye (Ger). In Boeck J, Ossoinig K. (eds.): *Ultrasonographia medica Verlag Wiener Med Akad 2*:209, 1971.

121. Oksala A. Ultrasonic findings in the vitreous body in patients with acute anterior uveitis. *Acta Ophthalmol 55*:287, 1977.

122. Oksala A. Ultrasonic findings in the vitreous space in patients with detachment of the retina. *Albrecht von Graefes Arch Klin Ophthalmol 202*:197, 1977.

123. Oksala A. Ultrasonography in the diagnosis of retinal detachment. *Bibl Ophthalmol 72*:218, 1967.

124. Oksala A, Pueroinen L. Experimental researches on the ultrasonic field and the point of departure of the echo from the scleral calotte using the sclera as a test piece. *Acta Ophthalmol* (Kobenhaven) *44*:549, 1966.

125. Oksala A, Varonen ER. Analysis of echoes from the rear eye wall with the aid of experimental and clinical research II. Effect of the absorption of the lens and of amplification. *Acta Ophthalmol* (Kobenhaven) *42*:782, 1964.

126. Oksala A, Varonen ER. The effect of the lens on the ultrasonic field in diagnosis of the eye by ultrasound. *Acta Ophthalmol* (Kobenhaven) *43*:260, 1965.

127. Oksala A, Varonen ER. The influence of the eyeball on the ultrasonic field of the transducer and its diagnostic significance. *Acta Ophthalmol* (Kobenhaven) *43*:268, 1965.

128. Orlowski WJ, Szczypinski J. Ultrasonography of subretinal space in rhegmatogenous retinal detachment. *Mod Probl Ophthalmol 18*:40, 1977.

129. Ossoinig K. Additional experience with phantoms as aids in ultrasonic diagnosis of intraocular tumors. *Acta Fac Med Univ Brunen 35*:207, 1968.

130. Ossoinig K. A-mode echography of intraocular tumors. *Klin Monatsbl Augenheilkd 146*:321, 1965.

131. Ossoinig K. Basics, methods and results of ultrasonography used in diagnosis of intraorbital tumors. In Gitter KA, Keeney AH, Sarin LK, Meyer D (eds): *Ophthalmic Ultrasound*. St. Louis, CV Mosby, 1969.

132. Ossoinig K. Clinical echo-ophthalmography I. Echography in intraocular diseases. In Boeck J, Ossoinig K, (eds): *Ultrasonographia medica Verlag Wiener Med Akad. 2*:333, 1971.

133. Ossoinig K. Clinical echo-ophthalmography II. Echography in orbital diseases. In Boeck J, Ossoinig K, (eds): *Ultrasonographia medica Verlag Wiener Med Akad. 2*:423, 1971.

134. Ossoinig K. Clinical echo-ophthalmology. In Blodi FC (ed): *Current Concepts of Ophthalmology*. St Louis, CV Mosby, 1972. Vol 3, pp 101–130.

135. Ossoinig K. Echography of orbital tumors; an A-mode study. *Klin Monatsbl Augenheilkd 149*:817, 1966.

136. Ossoinig K. Experimental and clinical investigations with the A-mode technique in ultrasonic diagnosis of ocular and orbital tumors. *Wiss Z Humboldt-Univ Berlin 14*:185, 1965.

137. Ossoinig K. Fundamentals of non-traumatic tissue differentiation by ultrasound I. Experimental and clinical investigations of the influence of technical parameters on the diagnostic values of the echograms. In Boeck J, Ossoinig K (eds): *Ultrasonographia medica Verlag Wiener Med Akad 1*:155, 1971.

138. Ossoinig K. Fundamentals of non-traumatic tissue differentiation by ultrasound II. The accoustic behavior of biological structures. In Boeck J, Ossoinig K (eds): *Ultrasonographia medica Verlag Wiener Med Akad 1*:419, 1971.

139. Ossoinig K. Fundamentals of non-traumatic tissue differentiation by ultrasound IV. Clinical standardization. In Boeck J, Ossoinig K (eds): *Ultrasonographia medica Verlag Wiener Med Akad 2*:83, 1971.

140. Ossoinig K. The echographic picture presented by healthy orbit (A-scan echograms). *Acta Fac Med Univ Brunen 35*:101, 1968.

141. Ossoinig K. The evaluation of kinetic properties of echo signals. *Ultrasonics in Ophthalmology*. Symposium Muenster, New York, 1966.

142. Ossoinig K. Routine ultrasonography of the orbit. In Wainstock MA (ed): *Ultrasonography in Ophthalmology. International Ophthalmology Clinics*. Boston, Little, Brown, 1969.

143. Ossoinig K. Ultrasonic diagnostics of ocular foreign bodies. *Ber 67 Fus Deutsche Ophthal Ges*. Heidelberg, Munich, Verlag Bergmann JF, 1965.

144. Ossoinig K. Ultrasonic diagnostics of orbital tumors, combined A-mode and B-scan examinations. *Graefe Arch Klin Exp Ophthalmol* *172*:364, 1967.

145. Ossoinig K. Ultrasonic diagnosis of orbital vascular processes. *Klin Monatsbl Augenheilkd* *158*:526, 1971.

146. Ossoinig K. Ultrasonic diagnosis of the eye. An aid for the clinic. *Ultrasonics in Ophthalmology.* Symposium Muenster, New York, 1966.

147. Ossoinig K, Kaufman F. Investigations of the origin of echoes in submacroscopical structures of tumors exposed to ultrasound II. An important phenomenon occurring in echography of citrated blood. *Graefe Arch Klin Exp Ophthalmol* *173*:327, 1967.

148. Ossoinig K, Seher K. Investigations of the origins in submacroscopical structures of tumors exposed to pulsed ultrasound I. Theoretical considerations. *Graefe Arch Klin Exp Ophthalmol* *171*:17, 1966.

149. Ossoinig K, Seher K. Results of the diagnosis of orbital tumors by means of ultrasound. *Acta Fac Med Univ Brunen* *35*:333, 1968.

150. Ossoinig K, Seher K. Ultrasonic diagnosis of intraocular foreign bodies. In Gitter KA, Keeney AH, Sarin LK, Meyer D (eds): *Ophthalmic Ultrasound.* St. Louis, CV Mosby, 1969.

151. Ossoinig K, Steiner H. Standardization problems in ultrasonic diagnostics of the eye. *Graefe Arch Klin Exp Ophthalmol* *199*:241, 1966.

152. Ossoinig K, Till P. Methods and results of ultrasonography in the diagnosis of ocular tumors. In Gitter KA, Keeney AH, Sarin LK, Meyer D (eds): *Ophthalmic Ultrasound.* St. Louis, CV Mosby, 1969.

153. Ossoinig K, Valencak E. Ultrasonography and other diagnostic methods: importance in orbital tumors. In Gitter KA, Keeney AH, Sarin LK, Meyer D (eds): *Ophthalmic Ultrasound.* St. Louis, CV Mosby, 1969.

154. Otsuka J, Tokoro T, Araki M. Comparative studies of phocometry with ultrasonic method on refractive elements of the human eyes. *Acta Soc Ophthalmol Jpn* *65*:1777, 1961.

155. Penner R, Passmore JW. Magnetic vs. nonmagnetic intraocular foreign bodies: An ultrasonic determination. *Arch Ophthalmol* *76*:676–677, 1966.

156. Poujol MJ. Clinical echography of intraocular tumors. In Boeck J, Ossoinig K (eds): *Ultrasonographia medica Verlag Wiener Med Akad* *2*:275, 1971.

157. Poujol MJ. Localization of intraocular lesions by ultrasonography. Experimental study. *Bull Soc Franc Ophthalmol* *68*:739, 1968.

158. Preisova J, Anton M, Vanysek J. Comparison of ultrasonic diagnosis with findings on enucleated bulbs. In Boeck J, Ossoinig K (eds): *Ultrasonographia medica Verlag Wiener Med Akad* *2*:357, 1971.

159. Pruett RC, Regan CDJ. *Retina Congress.* New York, Appleton-Century-Crofts, 1972.

160. Purnell EW. B-mode orbital ultrasonography. *Int Ophthalmol Clin* *9*:643, 1969.

161. Purnell EW. Intensity modulated B-scan ultrasonography. In Goldberg RE, Sarin LK (eds): *Ultrasonics in Ophthalmology.* Philadelphia, WB Saunders, pp 102–123, 1967.

162. Purnell EW. Orbital ultrasonography. In Gitter K, Keeney AH, Sarin LK, Meyer D (eds): *Ophthalmic Ultrasound.* St Louis, CV Mosby, 1969.

163. Purnell EW. Ultrasonic interpretation of orbital disease. In Gitter KA et al (eds): *Ophthalmic Ultrasound.* St. Louis, CV Mosby, pp 249–255, 1969.

164. Purnell EW Sokollu A. Ultrasonic measurement of eye length. *Acta Ophthalmol* (Kobenhaven) *40*:219, 1962.

165. Reese AB. *Tumors of the Eye.* 3rd Edition. New York, Harper and Row, 1975.

166. Roy FH. Ocular differential diagnosis. Philadelphia, Lea and Febiger, 1972.

167. Samuels B, Fuchs A. *Clinical Pathology of the Eye.* New York, Hoeber, 1952.

168. Sarin LK. Diagnostic uses of ultrasound. *Trans Penn Acad Ophthalmol* *20*:72, 1967.

169. Sawada A, Cornell SH. Computerized tomography with A-scan echography in detection of orbital disorders (Preliminary report). *Acta Ophthalmol Jpn* *80*:1090, 1976.

170. Schroeder M. Running time of ultrasound in the distal portion of the optic nerve. *Klin Monatsbl Augenheilkd* *169*:743, 1976.

171. Schroeder W. The use of A-scan echography in the clinical diagnosis of persistent hyperplastic primart vitreous (PHPV). *Klin Monatsbl Augenheilkd* *168*:210, 1976.

172. Schwab B, Nover A. Results of A-scan echography investigating intraocular tumors. *Klin Monatsbl Augenheilkd* *169*:576, 1976.

173. Shields JA, McDonald PR, Leonard BC et al. Ultrasonography and 32P test in diagnosis of malignant melanomas in eyes with hazy media. *Trans Am Ophthalmol Soc* *74*:261, 1977.

174. Shields JA, Tasman WS. B-scan ultrasonography of lesions simulating choroidal melanomas. *Mod Probl Ophthalmol* *18*:57, 1977.

175. Skalka HW. Ultrasonography in foreign body detection and localization. *Ophthalmic Surg* *7*:27, 1976.

176. Sokollu A. A critical evaluation of ultrasonic images of the eye obtained by various echoscopic scan modes. *Acta Fac Med Univ Brunen* *35*:35, 1968.

177. Sokollu A. Concise physics of ultrasound as ap-

plied in ophthalmology. *Int Ophthalmol Clin* 9:793, 1969.

178. Soriano H. A-mode echography in the diagnosis of uveal disease. *Can J Ophthalmol 12*:157, 1977.

179. Stallkamp H, Nover A. Diagnostic studies with ultrasonics on the healthy eye. *Graefe Arch Ophthalmol 164*:399, 1962.

180. Stepanik J, Ossoinig K. The behavior of the saggital axis of the human eye in vivo during corneal applanations of different strengths. *Graefe Arch Klin Exp Ophthalmol 173*:114, 1967.

181. Sugar HS. *Glaucomas. 2nd Edition.* New York, Hoeber, 1957.

182. Tane S, Funahashi T, Horiuchi T. Studies on an ultrasonic diagnosis in ophthalmology III. An ultrasound technique for the vitreous body of healthy and affected eyes. *Folia Ophthalmol Jpn 22*:79, 1071.

183. Tane S, Sakuma F, Sakuma Y et al. The studies on the ultrasonic diagnosis in ophthalmology (Report II). Ten year study on clinical ophthalmic echography Part I. Echographic results in the differential diagnosis and diagnostic criteria. *Acta Soc Ophthalmol Jpn 80*:1108, 1976.

184. Tasman W, Shields JA. Ultrasound in the differential diagnosis of juvenile retinal detachment. *Mod Probl Ophthalmol 18*:45, 1977.

185. Till P. Echography in post-traumatic orbital cases. In Boeck J, Ossoinig K (eds): *Ultrasonographia medica Verlag Wiener Med Akad 2*:437, 1971.

186. Till P. Ultrasonic diagnosis of retrobulbar hematomas. *Klin Monatbsl Augenheilkd 158*:723, 1971.

187. Till P, Neumann A. The reliability of biological standards. In Boeck J, Ossoinig K (eds): *Ultrasonographia medica Verlag Wiener Med Akad 2*:119, 1971.

188. Till P, Ossoinig K. Echography of retinablastoma. *Ber Deutsche Ophthalmol Ges 69*:203, 1969.

189. Tokoro T, Hayashi K, Muto M et al. Studies on the measurement of axial length of the eye by a new ultrasound system. Report III. Comparison with photographic technique. *Acta Soc Ophthalmol Jpn 80*:147, 1976.

190. Tokoro T, Manabe T, Hayashi K et al. Studies on the measurement of axial length of the eye by a new ultrasound system. Report III. Influence of postural change on measurement of axial length. *Acta Soc Ophthalmol Jpn 81*:216, 1977.

191. Tolentino FI, Schepens CI, Freeman HM. *Vitreoretinal disorders*. Philadelphia, Saunders, 1976.

192. Ursin KV. Ultrasonographic examination of the vitreous body before cataract extraction. *Duodecim 80*:422, 1964.

193. Valencak E. Comparison of echographical and clinical findings in orbital tumors. In Boeck J, Ossoinig K (eds): *Ultrasonographia medica Verlag Wiener Med Akad 2*:443, 1971.

194. Valencak E, Ossoinig K. Ultrasonic diagnostics in arteriovenous fistulas of the orbit using A-mode and B-scan echography. In Boeck J, Ossoinig K (eds): *Ultrasonographia medica Verlag Wiener Med Akad 2*:453, 1971.

195. Vanysek J, Obraz J, Preisova J. On the possibilities of an ultrasonic examination in ophthalmology. *Ophthalmologica* (Basel) *144*:20, 1962.

196. Veirs ER. The lacrimal system. *Proceedings of the First International Symposium.* Philadelphia, WB Saunders, 1976.

197. Volkov VV, Sukhopara NV, Neverova LG. Ultrasound and radioactive phosphorus in diagnosis of intraocular pathological processes with opacification of the optical eye medial. *Vestn Oftalmol 4*:75, 1976.

198. Wainstock MA. Ultrasonic presurgical diagnosis in ophthalmology. *Int Surg 62*:314, 1977.

199. Wainstock MA. Ultrasonography in ophthalmology. Conclusions and practical applications. *Int Ophthalmol Clin 9*:745, 1969.

200. Weale RA. *The Aging Eye.* New York, Hoeber, 1963.

201. Wild JJ, Neal D. Use of high frequency ultrasonic waves for detecting changes of texture in living tissues. *Lancet 1*:655, 1951.

202. Wild JJ, Reid JM. Further pilot echographic studies on the histologic structure of tumors of the living intact human breast. *Am J Pathol 28*:839, 1952.

203. Yamamoto Y, Hirano S, Manabe T et al. Supersonic observation of eyes in premature babies. Part I. Hemodynamics at eye-ground. *Acta Soc Ophthalmol Jpn 80*:1194, 1976.

index

C

Camera artifact, 181–183
Carotid artery, disease of, opthalmic effects, 43
Carotid-cavernous fistula, definition of, 188
Cataracts
    causes of, 81
    definition of, 188
    dislocated lens in, 86–88
    from foreign bodies, 75
    morgagnian, 192
    ultrasonography of, 24, 43, 44, 69, 80–88
        sonopathology, 82–88
Cathode-ray tube, 11–12
Cat's-eye pupil, description of, 193
Cavernous sinus, description of, 195
Central angiospastic retinopathy, definition of, 188
Centrocecal scotoma, definition of, 189
Cercinate retinopathy, definition of, 189
Cherry-red spot, definition of, 189
Chorioretinitis, ultrasonography of, 51
Choroid
    detachment of, 60, 78, 118, 132
        "kissing" type, 125, 126
        ultrasonography, 123–126
    hemangiomas of, 159
    nevi of, 51, 153, 159, 160
    thickening of, 77, 123
    tumors of, 157–161
    ultrasonography of, 108–132
Choroideremia, definition of, 189
Choroiditis, definition of, 189
Chromosomes, ultrasound effects on, 22
Ciliary body, anatomy of, 29
Coat's disease, subretinal exudates in, 130
Coloboma, 49
    definition of, 189
    ultrasonography of, 127, 128
Commotio retina, definition of, 189
Compound scan, 14
Compression technique, in oculosonotomography, 56
Congruous field defects, description of, 189
Conjunctivitis, definition of, 189
Consensual light reflex, definition of, 189
Contact lens, 189

Cornea
    anatomy of, 27–28
    bedewing of, 188
    calcification of, 172
    examination of, 47
    nebula of, 192
    staphylomas of, 126
Cortical blindness, definition of, 189
Cotton wool spots, definition of, 189
Coupling artifact, 184–185
Crohn's disease, 178
Cross-sectional image production, mechanism of, 10–11
Crystalline lens, definition of, 189
Crystals, in transducers, 17–18
Cyanosis retinea, definition of, 189
Cycle, of sound waves, 3, 9
Cyclitic membrane, 77, 114, 115, 121, 131, 132
Cycloplegia, definition of, 189
Cystic tumor, ultrasonography of, 39
Cysts, 162
    macular, 129–130
    retinal, 121–122
    in retinal detachment, 115
    ultrasonography of, 5, 25

D

Dacryoadenitis, definition of, 189
Damping system, 18
"Dead zone," 21
Descemet's membrane, 28
Diabetes
    asteroid hyalosis in, 104
    ocular lesions from, 174–177
    retinopathy from, 44, 49, 110, 127, 173, 175
Diopter, definition of, 189
Diplopia, definition of, 189
Disciform keratitis, definition of, 190
Disharmonious, definition of, 190
Distortion, artifacts from, 21
Doyne syndrome, description of, 195
Drusen
    definition of, 190
    of optic nerve head, 137, 138
Dysmetria, definition of, 190